Basic Dysrhythmias

interpretation & management

Basic Dysrhythmias

interpretation & management

Second Edition

Robert J. Huszar, M.D.

Former Medical Director
Emergency Medical Services Program
New York State Department of Health

with 355 illustrations

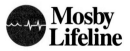

St. Louis Baltimore Berlin Boston Carlsbad Chicago London Madrid
Naples New York Philadelphia Sydney Tokyo Toronto

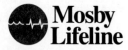

**Mosby
Lifeline**

Dedicated to Publishing Excellence

Publisher: David T. Culverwell
Executive Editor: Claire Merrick
Editorial Project Supervisor: Cecilia F. Reilly
Developmental Editor: Nancy Peterson
Project Manager: Karen Edwards
Production Editor: Richard Barber
Manufacturing Supervisor: John Babrick

Second Edition

Copyright © 1994 by Mosby–Year Book, Inc.
A Mosby Lifeline imprint of Mosby–Year Book, Inc.

Previous edition copyrighted 1988

Printed in the United States of America
Composition by Graphic World
Printing/binding by Von Hoffman Press

Mosby–Year Book, Inc.
11830 Westline Industrial Drive
St. Louis, Missouri 63146

Library of Congress Cataloging in Publication Data

Huszar, Robert J.
    Basic dysrhythmias : interpretation and management / Robert J.
Huszar. — 2nd ed.
      p.   cm.
    Includes index.
    ISBN 0-8016-7203-1
    1. Arrhythmia.   I. Title.
    [DNLM: 1. Arrhythmia—diagnosis. 2. Arrhythmia—therapy.
3. Electrocardiography.   WG 330 H972b 1994]
RC685.A65H89   1994
616.1′28—dc20
DNLM/DLC
for Library of Congress   93-49687
                                     CIP

94 95 96 97 98   9 8 7 6 5 4 3 2 1

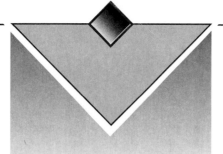

Introduction
to the Second Edition

Basic Dysrhythmias: Interpretation and Management, 2nd Edition, has been revised and expanded considerably to include the following new features:

- Extensive addition of new material to *Chapter 2, The Electrocardiogram,* which includes (1) an in-depth discussion of **12-lead electrocardiography** and the electrode placement for each lead, (2) the derivation of electrical axes and vectors and the lead axes, and (3) what is meant by a QRS axis, its determination using the hexaxial reference figure, and the significance of a QRS axis falling outside the normal range.

- Rearrangement of *Chapter 3, Components of the Electrocardiogram,* into a more logical format.

- Restructuring of *Chapter 5, Arrhythmia Identification* into five separate chapters, each devoted to a group of arrhythmias, i.e., sinus node, atrial, junctional, and ventricular arrhythmias and AV blocks.

- New *Chapter 10, Bundle Branch and Fascicular Blocks,* which includes the causes of bundle branch and fascicular blocks and detailed discussion and illustrations of the changes in the ECG typical of each block.

- New *Chapter 11, Myocardial Ischemia, Injury, and Infarction,* which includes a detailed discussion of the anatomy of the coronary artery circulation, the pathophysiology of coronary artery occlusion, and the regions of the heart affected by the occlusion of individual coronary arteries. The new material also includes the differentiation between myocardial ischemia, injury, and infarction; the effect each has on the ECG; and the timing of their appearance in the early and late phases of acute myocardial infarction. The correlation between the specific facing ECG leads in which the early and late changes of acute myocardial infarction appear, the area of the heart involved, and the coronary arteries occluded are graphically illustrated.

- New *Chapter 12, Miscellaneous ECG changes,* which includes the ECG changes present in various heart diseases (right and left atrial and ventricular enlargement or hypertrophy and pericarditis), pulmonary disease (acute pulmonary embolism, chronic obstructive pulmonary disease [COPD], and cor pulmonale), electrolyte imbalance (calcium and potassium), and drug effect (digitalis, procainamide, and quinidine).

- Update of *Chapter 13, Clinical Significance and Treatment of Arrhythmias,* to include changes, deletions, and additions in arrhythmia treatment based on the recommendations of the 1992 National Conference on Standards and Guidelines for Cardiopulmonary Resuscitation (CPR) and Emergency Cardiac Care (ECC) sponsored by the American College of Cardiology, the American Heart Association, the American Red Cross, and the National Heart, Lung and Blood Institute.

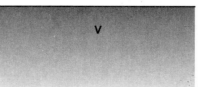

- Update of *Chapter 14, Arrhythmia Interpretation: Self-assessment* to include ECG strips based on the new material in **Chapters 2, 10, 11,** and **12,** as noted above.
- Update of the appendix to include various detailed methods of determining the QRS axis
- Update of the *Glossary* to include the new terminology.
- **Chapter objectives** for each chapter, which outline the contents of the chapter and help the instructor identify the material the student needs to study and know.
- **Chapter review questions.**

It is hoped that the new material on acute myocardial infarction presented in **Basic Dysrhythmias: Interpretation and Management, 2nd Ed.** will be useful to prehospital, emergency department, and other allied health personnel having to manage patients with acute myocardial infarction, to acquire the skills to analyze and identify the electrocardiographic changes typical of the early phases of AMI. This has become extremely important in view of the demonstrated need for early aggressive therapy in acute myocardial infarction, as early as in the prehospital phase of acute myocardial infarction by paramedics.

I wish to gratefully acknowledge the expertise of the following for their assistance in the revision of the second edition of this book:

Reviewers: Kevin B. Kraus, BS, EMT-P, New York State Disaster Preparedness Commission; **Arthur T. Otto, NREMT-P** (deceased), Operations Manager, Murphy Ambulance Service, Inc., St. Cloud, Minnesota; **Mikel Rothenberg, M.D.,** Emergency Care Educator, Executive Physician Editor of ACLS Alert, and Attending Emergency Physician, Lutheran Medical Center, Cleveland, Ohio; and **Judith Ruple, Assistant Professor,** Director of Emergency Medical Technology Programs, University of Toledo, Toledo, Ohio.

Mosby Lifeline Staff (Hanover, Maryland): Claire Merrick, Executive Editor: **Cecilia F. Reilly,** Editorial Project Supervisor; and **Nancy Peterson,** Developmental Editor.

Mosby Year Book Production and Manufacturing Staff (St. Louis, Missouri): Pat Stinecipher, Lin Dempsey, and **Rich Barber.**

Special acknowledgement and thanks is given to **Robert Elling, MPA, NREMT-P,** Syngerism Associates, Ltd., for providing the chapter review questions.

The new illustrations, graphics, and electrocardiograms incorporated in the second edition were prepared by the author using **Micrografx Designer 4.0.**

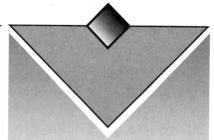

Preface
To the First Edition

Basic Dysrhythmias: Interpretation and Management is designed to help medical, nursing and paramedical personnel (physicians, nurses, residents, interns, medical students, paramedics, emergency medical technicians, cardiology technicians, and other allied health personnel) acquire the skills to analyze and identify common arrhythmias (or dysrhythmias). The term "arrhythmia," meaning an absence of rhythm, is used in this book by the author's preference instead of the more accurate term "dysrhythmia," meaning abnormality in rhythm. This choice was dictated by the fact that most medical editors prefer the term "arrhythmia."

The text is simply written, profusely illustrated with descriptive diagrams, and interspersed with numerous ECG drawings and tracings. Although the student who is being introduced to the interpretation of ECGs for the first time was continuously kept in mind during the preparation of the manuscript, the book should be of value as a reference to those already acquainted with the principles of electrocardiography.

The anatomy and electrophysiology of the heart is presented in Chapter 1 in a simplified manner yet, with sufficient detail to provide a sound basis for arrhythmia identification. In Chapter 2, the electrical basis of the electrocardiogram is discussed, and the ECG paper, leads, and artifacts are described. In the unique and detailed description of the components of the ECG in Chapter 3, numerous examples of the normal and abnormal waves, com-

plexes, segments, and intervals are included to help prepare the reader to recognize the numerous variations of these components found in clinical electrocardiography. In Chapter 4, a detailed step-by-step method for identifying an arrhythmia is presented. In the description of individual arrhythmias in Chapter 5, numerous examples of each arrhythmia are included so that the reader can appreciate the various appearances that an arrhythmia may have. Chapter 6 includes the treatment of common arrhythmias presented in a protocol format, based on the current American Heart Association/American Red Cross standards. The reader is given an opportunity for self-evaluation in Chapter 7, which includes all the ECGs presented in the previous chapters plus new ones.

I wish to gratefully acknowledge the assistance of Timothy Frank, Kevin Kraus, and Andrew Stern, who reviewed the manuscript, and the following who supplied many of the original ECG tracings: Ann Charlebois, R.N., M.S., Cardiac Resuscitation Corporation (Wilsonville, Oregon), Ronald Baker, EMT-Paramedic and Paramedic Instructor, Troy Fire Department (Troy, New York), Earl Evans, Regional Emergency Medical Organization (Albany, New York), Anne Ficarelli, EMT-Paramedic and Paramedic Trainer, Mary Immaculate Hospital (New York City, New York), Joan C. Hillgardner, EMT-Paramedic, New York City Emergency Medical Services, Health and Hospitals Corporation (New York City, New York), John Spoor, M.D., Imogene Bassett Hospital (Cooperstown, New York), and the staff of the Cardiology Departments of Leonard Hospital (Troy, New York) and Saint Peter's Hospital (Albany, New York).

Special acknowledgment is given Marta Huszar for her expertise in providing the original graphic design of the book, Jo Ann Jakiela for her invaluable assistance in preparing the manuscript, and Eric Boehm for his typesetting skills. The illustrations and graphics were prepared by the author.

*This book is dedicated
to my wife, Jean*

A Note to the Reader

The author and publisher have made every attempt to check dosages and advanced life support content for accuracy. The care procedures presented here represent accepted practices in the United States. They are not offered as a standard of care. Advanced life support level emergency care is performed under the authority of a licensed physician. It is the reader's responsibility to know and follow local care protocols as provided by their medical advisers. It is also the reader's responsibility to stay informed of emergency care procedure changes.

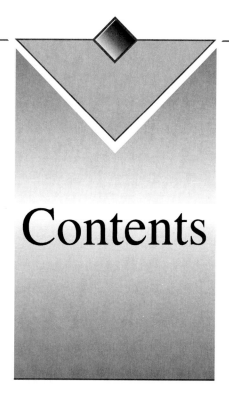

Contents

4 ECG Interpretation, 95

5 Sinus Node Arrhythmias, 121

CHAPTER 1

Anatomy and Physiology of the Heart

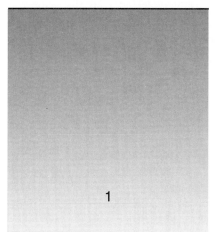

Upon completion of all or part of this chapter you should be able to complete the following objectives indicated by your instructor:

☐ 1. Name and identify the following anatomical features of the heart on an anatomical drawing:
   - ☐ The four chambers of the heart
   - ☐ The two main septa of the heart
   - ☐ The three layers of the ventricular walls
   - ☐ The base and apex of the heart

☐ 2. Name and identify the layers of the pericardium and its major space or cavity.

☐ 3. Define the right heart and left heart and the primary function of each with respect to the pulmonary and systemic circulations.

☐ 4. Name and locate on an anatomical drawing the following major structures of the circulatory system: the aorta, the pulmonary artery, the superior and inferior venae cavae, the coronary sinus, the pulmonary veins, and the four heart valves.

☐ 5. Define (a) atrial systole and diastole and (b) ventricular systole and diastole.

☐ 6. Name and identify the parts of the electrical conduction system of the heart.

☐ 7. Name the two basic kinds of cardiac cells and give their functions.

☐ 8. Name and define the four properties of cardiac cells.

☐ 9. Describe a resting, polarized cardiac cell and a depolarized cardiac cell.

☐ 10. Define the following:
   - ☐ Depolarization process
   - ☐ Repolarization process
   - ☐ Threshold potential

☐ 11. Name and locate on a schematic of a cardiac action potential the five phases of a cardiac potential.

☐ 12. Define and locate on an ECG the following:
   - ☐ Absolute refractory period
   - ☐ Relative refractory period
   - ☐ Vulnerable period of repolarization
   - ☐ Supernormal period

☐ 13. Explain the rationale behind the property of automaticity (spontaneous depolarization) and how the slope of phase 4 depolarization relates to the rate of impulse formation.

☐ 14. Define (a) dominant and latent pacemaker cells and (b) nonpacemaker cells.

☐ 15. Define and locate the primary, escape, and ectopic pacemakers of the heart.

☐ 16. Define inherent firing rate and give the inherent firing rates of the following:
   - ☐ SA node
   - ☐ AV junction
   - ☐ Ventricles

☐ 17. Give three conditions under which an escape pacemaker may assume the role of pacemaker of the heart.

☐ 18. List and define the three basic mechanisms that are responsible for ectopic beats and rhythms.

☐ 19. Describe the part of the autonomic nervous system controlling the heart.

☐ 20. List the effects on the heart produced by the stimulation of the sympathetic and parasympathetic nervous system.

Anatomy and Physiology of the Heart

The **heart,** whose sole purpose is to circulate blood through the **circulatory system** (the blood vessels of the body), consists of four hollow chambers (Figure 1-1). The upper two chambers, the **right** and **left atria,** are thin-walled; the lower two, the **right** and **left ventricles,** are thick-walled and muscular. The walls of the ventricles are composed of three layers of tissue: the innermost thin layer is called the **endocardium;** the middle thick, muscular layer, the **myocardium;** and the outermost thin layer, the **epicardium.** The myocardium is further divided into the **subendocardial area** just beneath the endocardium and the **subepicardial area** be-

neath the epicardium. The walls of the left ventricle are more muscular and about three times thicker than those of the right ventricle.

The atrial walls are also composed of three layers of tissue like those of the ventricles, but the middle muscular layer is much thinner. The two atria form the **base of the heart;** the ventricles form the **apex of the heart.**

Enclosing the heart is the **pericardium,** which consists of an outer tough, fibrous sac, the **fibrous pericardium,** and an inner, two-layered, fluid-secreting membrane, the **serous pericardium.** The outer, fibrous pericardium comes in direct contact with the covering of the lung, the **pleura.** The inner layer of the serous pericardium, the **visceral peri-**

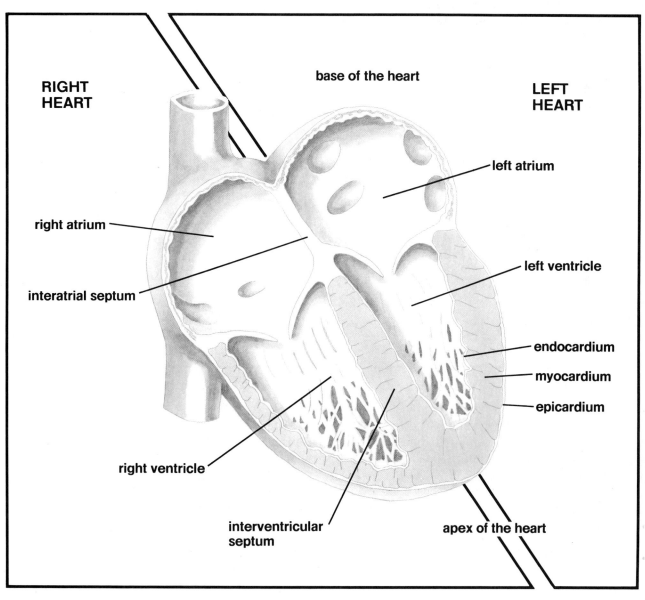

Figure 1-1. Anatomy of the heart.

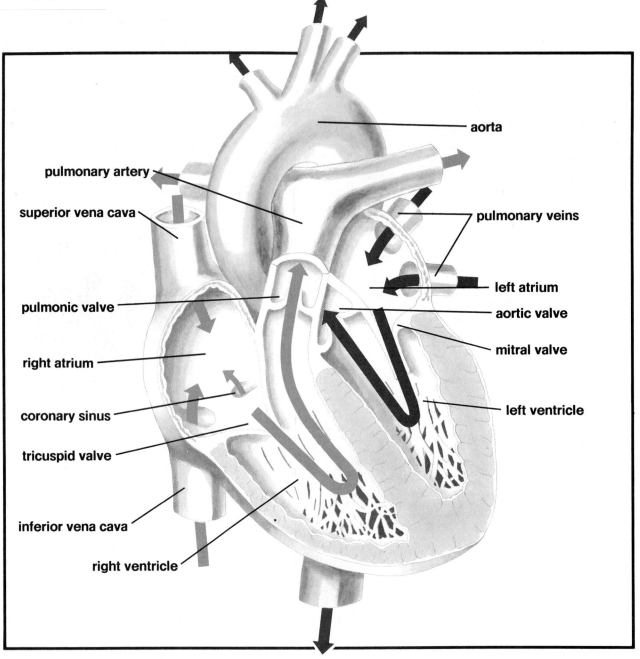

aorta

pulmonary artery

superior vena cava

pulmonary veins

left atrium

pulmonic valve

aortic valve

mitral valve

right atrium

coronary sinus

left ventricle

tricuspid valve

inferior vena cava

right ventricle

Figure 1-2. Circulation through the heart.

cardium or, as it is more commonly known, the **epicardium,** covers the heart itself, and the outer layer, the **parietal pericardium,** lines the fibrous pericardium. Between the two layers of the serous pericardium is the **pericardial space** or **cavity.** It contains up to 50 milliliters of fluid, the **pericardial fluid,** which helps to lubricate the movements of the heart within the pericardium.

The pericardium is attached to the center of the diaphragm inferiorly, to the sternum anteriorly, and to the esophagus, trachea, and main bronchi posteriorly. In this way, the pericardium anchors the heart to the chest and prevents it from shifting about.

The **interatrial septum** (a thin membranous wall) separates the two atria, and a thicker, more muscular wall, the **interventricular septum,** separates the two ventricles. The two septa, in effect, divide the heart into two pumping systems, the **right heart** and **left heart,** each one consisting of an atrium and a ventricle.

The right heart pumps blood into the **pulmonary circulation** (the blood vessels within the lungs and those carrying blood to and from the lungs). The left heart pumps blood into the **systemic circulation** (the blood vessels in the rest of the body and those carrying blood to and from the body).

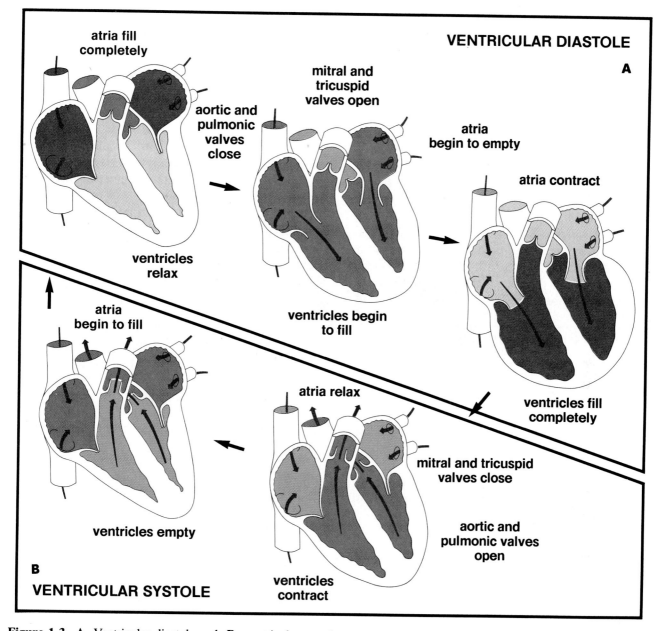

Figure 1-3. A, Ventricular diastole and, **B,** ventricular systole.

The right atrium receives unoxygenated blood from the body via two of the body's largest veins (the **superior vena cava** and **inferior vena cava**) and from the heart itself by way of the **coronary sinus** (Figure 1-2). The blood is delivered to the right ventricle through the **tricuspid valve.** The right ventricle then pumps the unoxygenated blood through the **pulmonic valve** and into the lungs via the **pulmonary artery.** In the lungs, the blood picks up oxygen and releases excess carbon dioxide.

The left atrium receives the newly oxygenated blood from the lungs via the **pulmonary veins** and delivers it to the left ventricle through the **mitral valve.** The left ventricle then pumps the oxygenated blood out through the **aortic valve** and into the **aorta,** the largest artery in the body. From the aorta, the blood is distributed throughout the body where the blood releases oxygen to the cells and collects carbon dioxide from them.

The heart performs its pumping action over and over in a rhythmic sequence. First, the atria relax **(atrial diastole),** allowing the blood to pour in from the body and lungs (Figure 1-3). As the atria fill with blood, the atrial pressure rises above that in the ventricles, forcing the tricuspid and mitral valves to open and allowing the blood to empty rapidly into the relaxed ventricles. Then, the atria contract **(atrial systole),** filling the ventricles to capacity.

The period of relaxation and filling of the ventricles with blood is called **ventricular diastole.**

Following the contraction of the atria, the pressures in the atria and ventricles equalize, and the tricuspid and mitral valves begin to close. Then, the ventricles contract vigorously, causing the ventricular pressure to rise sharply. The tricuspid and mitral valves close completely, and the aortic and pulmonic valves snap open, allowing the blood to be ejected forcefully into the pulmonary and systemic circulations. The period during which the ventricles contract and empty of blood is called **ventricular systole.**

Meanwhile, the atria are again relaxing and filling with blood. As soon as the ventricles empty of blood and begin to relax, the ventricular pressure falls, the aortic and pulmonic valves shut tightly, the tricuspid and mitral valves open, and the rhythmic cardiac sequence begins anew.

Electrical Conduction System of the Heart

The **electrical conduction system** of the heart (Figure 1-4) is composed of the following structures:
- **Sinoatrial (SA) node**
- **Internodal atrial conduction tracts** and the **interatrial conduction tract (Bachmann's bundle)**
- **Atrioventricular (AV) junction** consisting of the **atrioventricular (AV) node** and **bundle of His**
- **Right bundle branch, left bundle branch,** and **left anterior** and **posterior fascicles**
- **Purkinje network**

The prime function of the **electrical conduction system of the heart** is to transmit minute **electrical impulses** from the SA node (where they are normally generated) to the atria and ventricles, causing them to contract (Figure 1-5).

The **SA node** lies in the wall of the right atrium near the inlet of the superior vena cava. It consists of pacemaker cells that generate electrical impulses automatically and regularly.

The three **internodal atrial conduction tracts,** running through the walls of the right atrium between the SA node and the AV node, conduct the electrical impulses rapidly from the SA node to the AV node in about **0.03 second.** The **interatrial conduction tract (Bachmann's bundle),** a branch of one of the internodal atrial conduction tracts, extends across the atria, conducting the electrical impulses from the SA node to the left atrium.

The **AV node,** the proximal part of the atrioventricular (AV) junction, lies partly in the right side of the interatrial septum in front of the opening of the coronary sinus and in the upper part of the interventricular septum above the base of the tricuspid valve. The primary function of the AV node is to relay the electrical impulses from the atria into the ventricles in an orderly and timely way. A ring of fibrous tissue insulates the remainder of the atria from the ventricles, preventing electrical impulses

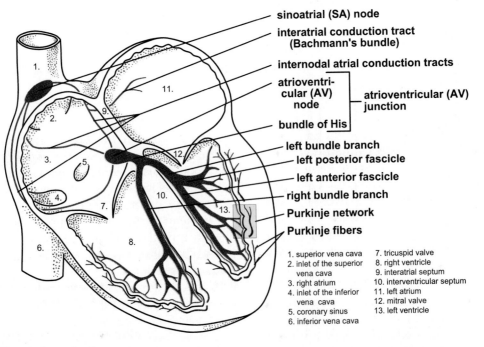

sinoatrial (SA) node
interatrial conduction tract (Bachmann's bundle)
internodal atrial conduction tracts
atrioventricular (AV) node
bundle of His
atrioventricular (AV) junction
left bundle branch
left posterior fascicle
left anterior fascicle
right bundle branch
Purkinje network
Purkinje fibers

1. superior vena cava
2. inlet of the superior vena cava
3. right atrium
4. inlet of the inferior vena cava
5. coronary sinus
6. inferior vena cava
7. tricuspid valve
8. right ventricle
9. interatrial septum
10. interventricular septum
11. left atrium
12. mitral valve
13. left ventricle

Figure 1-4. Electrical conduction system.

from entering the ventricles except through the AV node.

The electrical impulses slow as they travel through the AV node, taking about **0.06 to 0.12 second** to reach the bundle of His. The delay is such that the atria can contract and empty, and the ventricles fill before they are stimulated to contract.

The **bundle of His,** the distal part of the AV junction, lies in the upper part of the interventricular septum, connecting the AV node with the two bundle branches. Once the electrical impulses enter the bundle of His, they travel more rapidly on their way to the bundle branches, taking **0.03 to 0.05 second.**

The right bundle branch and the **left common bundle branch** arise from the bundle of His, straddle the interventricular septum, and continue down both sides of the septum. The left common bundle

branch further divides into two major divisions: the **left anterior fascicle** and the **left posterior fascicle.** The bundle branches subdivide into smaller and smaller branches, the smallest ones connecting with the **Purkinje network,** an intricate web of tiny **Purkinje fibers** spread widely throughout the ventricles beneath the endocardium. The ends of the Purkinje fibers finally terminate at the myocardial cells. The bundle of His, the right and left bundle branches, and the Purkinje network are also known as the **His-Purkinje system of the ventricles.**

The electrical impulses travel very rapidly to the Purkinje network through the bundle branches in less than **0.01 second.** All in all, it normally takes the electrical impulses less than **0.2 second** to travel from the SA node to the Purkinje network in the ventricles.

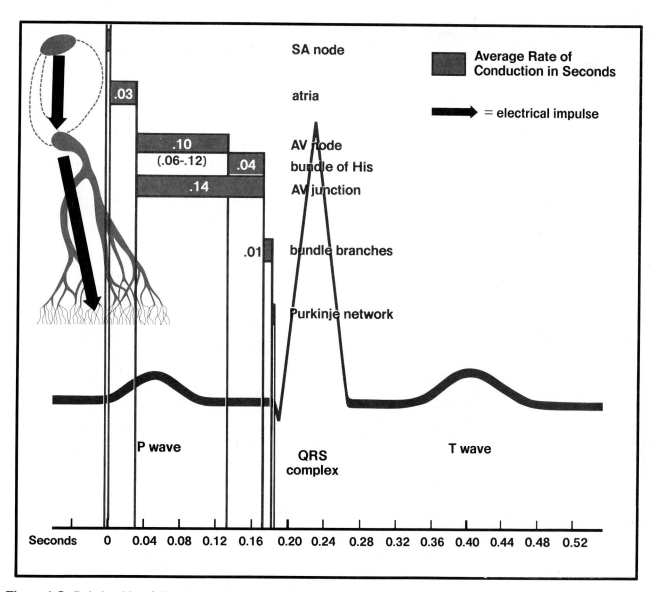

Figure 1-5. Relationship of the electrical impulse to the electrical conduction system.

Cardiac Cells

The heart is composed of cylindrical **cardiac cells** (Figure 1-6), which partially divide at their ends into two or more branches. These connect with the branches of adjacent cells, forming a branching and anastomosing network of cells called a **syncytium.** At the junctions where the branches join together are specialized cellular membranes not found in any other cells—the **intercalated disks.** These membranes contain areas of low electrical resistance called **"gap junctions,"** which permit very rapid conduction of electrical impulses from one cell to another. The ability of cardiac cells to conduct electrical impulses is called the **property of conductivity.**

Cardiac cells are enclosed in a semipermeable cell membrane, which allows certain charged chemical particles **(ions),** such as sodium, potassium, and calcium ions, to flow in and out of the cells, making the contraction and relaxation of the heart and the generation and conduction of electrical impulses possible.

There are two basic kinds of cardiac cells in the heart—the **myocardial** (or **"working"**) **cells** and the **specialized cells of the electrical conduction system** of the heart.

The **myocardial cells** contain numerous thin **myofibrils** that consist of contractile protein filaments called **actin** and **myosin.** These myofibrils give the myocardial cells the **property of contractility**—the ability to shorten and return to their original length when stimulated by an electrical impulse. The myocardial cells form the thin muscular layer of the atrial wall and the much thicker muscular layer of the ventricular wall—the **myocardium**.

The force of myocardial contractility increases in response to certain drugs (e.g., bretylium, digitalis, sympathomimetics) and physiologic conditions (e.g., increased venous return to the heart, exercise, emotion, hypovolemia, anemia). In contrast, other drugs (e.g., procainamide, quinidine, beta-blockers, potassium) and pathophysiologic conditions (e.g., shock, hypocalcemia, hypothyroidism) decrease the force of myocardial contractility.

The **specialized cells of the electrical conduction system** do not contain myofibrils and, therefore, cannot contract. They do, however, contain more gap junctions than do myocardial cells, permitting them to conduct electrical impulses ex-

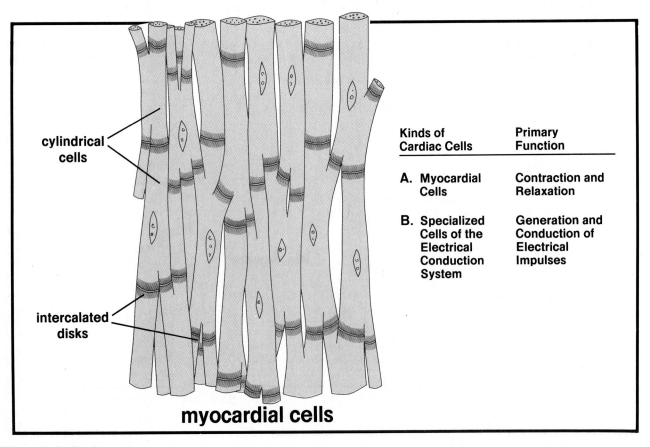

cylindrical cells

intercalated disks

myocardial cells

Kinds of Cardiac Cells	Primary Function
A. Myocardial Cells	Contraction and Relaxation
B. Specialized Cells of the Electrical Conduction System	Generation and Conduction of Electrical Impulses

Figure 1-6. Cardiac cells.

tremely rapidly (at least six times faster than do myocardial cells). Certain of the specialized cells of the electrical conduction system—the **pacemaker cells**—are also capable of generating electrical impulses spontaneously. This capability, the **property of automaticity,** will be discussed in greater detail later in this chapter.

Electrophysiology of the Heart

Cardiac cells are capable of generating and conducting electrical impulses that are responsible for the contraction and relaxation of myocardial cells. These electrical impulses are the result of brief but rapid flow of positively charged ions (primarily sodium and potassium ions and, to a lesser extent, calcium ions) back and forth across the cardiac **cell membrane.** The difference in the concentration of such ions across the cell membrane at any given instant is called the **electrical potential (or voltage)** and is measured in **millivolts (mV).**

Resting State of the Cardiac Cell

When a myocardial cell, for example, is in the **resting state,** a high concentration of positively charged sodium ions (Na +) **(cations)** is present *out-side* the cell. At the same time, a high-concentration of both positively charged potassium ions (K +) and a mixture of negatively charged ions (especially organic phosphate ions, organic sulfate ions, and protein ions) **(anions)** is present *inside* the cell. Under these conditions, where the interior of the cell is electrically negative with reference to its positive exterior, a **negative electrical potential** exists across the cell membrane. This is made possible by the cell membrane being impermeable to (1) positively charged sodium ions during the resting state and (2) negatively charged phosphate, sulfate, and protein ions at all times (Figure 1-7). When a cell membrane is impermeable to an ion, it does not permit the free flow of that ion across it.

The resting myocardial cell can be depicted as having a layer of positive ions surrounding the cell membrane and an equal number of negative ions lining the inside of the cell membrane directly opposite each positive ion. When the ions are so aligned, the resting cell is called **"polarized."**

The electrical potential across the membrane of a resting cardiac cell is called the **resting membrane potential.** The resting membrane potential in atrial and ventricular myocardial cells and the specialized cells of the electrical conduction system (except those of the SA and AV nodes) is normally

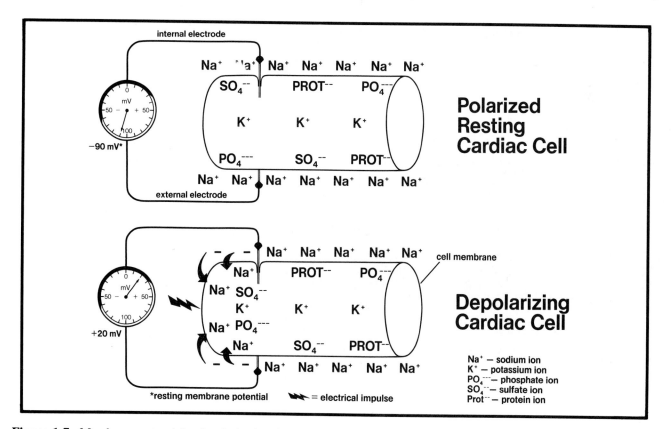

Figure 1-7. Membrane potentials of polarized and depolarized cardiac cells.

−90 mV. It is somewhat less in the SA and AV nodal cells, −70 mV.

Depolarization and Repolarization

Upon stimulation by an electrical impulse, the membrane of a polarized myocardial cell, for example, becomes permeable to positively charged sodium ions, allowing sodium to flow into the cell. This causes the interior of the cell to become less negative. When the membrane potential drops to about −60 mV from its resting potential of −90 mV, large pores in the membrane (the **fast sodium channels**) momentarily open. These channels facil-

itate the rapid, free flow of sodium across the cell membrane, resulting in a sudden large influx of positively charged sodium ions into the cell. This causes the exterior of the cell to become rapidly negative with respect to the now positive interior. At the moment when the interior of the cell becomes maximally positive and the exterior maximally negative, the cell is **"depolarized."** The process by which the cell's resting, polarized state is reversed is called **depolarization** (Figure 1-8).

The fast sodium channels are typically found in the myocardial cells and the specialized cells of the electrical conduction system other than those of the

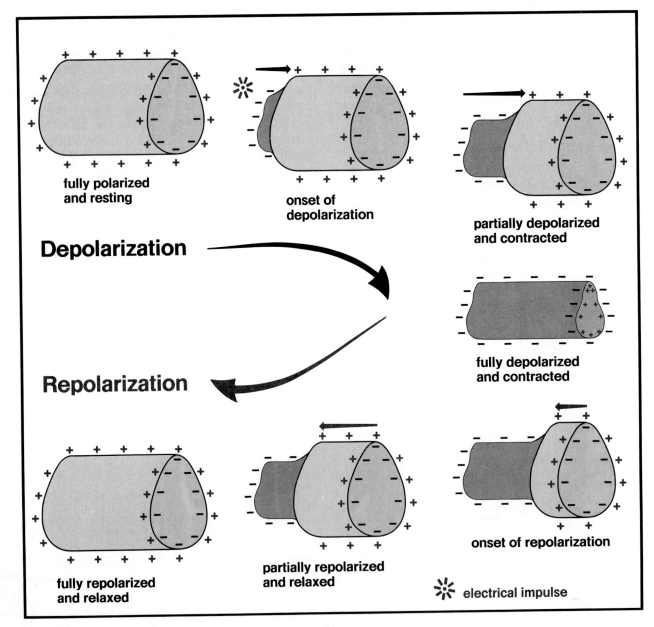

Figure 1-8. Depolarization and repolarization of a muscle fiber.

SA and AV nodes. The cells of the SA and AV nodes have, instead of fast sodium channels, **slow calcium-sodium channels** that open when the membrane potential drops to about −50 mV. They permit the entry of positively charged calcium and sodium ions into the cells during depolarization at a slow and gradual rate. The result is a slower rate of depolarization as compared to the depolarization of cardiac cells with fast sodium channels.

As soon as a cardiac cell depolarizes, positively charged potassium ions flow out of the cell, initiating a process by which the cell returns to its resting, polarized state. This process, called **repolarization,** (Figure 1-8), involves a complex exchange of sodium, calcium, and potassium ions across the cell membrane.

Depolarization of one cardiac cell acts as an electrical impulse (or stimulus) on adjacent cells and causes them to depolarize. The propagation of the electrical impulse from cell to cell produces an electric current, which flows in the direction of depolarization. As the cells repolarize, another electric current is produced, similar to, but opposite in direction to, the first one. The direction of flow and magnitude of the currents generated by depolarization and repolarization of the myocardial cells of the atria and ventricles can be detected by surface electrodes and recorded as the **electrocardiogram (ECG).** Depolarization of the myocardial

cells produces the **QRS complex,** and repolarization of the cells results in the **T wave** in the electrocardiogram.

Threshold Potential

A cell need not be repolarized completely to its resting, polarized state (-90 mV) before it can be stimulated to depolarize again. The cells of the SA and AV nodes can be depolarized when they have been repolarized to about −30 to −40 mV. The rest of the cells of the electrical conduction system of the heart and the myocardial cells can be depolarized when they have been repolarized to about −60 to −70 mV. The level to which a cell must be repolarized before it can be depolarized again is called the **threshold potential.**

It is important to note that a cardiac cell cannot be stimulated to generate or conduct an electrical impulse or to contract until it has been repolarized to its threshold potential.

Cardiac Action Potential

A **cardiac action potential** is a schematic representation of the changes in the membrane potential of a cardiac cell during depolarization and repolarization (Figure 1-9). The cardiac action potential is divided into five phases—**phase 0** to **phase 4.**

The following are the five phases of the cardiac action potential of a typical myocardial cell.

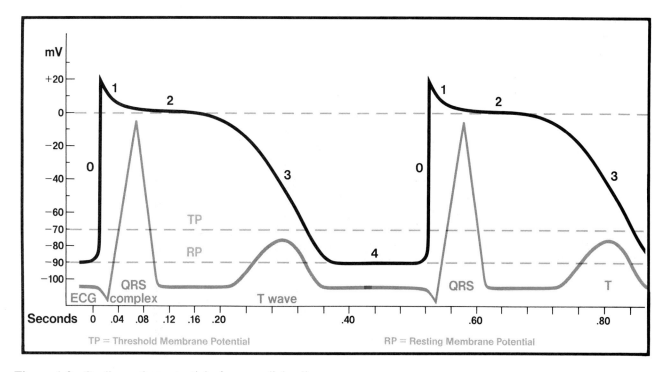

Figure 1-9. Cardiac action potential of myocardial cells.

Phase 0: Phase 0 **(depolarization phase)** is the sharp, tall upstroke of the action potential during which the cell membrane reaches the threshold potential, triggering the fast sodium channels to open momentarily and permit the rapid entry of sodium into the cell. As the positively charged ions flow into the cell, the interior of the cell becomes electrically positive to about +20 mV with respect to its exterior. During the upstroke, the cell depolarizes and begins to contract.

Phase 1: During this phase **(early rapid repolarization phase),** the fast sodium channels close, terminating the rapid flow of sodium into the cell, followed by a loss of potassium from the cell. The net result is a decrease in the number of positive electrical charges within the cell and a drop in the membrane potential to about 0 mV.

Phase 2: This is the prolonged phase of slow repolarization **(plateau phase)** of the action potential of the myocardial cell, allowing it to finish contracting and begin relaxing. During phase 2, the membrane potential remains about 0 mV because of a very slow rate of repolarization. In a complicated exchange of ions across the cell membrane, calcium slowly enters the cell through the slow calcium channels as potassium continues to leave the cell and sodium to enter it.

Phase 3: Phase 3 is the **terminal phase of rapid repolarization,** during which the inside of the cell becomes markedly negative and the membrane potential once again returns to about −90 mV, its resting level. This is caused primarily by the flow of potassium from the cell. Repolarization is completed by the end of phase 3.

Phase 4: At the onset of phase 4 **(the period between action potentials),** the membrane has returned to its resting potential and the inside of the cell is once again negative (−90 mV) with respect to the outside. But there is still an excess of sodium in the cell and an excess of potassium outside. At this point, a mechanism known as the **"sodium-potassium pump"** is activated, transporting the excess sodium out of the cell and potassium back in. Because of this mechanism and the impermeability of the cell membrane to sodium during phase 4, the myocardial cell normally maintains a stable membrane potential between action potentials.

Refractory and Supernormal Periods

The time between the onset of depolarization and the end of repolarization is customarily divided into periods during which the cardiac cells can or cannot be stimulated to depolarize. These are the **refractory periods (absolute and relative)** and the **supernormal period** (Figure 1-10).

The **refractory period** of cardiac cells (for example, those of the ventricles) begins with the onset of phase 0 of the cardiac action potential and ends

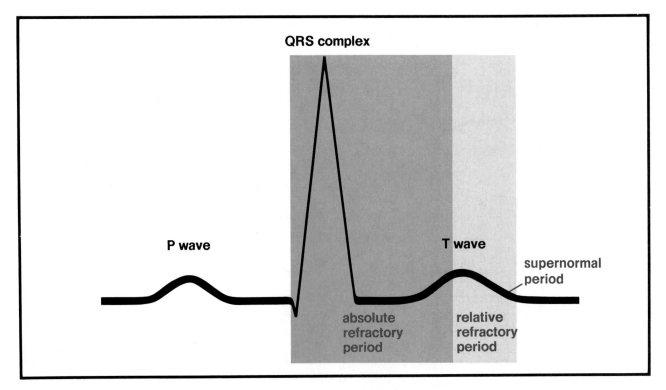

Figure 1-10. Refractory and supernormal periods.

with the end of phase 3. On the ECG, it extends from the onset of the QRS complex to the end of the T wave.

The refractory period is further divided into the **absolute** and **relative refractory periods.** The **absolute refractory period (ARP)** begins with the onset of phase 0 and ends midway through phase 3 at about the peak of the T wave. During this period, the cardiac cells, having completely depolarized, are in the process of repolarizing. Because they have not repolarized to their threshold potential, the cardiac cells cannot be stimulated to depolarize. In other words, myocardial cells cannot contract, and the cells of the electrical conduction system cannot conduct an electrical impulse during the absolute refractory period.

The **relative refractory period (RRP)** extends through the second half of phase 3, corresponding to the downslope of the T wave. During this period, the cardiac cells, having repolarized to their threshold potential, can be stimulated to depolarize if the stimulus is strong enough. This period is also called the **vulnerable period of repolarization.**

During a short portion of phase 3 near the end of the T wave, just before the cells return to their resting potential, a stimulus weaker than is normally required can depolarize cardiac cells. This portion of repolarization is called the **supernormal period.**

Excitability and Automaticity

The capability of a resting, polarized cardiac cell to depolarize in response to an electrical stimulus is called the **property of excitability.** All cardiac cells have this property.

The capability of a cardiac cell to depolarize spontaneously during phase 4—to reach threshold potential and to depolarize completely without being externally stimulated—is called the **property of automaticity.** (This could also be called the **property of self-excitation.**)

Spontaneous depolarization depends on the ability of the cell membrane to become permeable to sodium during phase 4, thus allowing a steady leakage of sodium ions into the cell. This causes the resting membrane potential to become progressively less negative. As soon as the threshold potential is reached, rapid depolarization of the cell (phase 0) occurs. The rate of spontaneous depolarization is dependent on the **slope of phase 4 depolarization** (Figure 1-11). The steeper the slope of phase 4 de-

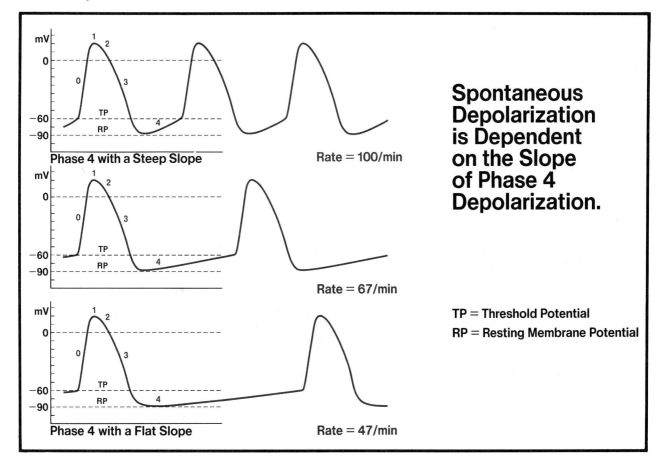

Spontaneous Depolarization is Dependent on the Slope of Phase 4 Depolarization.

TP = Threshold Potential
RP = Resting Membrane Potential

Figure 1-11. Cardiac action potential of pacemaker cells.

polarization, the faster is the rate of spontaneous depolarization and the **rate of impulse formation (the firing rate).** The flatter the slope, the slower the firing rate.

Certain of the specialized cells of the electrical conduction system normally have the property of automaticity. These cells, the **pacemaker cells,** are located in the SA node, in some areas of the internodal atrial conduction tracts and AV node, and throughout the bundle of His, bundle branches, and Purkinje network. The pacemaker cells of the SA node are normally the **dominant (or primary) pacemaker cells of the heart.** The pacemaker cells in the rest of the electrical conduction system hold the property of automaticity in reserve should the SA node fail to function properly or electrical impulses fail to reach them for any reason, such as a disruption in the electrical conduction system. For this reason, these pacemaker cells are called **latent (or subsidiary) pacemaker cells.** Myocardial cells, which do not normally have the capability to depolarize spontaneously during phase 4, are called **nonpacemaker cells.**

Increase in **sympathetic activity** and administration of **catecholamines** increase the **slope of phase 4 depolarization,** resulting in an increase in the automaticity of the pacemaker cells and their firing rate. On the other hand, an increase in **parasympathetic activity** and administration of such drugs as lidocaine, procainamide, and quinidine decrease the **slope of phase 4 depolarization,** causing a decrease in the automaticity and firing rate of the pacemaker cells.

Dominant and Escape Pacemakers of the Heart

Normally, the pacemaker cells with the fastest firing rate control the heart rate at any given time. Each time these pacemaker cells generate an elec-

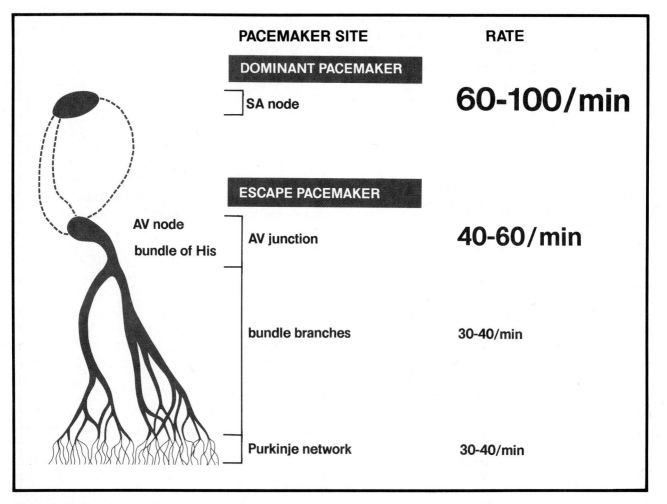

Figure 1-12. Dominant and escape pacemakers.

trical impulse, the slower-firing latent pacemaker cells are depolarized before they can do so spontaneously. This phenomenon is called **overdrive suppression.**

The **SA node** is normally the **dominant and primary pacemaker of the heart** (Figure 1-12) because it possesses the highest level of automaticity; that is, its rate of automatic firing (60 to 100 times a minute) is normally greater than that of the latent pacemaker cells. If the SA node fails to generate electrical impulses at its normal rate or stops functioning entirely or if the conduction of the electrical impulses is blocked for any reason (in the AV node, for example), latent pacemaker cells in the **AV junction** will usually assume the role of pacemaker of the heart but at a slower rate (40 to 60 times a minute). Such a pacemaker is called an **escape pacemaker.** If the AV junction is unable to take over as the pacemaker because of disease, an escape pacemaker in the electrical conduction system below the AV junction (i.e., in the **bundle branches** or **Purkinje network**) may take over at a still slower rate (less than 40 times a minute). In general, the farther the escape pacemaker is from the SA node, the slower it generates electrical impulses.

The rate at which the SA node or an escape pacemaker normally generates electrical impulses is called the pacemaker's **inherent firing rate.** A beat or a series of beats arising from an escape pacemaker is called an **escape beat** or **rhythm** and is identified according to its site of origin (e.g., junctional, ventricular).

Mechanisms of Abnormal Electrical Impulse Formation

Under certain circumstances, cardiac cells in any part of the heart, whether they are latent pacemaker cells or nonpacemaker, myocardial cells, may take on the role of a pacemaker and start generating extraneous electrical impulses. Such pacemakers are called **ectopic pacemakers.** The result can be abnormal **ectopic beats** and **rhythms,** such as **premature contractions, tachycardias, flutters,** and **fibrillations.** These arrhythmias* are identified according to the location of the ectopic pacemaker (e.g., atrial, junctional, ventricular). The three basic mechanisms that are responsible for ectopic beats

*The term *arrhythmia,* meaning an absence of rhythm, is used in this book by preference instead of the more accurate term *dysrhythmias,* meaning abnormality in rhythm. This choice was dictated by the fact that most medical editors prefer the term *arrhythmia.* The terms, however, can be used interchangeably.

and rhythms are **(1) enhanced automaticity, (2) reentry,** and **(3) triggered activity.**

Enhanced Automaticity

Enhanced automaticity is an abnormal condition of latent pacemaker cells in which their firing rate is increased beyond their inherent rate. This occurs when the cell membrane becomes abnormally permeable to sodium during phase 4. The result is an abnormally high leakage of sodium ions into the cells and, consequently, a sharp rise in the phase 4 slope of spontaneous depolarization. Even myocardial cells that do not ordinarily possess automaticity (nonpacemaker cells) may acquire this property under certain conditions and depolarize spontaneously. Enhanced automaticity can cause atrial, junctional, and ventricular ectopic beats and rhythms.

Common causes of enhanced automaticity are an increase in catecholamines, digitalis toxicity, and administration of atropine. In addition, hypoxia, hypercapnia, myocardial ischemia or infarction, stretching of the heart, hypokalemia, hypocalcemia, or heating or cooling of the heart may also cause enhanced automaticity.

Reentry

Reentry is a condition in which the progression of an electrical impulse is delayed or blocked (or both) (Figure 1-13) in one or more segments of the electrical conduction system while being conducted normally through the rest of the conduction system. This results in the delayed electrical impulse entering cardiac cells, which have just been depolarized by the normally conducted impulse. If these cardiac cells have repolarized sufficiently, the delayed electrical impulse depolarizes them prematurely, producing ectopic beats and rhythms.

The reentry mechanism can result in the abnormal generation of single or repetitive electrical impulses in the atria, AV junction, bundle branches, and Purkinje network. This produces atrial, junctional, or ventricular ectopic beats and rhythms, such as atrial, junctional, and ventricular tachycardias. Such reentry tachycardias typically start and stop abruptly. If the delay in the conduction of the electrical impulse is constant for each conduction cycle, the abnormal beat will always follow the normal one at exactly the same interval of time. This is called **fixed coupling** and **bigeminal rhythm,** or simply **bigeminy.**

Myocardial ischemia and hyperkalemia are the two most common causes of delay or block in the conduction of an electrical impulse through the electrical conduction system responsible for the reentry mechanism.

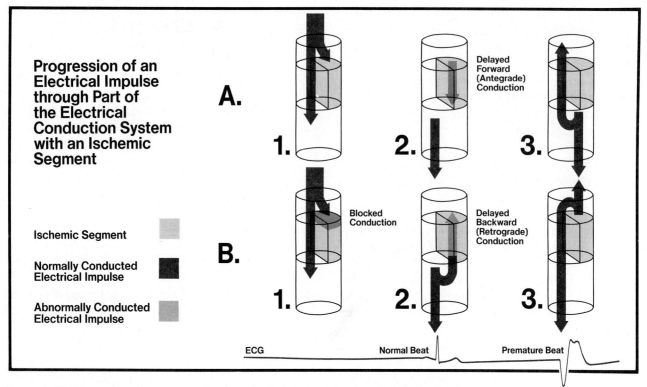

Figure 1-13. Examples of reentry mechanism. **A,** Delayed conduction. **B,** Blocked and delayed conduction.

Triggered Activity

Triggered activity is an abnormal condition of latent pacemaker and myocardial cells (nonpacemaker cells) in which the cells may depolarize more than once following stimulation by a single electrical impulse. The level of membrane action potential spontaneously and rhythmically increases after the first depolarization until it reaches threshold potential, causing the cells to depolarize. This phenomenon, called **afterdepolarization,** can occur immediately following repolarization early, in phase 3 **(early afterdepolarization),** or late in phase 4 **(delayed afterdepolarization).**

Triggered activity can result in atrial or ventricular ectopic beats occurring singly, in groups of two **(paired** or **coupled beats),** or in bursts of three or more beats **(paroxysms of beats** or **tachycardia).**

Common causes of triggered activity, like those of enhanced automaticity, include an increase in catecholamines, digitalis toxicity, hypoxia, myocardial ischemia or injury, and stretching or cooling of the heart.

Nervous Control of the Heart

The heart is under constant control of the **autonomic nervous system,** which includes the **sympathetic (adrenergic)** and **parasympathetic (cho-** linergic or vagal) nervous systems (Figure 1-14), each producing opposite effects when stimulated. These two systems work together to cause changes in **cardiac output** (by regulating the heart rate and stroke volume) and **blood pressure.**

Nervous control of the heart originates in two separate nerve centers located in the **medulla oblongata,** a part of the brain stem. One is the **cardioaccelerator center,** a part of the sympathetic nervous system; the other, the **cardioinhibitor center,** is a part of the parasympathetic nervous system. Impulses from the cardioaccelerator center reach the electrical conduction system of the heart and the atria and ventricles by way of the **sympathetic nerves.** Impulses from the cardioinhibitor center innervate the atria, SA node, and AV junction and to a small extent the ventricles by way of the **right** and **left vagus nerves.**

Another important cardioinhibitor (parasympathetic) nerve center is the **carotid sinus,** a slight dilatation of the common carotid artery, located at the point where it branches into the internal and external carotid arteries. It contains sensory nerve endings important in the regulation of blood pressure and heart rate.

As the blood requirements of the body change, multiple sensors in the body relay impulses to the cardioinhibitor and cardioaccelerator centers for

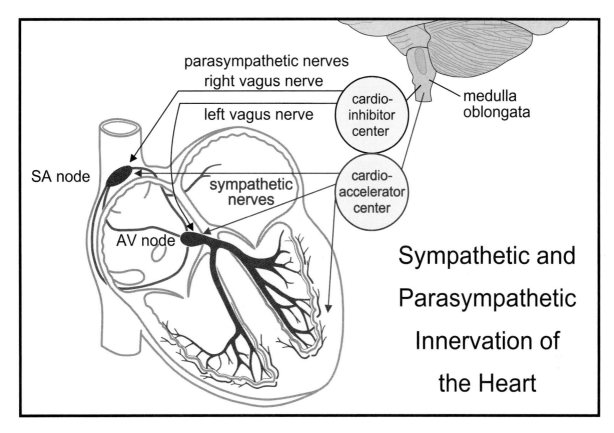

Figure 1-14. Sympathetic and parasympathetic innervation of the heart.

analysis. From here, the sympathetic and parasympathetic nerves transmit the appropriate impulses to the electrical conduction system of the heart and the atrial and ventricular myocardium where they influence the **automaticity, excitability, conductivity,** and **contractility** of the heart's cardiac cells.

Stimulation of the sympathetic nervous system produces the following adrenergic effects on the cardiovascular system:

- An increase in the firing rate of the SA node and escape and ectopic pacemakers throughout the heart by increasing their automaticity and excitability
- An increase in the conductivity of electrical impulses through the atria and ventricles, especially through the AV node
- An increase in the force of atrial and ventricular contractions

The result is an increase in heart rate, cardiac output, and blood pressure. This is accomplished by direct stimulation of the cardiac cells and indirectly by the secretion of **catecholamines,** such as **epinephrine (Adrenalin),** and their effect on the cardiac cells.

Stimulation of the parasympathetic nervous system produces the following cholinergic (vagal) effects on the cardiovascular system:

- A decrease in the firing rate of the SA node and escape and ectopic pacemakers in the atria and AV junction by decreasing their automaticity and excitability
- A slowing of conduction of electrical impulses through the AV node

The result is a decrease in heart rate, cardiac output, and blood pressure and, sometimes, an AV block.

The following maneuvers and bodily functions stimulate the parasympathetic nervous system:

- Pressure on the carotid sinus
- The Valsalva maneuver (the action of straining against a closed glottis or taking a deep breath while in a head-down tilt position)
- Straining to move the bowels
- Distention of the urinary bladder

Nausea, vomiting, bronchial spasm, sweating, faintness, and hypersalivation are examples of excessive parasympathetic activity. The drug **atropine,** a parasympathetic blocking agent, effectively blocks parasympathetic activity.

1. The visceral pericardium, the inner layer of the serous pericardium, which covers the heart itself, is more commonly called the:
   A. myocardium   C. endocardium
   B. epicardium   D. pericardium

2. The _____ heart pumps blood into the _____ circulation, while the _____ heart pumps blood into the _____ circulation.
   A. right, systemic: C. right, pulmonary:
      left, pulmonic   left, systemic
   B. left, pulmonary: D. left, systemic:
      right, systemic   right, pulmonic

3. The right ventricle pumps unoxygenated blood through the _____ valve and into the lungs through the _____ artery.
   A. pulmonic: pulmo-   C. aortic: mitral
      nary   D. tricuspid: pulmo-
   B. mitral: tricuspid   nary

4. The period of relaxation and filling of the ventricles with blood is called:
   A. atrial diastole   C. ventricular dias-
   B. ventricular systole   tole
                           D. atrial systole

5. Which structure is not a component of the electrical conduction system?
   A. Purkinje network   C. right bundle
   B. coronary sinus   branch
                           D. sinoatrial node

6. The ability of cardiac cells to conduct electrical impulses is called the property of:
   A. conductivity   C. self-excitation
   B. automaticity   D. contractility

7. In the resting state a myocardial cell has a high concentration of _____ charged _____ ions present outside the cell.
   A. negatively: sodium   C. negatively: potas-
   B. positively: potas-   sium
      sium   C. positively: sodium

8. Cardiac cells cannot be stimulated to depolarize during the:
   A. relative refractory C. supernormal pe-
      period   riod
   B. absolute refractory D. downstroke of the
      period   T wave

9. The normal and dominant pacemaker of the heart is the _____.
   A. Purkinje fibers   C. SA node
   B. AV node   D. Bundle of His

10. A condition in which the progression of an electrical impulse is delayed or blocked in one or more segments of the electrical conduction system while being conducted normally through the rest of the electrical conduction system is called:
    A. automaticity   C. bigeminy
    B. reentry   D. triggered activity

The Electrocardiogram

19

Upon completion of all or part of this chapter you should be able to complete the following objectives indicated by your instructor:

☐ **1.** Explain what the electrocardiogram (ECG) represents.

☐ **2.** Name and identify the components of the ECG, including the waves, complexes, segments, and intervals on an ECG.

☐ **3.** List at least four causes of artifacts in the ECG.

☐ **4.** Identify the measurements of time and distance as represented by the dark and light vertical and horizontal lines on an ECG grid.

☐ **5.** Define an ECG lead, a bipolar lead, and a unipolar lead.

☐ **6.** Describe how a monitoring ECG lead II is obtained.

☐ **7.** Describe the sequence and direction of normal ventricular depolarization and its relation to the QRS complex in lead II.

☐ **8.** Explain what a monitoring ECG lead MCL_1 is, under what circumstances it is useful, and how it is obtained.

☐ **9.** List the leads of a 12-lead ECG and indicate which are unipolar and which are bipolar.

☐ **10.** Define the following terms:
   ☐ Lead
   ☐ Lead axis
   ☐ Perpendicular axis
   ☐ Frontal and horizontal planes

☐ **11.** Describe how the six limb leads of a 12-lead ECG are obtained.

☐ **12.** Identify the site of attachment of the electrodes for the six precordial leads of a 12-lead ECG on an anatomical drawing of the chest and indicate over which region of the heart each electrode lies.

☐ **13.** Explain how (1) the triaxial reference figures for the standard (bipolar) limb leads and the augmented (unipolar) leads, (2) the hexaxial reference figure, and (3) the precordial reference figure are derived.

☐ **14.** List the facing leads that view the following surfaces of the heart:
   ☐ Anterior
   ☐ Lateral
   ☐ Inferior (or diaphragmatic)

☐ **15.** Define the following terms:
   ☐ Vector
   ☐ Mean vector
   ☐ Biphasic deflection
   ☐ Equiphasic deflection
   ☐ Predominantly positive deflection
   ☐ Predominantly negative deflection

☐ **16.** Define the following terms:
   ☐ Instantaneous electrical axis or vector
   ☐ Cardiac vector
   ☐ Mean QRS axis
   ☐ P axis
   ☐ T axis

☐ **17.** Identify and label on a hexaxial figure (1) the twelve spokes of the hexaxial figure according to their polarity and degree and (2) the four quadrants.

☐ **18.** Identify and label the lead axes of the six limb leads, their negative and positive poles, their direction in degrees, and their perpendiculars on a hexaxial figure in the frontal plane.

☐ **19.** Define the following terms:
   ☐ Normal QRS axis
   ☐ Left axis deviation (LAD)
   ☐ Right axis deviation (RAD)

☐ **20.** List the cardiac and pulmonary causes of left and right axis deviation.

☐ **21.** List three major reasons for determining the QRS axis in an emergency situation.

☐ **22.** List the basic steps in determining the QRS axis using leads I, II, III, and aVF.

Electrical Basis of the Electrocardiogram

The **electrocardiogram (ECG)** is a graphic record of the changes in magnitude and direction of the **electrical activity,** or, more specifically, the **electric** current, that is generated by the **depolarization** and **repolarization** of the atria and ventricles (Figure 2-1). This electrical activity is readily detected by electrodes attached to the skin. But neither the electrical activity that results from the generation and transmission of **electrical impulses** (which are too

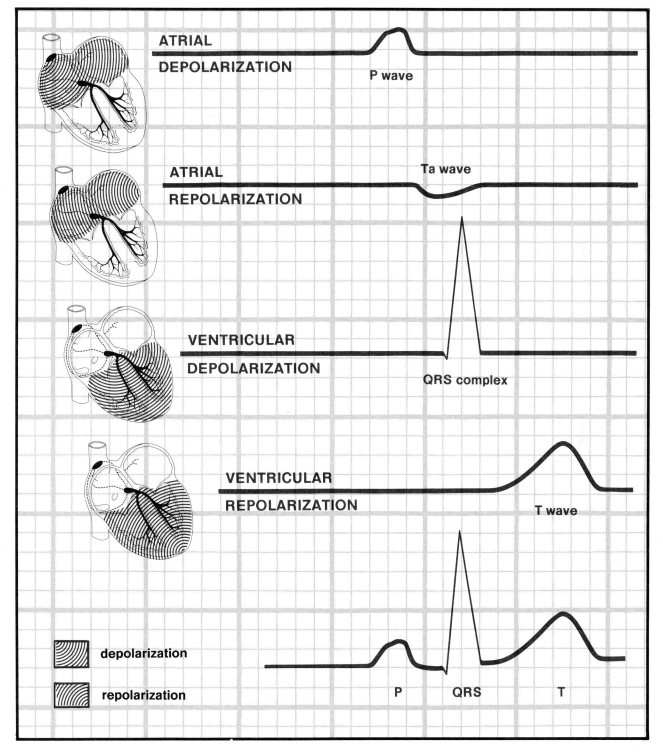

Figure 2-1. Electrical basis of the ECG.

feeble to be detected by skin electrodes) nor the mechanical contractions and relaxations of the atria and ventricles (which do not generate electrical activity) appear in the electrocardiogram.

Components of the Electrocardiogram

After the electric current generated by depolarization and repolarization of the atria and ventricles is detected by electrodes, it is amplified, displayed on an oscilloscope, and recorded on ECG paper as waves and complexes. The electric current gener-

ated by atrial depolarization is recorded as the **P wave,** and that generated by ventricular depolarization is recorded as the **Q, R,** and **S waves:** the **QRS complex.** Atrial repolarization is recorded as the **atrial T wave (Ta),** and ventricular repolarization, as the **ventricular T wave,** or simply, the **T wave.** Because atrial repolarization normally occurs during ventricular depolarization, the atrial T wave is buried or hidden in the QRS complex.

In a normal cardiac cycle, the P wave occurs first, followed by the QRS complex and the T wave (Figure 2-2).

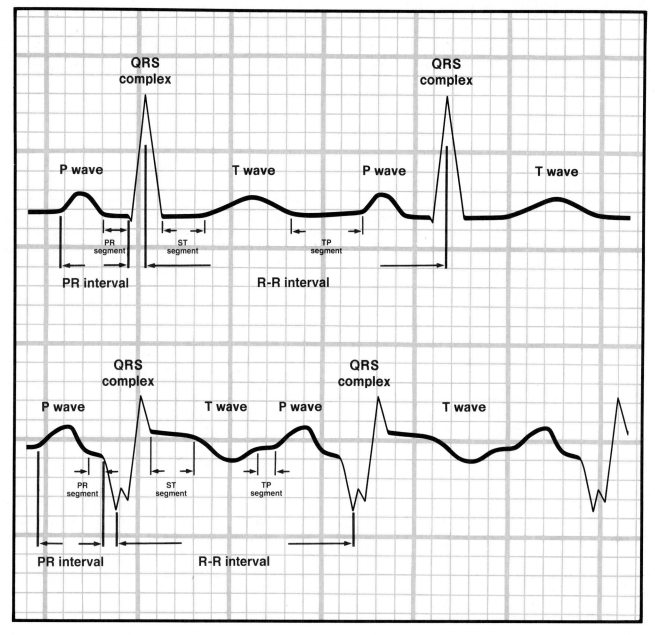

Figure 2-2. Components of the ECG.

The sections of the ECG between the waves and complexes are called **segments** and **intervals:** the **PR segment,** the **ST segment,** the **TP segment,** the **PR interval,** the **QT interval,** and the **R-R interval** (see Chapter 3). Intervals include waves and complexes, whereas segments do not.

When electrical activity of the heart is not being detected, the ECG is a straight, flat line—the **isoelectric line** or **baseline.**

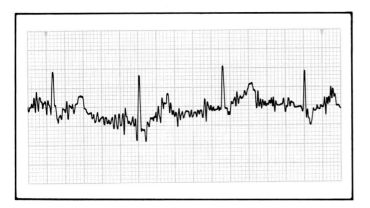

Figure 2-3. Muscle tremor.

AC interference (Figure 2-4) can occur when an improperly grounded, AC-operated ECG machine is used or when an ECG is obtained near high-tension wires, transformers, or electric appliances. This results in a thick baseline composed of 60-cycle waves.

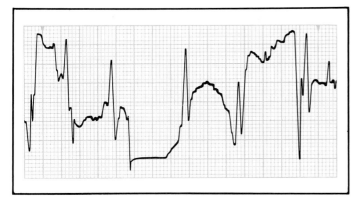

Figure 2-5. Loose electrodes.

Artifacts

Abnormal waves and spikes in an ECG that result from sources other than the electrical activity of the heart and interfere with or distort the components of the ECG are called **artifacts.** The causes of artifacts are muscle tremor, alternating current (AC) interference, loose electrodes, interference related to biotelemetry, and external chest compression.

Muscle tremor (Figure 2-3) can occur in tense or nervous patients or those shivering from cold and give the ECG a finely or coarsely jagged appearance.

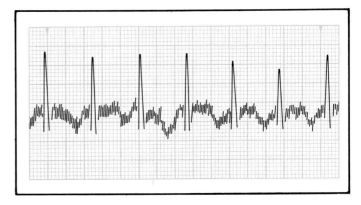

Figure 2-4. AC interference.

Loose electrodes (Figure 2-5) or electrodes that are in poor electrical contact with the skin because of insufficient or dried electrode paste or jelly can cause multiple, sharp spikes and waves in the ECG.

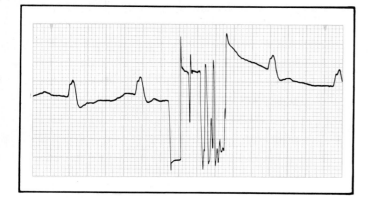

Figure 2-6. Biotelemetry.

Biotelemetry-related interference (Figure 2-6) that occurs when ECG signals are poorly received over a biotelemetry system can result in sharp spikes and waves and a jagged appearance of the ECG. Such interference can occur when the ECG transmitter's power is low because of weak batteries or when the ECG transmitter is used in the outer fringes of the reception area of the base station receiver.

External chest compressions (Figure 2-7) during cardiopulmonary resuscitation cause regularly spaced, wide, upright waves, synchronous with the downward compressions of the chest.

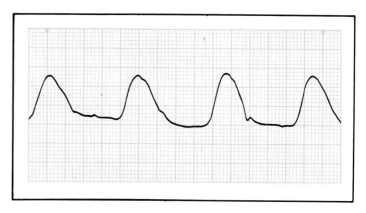

Figure 2-7. External chest compression.

ECG Paper

The paper used in recording electrocardiograms has a **grid** to permit the measurement of **time in seconds (sec)** and **distance in millimeters (mm)** along the horizontal lines and **voltage (amplitude) in millimeters (mm)** along the vertical lines (Figure 2-8).

The grid consists of intersecting dark and light vertical and horizontal lines that form large and small squares. When the ECG is recorded at the standard paper speed of 25 mm/sec:

- The **dark vertical lines** are **0.20 second (5 mm)** apart.
- The **light vertical lines** are **0.04 second (1 mm)** apart.

- The **dark horizontal lines** are **5 mm** apart.
- The **light horizontal lines** are **1 mm** apart.
- One **large square** is **5 × 5 mm.**
- One **small square** is **1 × 1 mm.**

Conventionally, the sensitivity of the ECG machine is adjusted, i.e., **calibrated** (or standardized), so that a **1-millivolt (mV)** electrical signal produces a **10-mm** deflection (two large squares) on the ECG.

Printed along one edge of the ECG paper, usually the upper one, are regularly spaced short, vertical lines denoting intervals of time. When the ECG is recorded at the **standard paper speed,** the distance between two consecutive short vertical lines is **75 mm (3 sec),** and that between every third short vertical line is **150 mm (6 sec).**

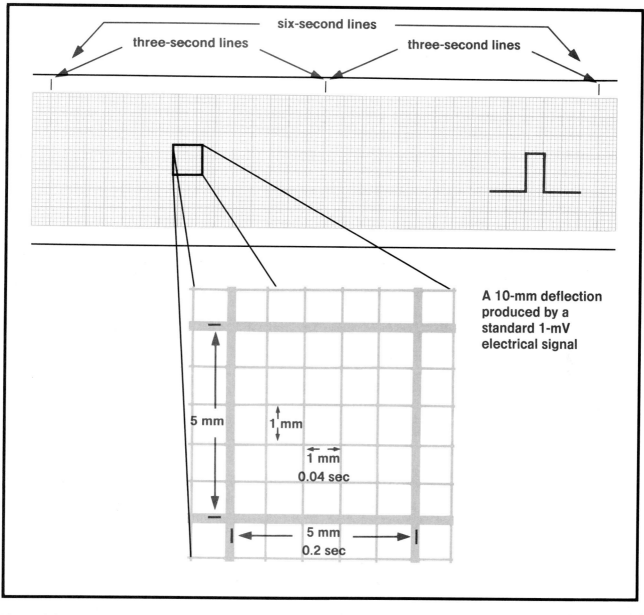

Figure 2-8. ECG paper.

ECG Leads

An **ECG lead** is a record of the electrical activity generated by the heart that is sensed by either one of two ways: (1) two electrodes of opposite polarity (one **positive** and the other **negative**) or (2) one **positive electrode** and an **"indifferent," zero reference point.** A lead composed of two electrodes of opposite polarity is called a **bipolar lead;** a lead composed of a single positive electrode and a zero reference point is a **unipolar lead.**

Depending on the ECG lead being recorded, the positive electrode may be attached to the right or left arm, the left leg, or one of several locations on the anterior chest wall. The negative electrode is usually attached to an opposite arm or leg or to a reference point made by connecting the limb electrodes together.

For a detailed analysis of the heart's electrical activity, usually in the hospital setting, an ECG recorded from 12 separate leads (the **12-lead ECG**) is used (Figure 2-9). The 12-lead ECG is also used in the prehospital phase of emergency care in certain advanced life support services to diagnose acute myocardial infarction and to help in the identification of certain arrhythmias. A **12-lead ECG** consists of **three standard (bipolar) limb leads (leads I, II, and III), three augmented (unipolar) leads (leads aVR, aVL, and aVF),** and **six precordial (unipolar) leads (V₁, V₂, V₃, V₄, V₅, and V₆).**

When monitoring the heart solely for arrhythmias, a single ECG lead, such as the **standard limb lead II,** is commonly used, especially in the prehospital phase of emergency care. A bipolar **lead MCL₁** is also used, especially in the monitoring of arrhythmias in the hospital.

Monitoring ECG Lead II

Lead II is obtained by attaching the negative electrode to the right arm and the positive electrode to the left leg (Figure 2-10). In the prehospital phase of emergency care, lead II is usually obtained by attaching the negative electrode to the upper right anterior chest wall and the positive electrode to the lower left anterior chest wall at the intersection of the fourth intercostal space and the midclavicular line. To eliminate or reduce electrical interference (**"noise"**) in the electrocardiogram when using lead II for monitoring, a third, electrically neutral electrode (or **ground electrode**) is commonly attached

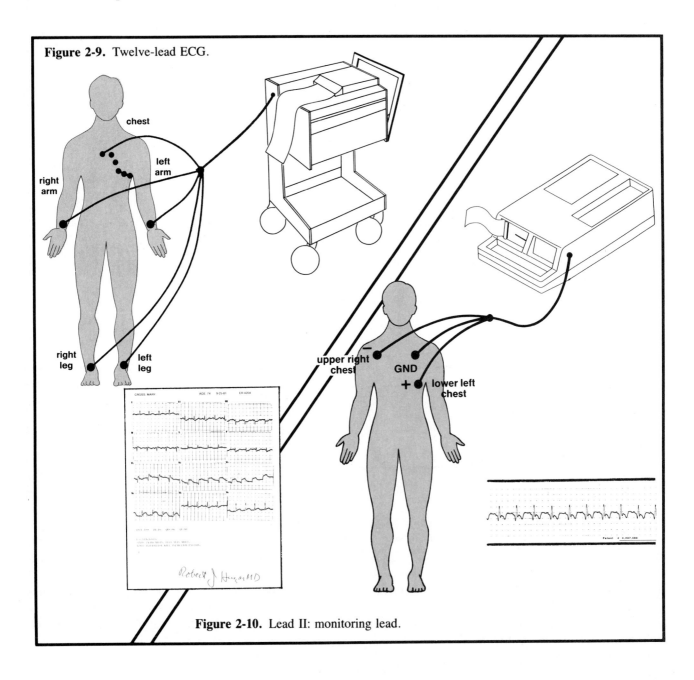

Figure 2-9. Twelve-lead ECG.

Figure 2-10. Lead II: monitoring lead.

to the upper left chest, to an extremity (the left arm or right leg), or, for that matter, to any part of the body.

When an electric current flows toward the positive electrode of a lead, a positive (upright) deflection is recorded on the electrocardiogram. Conversely, a negative (downward) deflection is recorded when an electric current flows away from the positive electrode. If the positive ECG electrode is attached to the left leg, all the electric currents generated in the heart that flow toward the left leg will be recorded as positive (upright) deflections; that which flow away from the left leg will be recorded as negative (downward) deflections.

It should be noted here that since normal depolarization of the atria and ventricles generally progresses from the right upper chest downward toward the left leg, the electric currents generated during normal depolarization of the heart will, for the most part, flow toward the left leg and be recorded as two positive (upright) deflections—a positive **P wave** and a large positive **R wave**—in lead II.

Since normal depolarization of the ventricles initially may progress away from the left leg for a short period of time, a small negative (inverted) deflection may occur before the R wave—the **Q wave** in lead II. In addition, depending on the position of the heart in the chest, the size of the ventricles, and the rotation of the heart, normal ventricular depolarization may also progress away from the left leg during the last phase of ventricular depolarization, producing a small negative (inverted) deflection after the R wave—the **S wave** (Figure 2-11).

Note: The ECG components and strips shown in this book are depicted as they would appear in lead II unless otherwise noted.

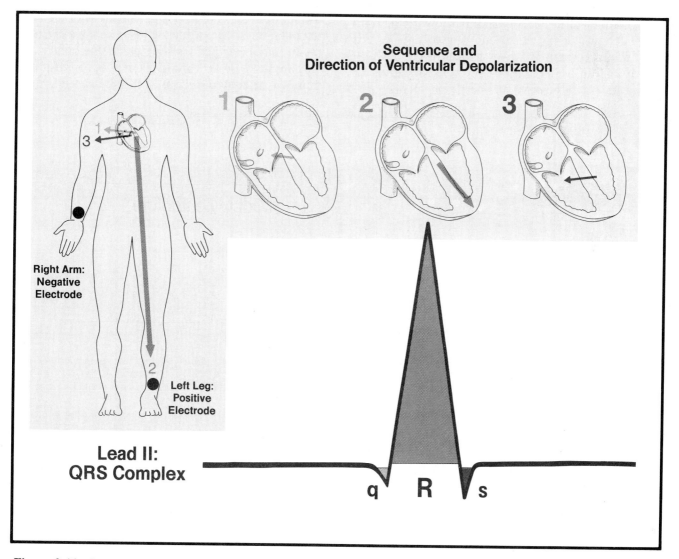

Figure 2-11. Sequence and direction of normal ventricular depolarization and the QRS complex in lead II.

Monitoring ECG Lead MCL$_1$

Lead MCL$_1$ is obtained by attaching the positive electrode to the right side of the anterior chest in the fourth intercostal space just right of the sternum (Figure 2-12). The negative electrode is attached to the left chest in the midclavicular line below the clavicle. The result is a bipolar lead simulating V$_1$ of the 12-lead ECG. Lead MCL$_1$ is helpful in identifying the origin of certain arrhythmias with wide QRS complexes. This will be discussed later in the book.

Unlike in lead II where a predominantly positive QRS complex with a **large R wave** is normally present, the electric current generated during normal ventricular depolarization will flow away from the positive electrode on the right chest toward the left leg, producing a predominantly negative QRS complex with a **large negative S wave** in lead MCL$_1$. The small electric current that flows toward the right shoulder producing the Q and S waves in lead II will produce small R waves in lead MCL$_1$. The P wave in lead MCL$_1$ may be positive, negative, or biphasic (partly positive and partly negative).

12-Lead ECG

A **12-lead** (or **conventional**) ECG consists of:

- **Six limb or extremity leads**
  - **Three standard (bipolar) limb leads:** leads I, II, and III
  - **Three augmented (unipolar) leads:** leads aVR, aVL, and aVF
- **Six precordial (unipolar) leads:** leads V$_1$, V$_2$, V$_3$, V$_4$, V$_5$, and V$_6$

Each lead is obtained using a **positive ("sensing" or "probing") electrode** and a **negative electrode.** An additional electrode, the **ground electrode,** is attached to the right leg (or any other location on the body) to provide a path of least resistance for electrical interference in the body.

The **positive electrode** may be attached to the extremities (right arm, left arm, or left leg) to obtain the six limb leads or to designated areas of the chest to obtain the six precordial leads. The **negative electrode** may be either a **single electrode** attached to an extremity or an **"indifferent," zero reference point**—the **central terminal (CT),** formed by con-

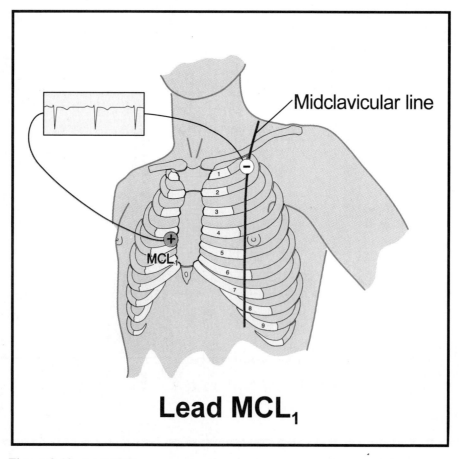

Lead MCL$_1$

Figure 2-12. Lead MCL$_1$.

necting the extremity electrodes together. The central terminal is a common negative electrode with an **electrical potential** of **zero.** It is hypothetically located in the heart, left of the interventricular septum and below the AV junction where the electrical center of the heart is located.

A lead obtained using a **positive electrode** and a **single negative electrode** is called a **bipolar lead** (Figure 2-13, *A*). Bipolar leads include the **standard leads I, II, and III.**

A lead obtained using a **positive electrode** and a **central terminal** is called a **unipolar** (or "V") **lead** (Figure 2-13, *B*). Unipolar leads include the **three augmented leads** (**leads aVR, aVL,** and **aVF**) and the **six precordial leads** (**leads** V_1, V_2, V_3, V_4, V_5, and V_6).

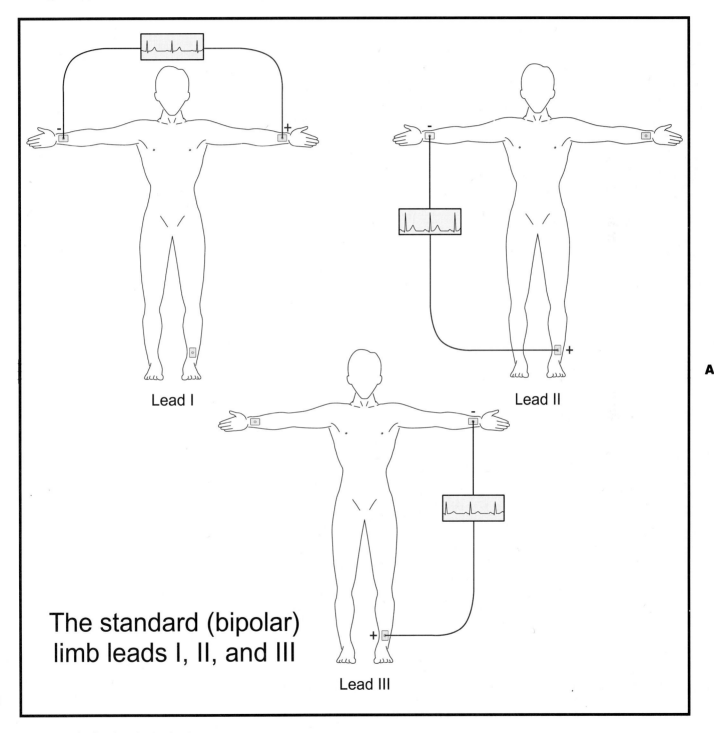

Lead I

Lead II

A

The standard (bipolar) limb leads I, II, and III

Lead III

Figure 2-13. A, Bipolar leads.

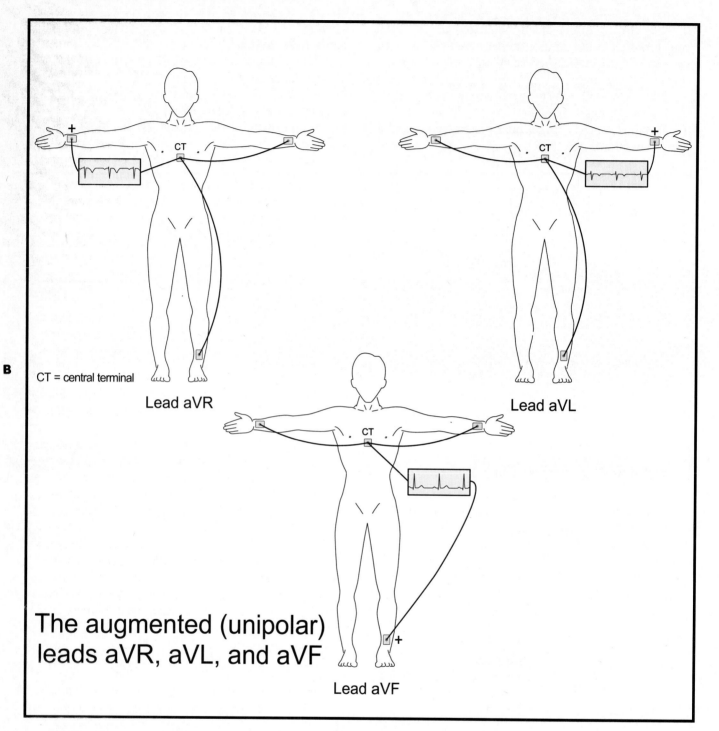

CT = central terminal

Lead aVR

Lead aVL

Lead aVF

The augmented (unipolar) leads aVR, aVL, and aVF

B

Figure 2-13, cont. B, Unipolar leads.

Lead Axis

Each lead of the 12-lead ECG measures the difference in **electrical potential** between the positive and negative electrodes (or **poles**). Thus, each lead has a **positive** and **negative pole.**

A hypothetical line joining the poles of a lead is known as the **axis of the lead** (or **lead axis**). The location of the positive and negative poles in a lead determines the **orientation** (or **direction**) of the axis of the lead. Thus, a lead axis has a **direction** and **polarity.**

In addition, each lead axis has a **perpendicular axis,** or, simply, the **perpendicular** (Figure 2-14). It is usually depicted as a line intersecting or connecting with the lead axis at ± 90° (or a right angle), at its electrically **"zero"** point.

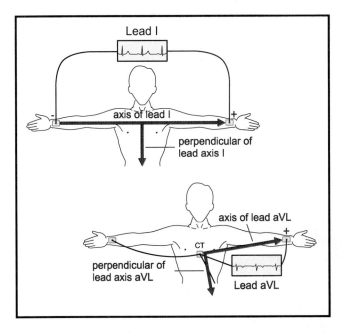

Figure 2-14. The axis of a lead and its perpendicular.

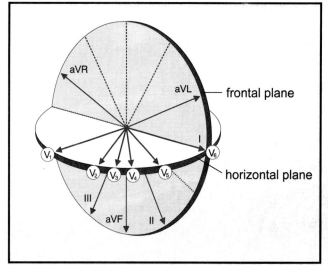

Figure 2-15. The frontal and horizontal planes.

Frontal and Horizontal Planes

The three standard limb leads (I, II, and III) and the three augmented leads (aVR, aVL, and aVF) measure the electrical activity of the heart in the **frontal plane,** that is, as viewed from the front of the patient's body (Figure 2-15). The six precordial leads (V_1, V_2, V_3, V_4, V_5, and V_6) measure the electrical activity of the heart at a right angle to the frontal plane, the **horizontal plane.**

Standard (Bipolar) Limb Leads

Each of the **standard limb leads I, II, and III** is obtained using a **positive electrode** attached to one of two extremities (left arm or left leg) and a single **negative electrode** to another extremity (right or left arm) (Figure 2-16). Thus, each **standard limb lead** measures the difference in electrical potential between two extremity electrodes. The **lead axis** for each standard limb lead is a line drawn between the two extremity electrodes, with one electrode designated as the negative pole, and the other as the positive pole. The perpendicular divides the lead axis into a positive and a negative half.

The electrodes are attached as follows to obtain the three standard limb leads:

Lead I	The **positive electrode** is attached to the **left arm** and the **negative electrode** to the **right arm.**
Lead II	The **positive electrode** is attached to the **left leg** and the **negative electrode** to the **right arm.**
Lead III	The **positive electrode** is attached to the **left leg** and the **negative electrode** to the **left arm.**

The relationships of the standard limb leads are such that the sum of the electric currents recorded in leads I and III equals the sum of the electric current recorded in lead II. This is called **Einthoven's law,** named after the developer of three-lead electrocardiography. The law is expressed mathematically as follows:

Lead I + Lead III = Lead II

Since the positive electrodes of the three standard limb leads are electrically about the same distance from the zero reference point in the heart, an equilateral triangle (**Einthoven's equilateral triangle**) can be depicted in the frontal plane using the three lead axes with the heart and its zero reference point in the center (Figure 2-17). The three sides of the equilateral triangle can be shifted to the right, left, and down without changing the angle of their orientation until their midpoints intersect at the same point. This creates a **triaxial reference figure** with each of the lead axes forming a 60-degree angle with its neighbors.

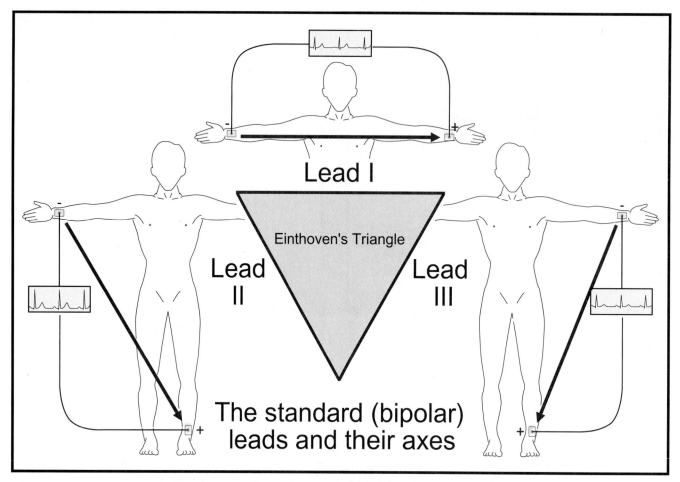

Figure 2-16. The standard (bipolar) limb leads I, II, and III and their axes.

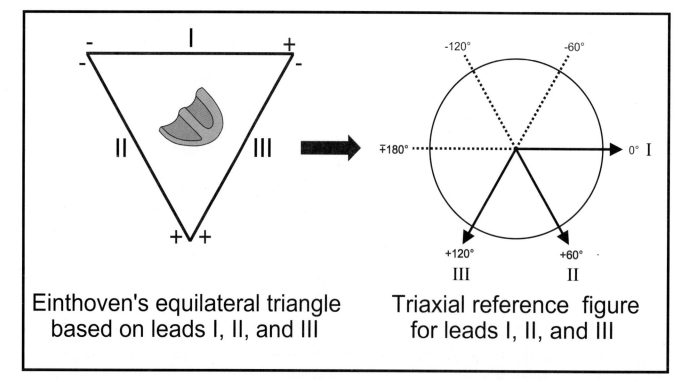

Figure 2-17. Einthoven's triangle and triaxial reference figure.

Augmented (Unipolar) Leads

The **augmented leads aVR, aVL, and aVF** are obtained using a **positive electrode** attached to one of three extremities (right arm, left arm, or right leg) and a **central terminal** made by connecting the other two extremity electrodes (Figure 2-18, *A*). Thus, an **augmented lead** measures the difference in electrical potential between one of three extremity electrodes and the central terminal. The **lead axis** for a particular augmented lead is a line drawn between the central terminal and its extremity electrode, with the central terminal labeled as the negative pole and the extremity electrode as the positive pole. The augmented lead axis is usually shown with its negative half extended as a dotted, dashed, or shaded line.

The three extremity electrodes are attached as follows to obtain the three augmented leads:

Lead aVR The **positive electrode** is attached to the **right arm** and the **negative electrode** to the **central terminal** (**left arm** and **left leg**).

Lead aVL The **positive electrode** is attached to the **left arm** and the **negative electrode** to the **central terminal** (**right arm** and **left leg**).

Lead aVF The **positive electrode** is attached to the **left leg** and the **negative electrode** to the **central terminal** (**right** and **left arms**).

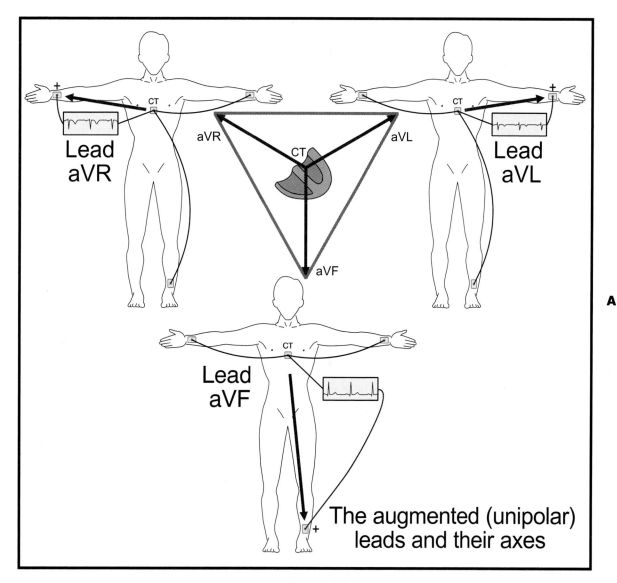

Figure 2-18. **A,** The augmented leads aVR, aVL, and aVF and their axes.

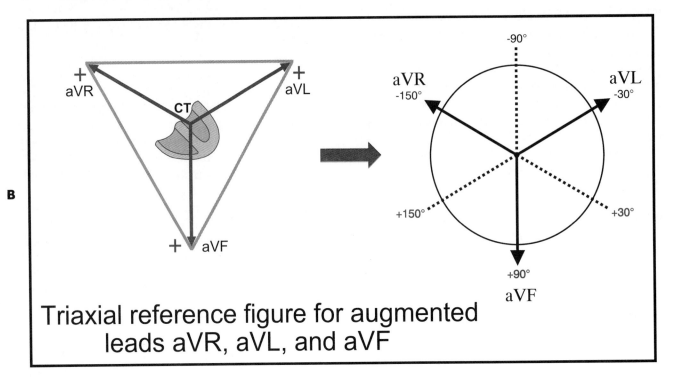

Triaxial reference figure for augmented leads aVR, aVL, and aVF

Figure 2-18, cont. B, The triaxial reference figure for the augmented leads.

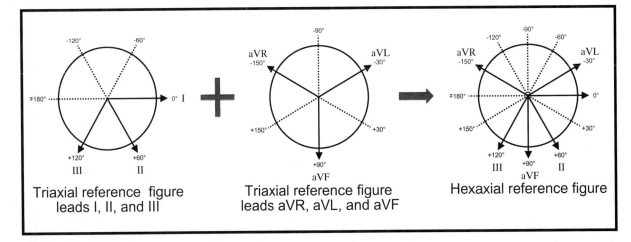

Figure 2-19. The hexaxial reference figure.

It must be noted that originally the central terminal for these unipolar leads was obtained by connecting the right arm, left arm, and left leg together. Because this hookup resulted in a small electric current, and consequently small waves and complexes, in the VR, VL, and VF leads, as they were originally called, the lead that was actually being taken was disconnected from the central terminal. Since this increased the electric current (and size) of the waves and complexes in the ECG, the unipolar leads were renamed **"augmented,"** thus the **"a"** in **aVR, aVL, and aVF.**

The positive electrodes of the three augmented leads, like those of the three standard limb leads, are also electrically equidistant from the zero reference point in the heart. The **triaxial reference figure** (Figure 2-18, *B*) formed in the frontal plane by the axes of the three augmented leads is similar to that of the standard limb leads, with its lead axes 60° apart but oriented around the zero reference point at slightly different angles.

When the triaxial reference figures of the standard limb leads and the augmented leads are superimposed, they form a **hexaxial reference figure** (Figure 2-19). Each augmented lead axis is perpendicular to a standard limb lead axis, so that each lead axis is spaced 30° apart. The hexaxial reference figure's use in determining the major direction of the heart's electrical activity (e.g., the **QRS axis**) in the frontal plane will be discussed later.

Precordial (Unipolar) Leads

The **precordial leads** V_1, V_2, V_3, V_4, V_5, and V_6 are unipolar leads obtained by attaching the **positive electrode** to prescribed areas over the anterior chest wall and the **negative lead** to the **central terminal,** which, in this case, is made by connecting all three extremity electrodes: the right and left arm electrodes and the left leg electrode (Figure 2-20, *A, B*). A precordial lead thus measures the difference in electrical potential between a chest electrode and the central terminal. The **lead axis** for each precordial lead is drawn from the central terminal to the specific chest electrode, with the central terminal designated as the negative pole and the chest electrode as the positive pole.

The individual chest electrodes are positioned across the anterior chest wall from right to left so that they overlie the right ventricle, the interventricular septum, and the anterior and lateral surfaces of the left ventricle.

The placement of the positive chest electrodes is as follows:

V_1 Right side of the sternum in the fourth intercostal space.

V_2 Left side of the sternum in the fourth intercostal space.

V_3 Midway between V_2 and V_4.

V_4 Midclavicular line in the fifth intercostal space.

V_5 Anterior axillary line at the same level as V_4.

V_6 Midaxillary line at the same level as V_4.

Electrodes V_1 and V_2 (the **right precordial [or septal] leads**) overlie the right ventricle; electrodes V_3 and V_4 (the **midprecordial [or anterior] leads**) overlie the interventricular septum and part of the left ventricle; and V_5 and V_6 (the **left precordial [or lateral] leads**) overlie the left ventricle.

A transverse (cross-sectional) outline of the chest wall showing the central terminal, the six chest elec-

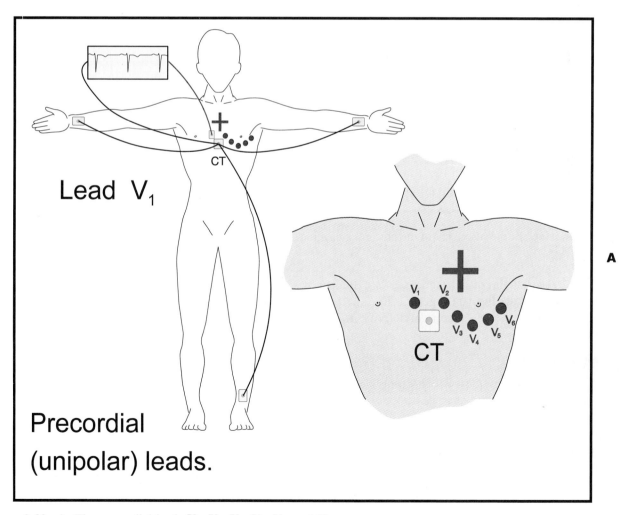

Lead V_1

Precordial (unipolar) leads.

A

Figure 2-20. A, The precordial leads V_1, V_2, V_3, V_4, V_5, and V_6.

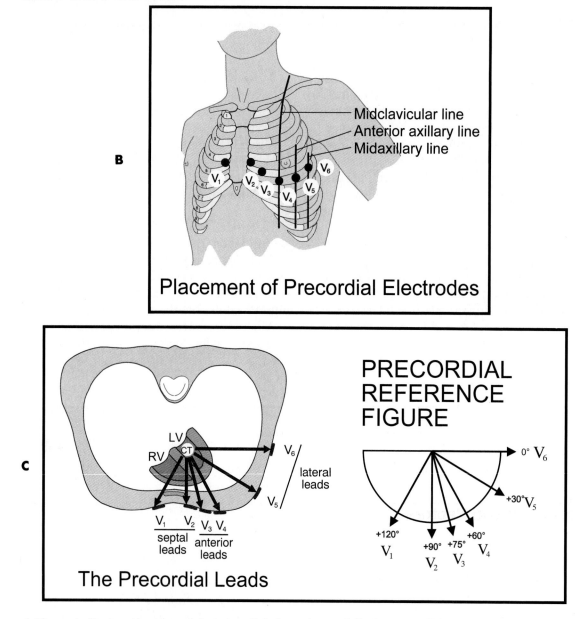

Figure 2-20, cont. B, the placement of the precordial electrodes; and **C,** the precordial reference figure.

trodes, and the six precordial lead axes is called a **precordial reference figure** (Figure 2-20, *C*). It is used in plotting the heart's electrical activity in the horizontal plane.

Facing Leads

A 12-lead ECG provides 12 different views of the electrical activity of the heart, each view looking from the outside of the chest toward the zero reference point within the chest. Leads I and aVL and the precordial leads V_5 and V_6 view the lateral surface of the heart; leads II, III, and aVF, the inferior (diaphragmatic) surface; and leads V_1 through V_4, the anterior surface of the heart. No leads face the posterior surface of the heart.

The leads that view specific surfaces of the heart are termed **"facing" leads** in this book (Figure 2-21). These include all the leads except aVR, which faces the interior, endocardial surface of the ventricles.

It is important to know the facing leads in determining the location of an acute myocardial infarction!

Facing leads	Surface of the heart viewed
V_1-V_4	Anterior
I, aVL, V_5-V_6	Lateral
II, III, aVF	Inferior (or diaphragmatic)

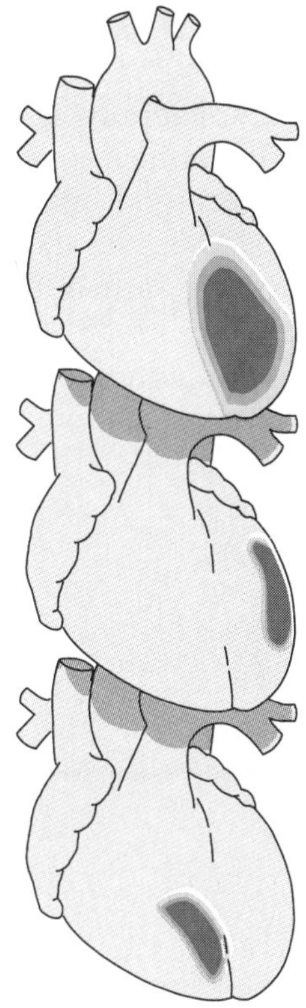

Surface of the Heart Viewed	Facing Leads
Anterior	V_1-V_4
Lateral	I, aVL, V_5-V_6
Inferior	II, III. aVF

Figure 2-21. The facing leads.

Electrical Axes and Vectors

The electric current generated by the depolarization or repolarization of the atria and ventricles at any given moment is called an **instantaneous electrical axis** or **vector** (Figure 2-22). These two terms *vector* and *axis* are synonymous and are often used interchangeably. Electrical axis is not to be confused with an axis of a lead.

A vector is commonly visualized graphically as an **arrow** that has **magnitude, direction,** and **polarity.** The length of the shaft of the arrow represents the magnitude of the electric current; the orientation or position of the arrow, the direction of flow of the electric current; and the tip of the arrow, the positive end, and the tail, the negative end.

The instantaneous electric currents produced by the ventricles during one cardiac cycle can be depicted as a series of **cardiac vectors,** each representing the moment-to-moment electric current generated by depolarization of a small segment of the ventricular wall.

The initial cardiac vector represents the depolarization of the interventricular septum and is directed from left to right. This is followed immediately by

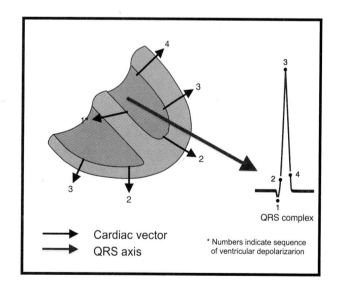

Figure 2-22. Cardiac vectors and the QRS axis.

a sequence of vectors produced by the endocardial to epicardial depolarization of segments of the ventricular wall, beginning in the right and left ventricles near the septum and ending in the lateral and posterior aspect of the left ventricle.

The vectors arising in the right ventricle are directed mostly to the right when viewed in the frontal plane; those in the left ventricle, to the left. The left ventricular vectors are larger and persist longer than those of the smaller right ventricle, primarily because of the much greater thickness of the left ventricular wall. The mean (or average) of all the ventricular vectors is a single large vector—the **mean QRS axis** or, simply, the **QRS axis**—pointing to the left and downward, reflecting the dominance of the left ventricle over the right ventricle.

The mean of all the vectors generated during the depolarization of the atria is the **P axis** and that during the repolarization of the ventricles, the **ST axis** and **T axis** (Figure 2-23).

The **P axis** is rarely determined. The **T axis** is determined in certain conditions, such as myocardial ischemia and acute myocardial infarction, in which there is a significant shift in the direction of the T axis. Determination of the shift in the T axis helps to localize the affected area of the myocardium. The **QRS axis** is the most important and also the most frequently determined axis. Commonly, when the term *axis* is used alone, it refers to the QRS axis.

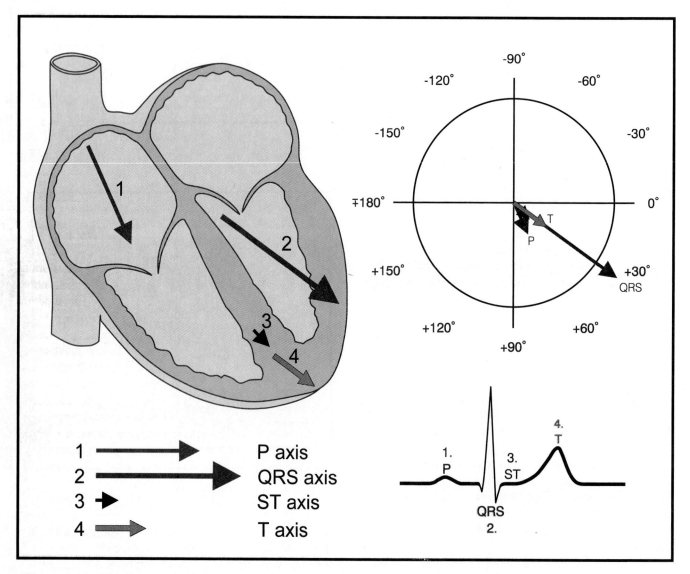

Figure 2-23. The P axis, the QRS axis, the ST axis, and the T axis.

The Electric Current, Vectors, and the Lead Axis

An electric current flowing **parallel** to the axis of a lead produces either a positive or a negative deflection on an ECG strip recorder or an ECG screen depending on the direction of its flow. An electric current flowing **toward the positive pole** produces a **positive deflection;** an electric current flowing **toward the negative pole,** a **negative deflection.** The greater the magnitude of the electric current, the larger the deflection, and vice versa. When the flow of electric current is **perpendicular** to the axis of a lead, no deflection is produced. Figure 2-24, *A,* shows the relationship between the direction of flow of an electric current, as represented by a **vector,** and the deflection it produces on an ECG.

When an electric current flows in a direction that is somewhat between being parallel and perpendicular (i.e., oblique), the deflection is smaller than when the same electric current flows parallel to the axis of a lead. The more parallel the electric current

is to the axis of the lead, the larger is the deflection; the more perpendicular, the smaller the deflection. This is true whether the electric current is flowing toward or away from the positive pole (Figure 2-24, *B*).

When an electric current flows partly toward and partly away from the positive pole, a **bidirectional** electric current is present. It is represented by a single **mean vector** that is an average of all the positive and negative electric currents present. Such an electric current produces a **biphasic deflection** on the ECG, one that is partly positive and partly negative. The size of the components of the deflection depends on the magnitude of the individual electric currents. If the **mean (or average) direction** of the biphasic deflection is positive, no matter by how much, the deflection is **predominantly positive;** if the mean direction is negative, the deflection is **predominantly negative.** Figure 2-24, *C,* shows the relationship between a bidirectional electric current, as represented by a **mean vector,** and the biphasic deflections on an ECG.

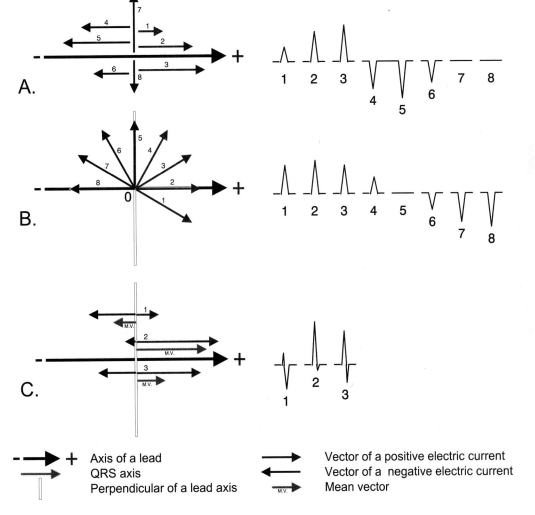

Figure 2-24. The axis of a lead, its perpendicular, and direction of flow of electric currents.

The more parallel the mean vector of a biphasic deflection is to the axis of the lead, the more positive is the biphasic deflection; the closer the orientation of the mean vector is to the perpendicular, the less positive is the biphasic deflection. When the positive and negative deflections are equal in magnitude, an **equiphasic deflection** is present, and the sum of the deflections is **zero.** In this case, the mean vector is **perpendicular** to the lead axis (Figure 2-24, *D*).

It is important to understand the significance of the relationship between the predominant direction of the deflections of the QRS complexes in a given

lead, the perpendicular of the related lead axis, and the QRS axis. A **predominantly positive QRS complex** in a given lead indicates that the positive pole of the vector of the QRS axis lies somewhere on the **positive side** of the perpendicular to that lead axis. Conversely, a **predominantly negative QRS complex** in a lead indicates that the positive pole of the vector of the QRS axis lies somewhere on the **negative side** of the perpendicular (Figure 2-24, *E*).

Thus, the perpendicular to an axis of a lead serves as a boundary between the predominantly positive and predominantly negative deflections in any given lead.

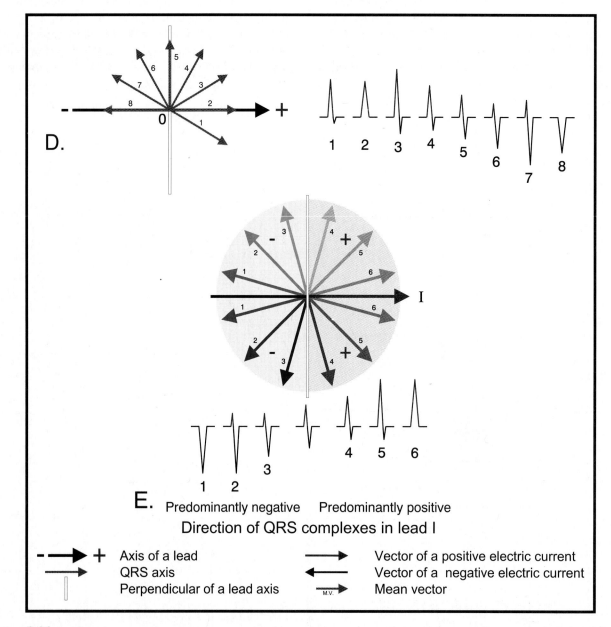

E. Predominantly negative   Predominantly positive
Direction of QRS complexes in lead I

Figure 2-24, cont.

Hexaxial Reference Figure

The **hexaxial reference figure,** as noted earlier, is a composite of the two triaxials formed by combining the axes of the three standard limb leads (I, II, III) and the three augmented leads (aVR, aVL, aVF) (Figure 2-25, *A*). The primary purpose of the hexaxial reference figure is to aid in the determination of the direction of the **QRS axis** in the frontal plane with some degree of precision.

Viewed from the front, the six lead axes are arranged like **spokes within a wheel** through a **central point** representing the potentially **"zero" center of the heart.** The axes of the leads are positioned within the wheel consistent with their actual direction and polarity in the frontal plane so that their positive and negative poles are spaced 30° apart around the rim of the wheel.

Each positive and negative pole is assigned a degree number ranging from 0° to 180°. The poles around the rim of the **upper half** of the wheel of the hexaxial reference figure are given negative degree numbers (− 30°, − 60°, − 90°, − 120°, − 150°, and − 180°); those around the **lower half** of the rim are given positive degree numbers (**+ 30°, + 60°, + 90°, + 120°, + 150°, and + 180°).** The

negative and positive degrees should not be confused with the negative and positive poles of the lead axes.

The **positive** and **negative poles** of the axes of the **three standard limb leads** and the **three augmented leads** are assigned the following degree numbers:

Standard leads	− Pole	+ Pole
Lead I	± 180°	0°
Lead II	− 120°	+ 60°
Lead III	− 60°	+ 120°
Augmented leads		
Lead aVR	+ 30°	− 150°
Lead aVL	+ 150°	− 30°
Lead aVF	− 90°	+ 90°

The hexaxial reference figure is divided into **four quadrants** (Figure 2-25, *B*) by the bisection of lead axes I and aVF. Although there are several different ways to designate the quadrants, the following designation is used in this chapter.

Quadrant	Number
0° to − 90°	I
0° to + 90°	II
+ 90° to + 180	III
− 90° to − 180°	IV

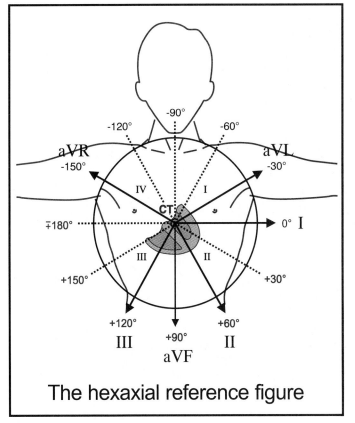

The hexaxial reference figure

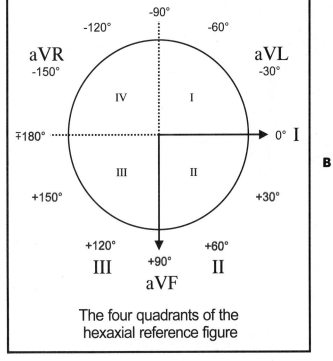

B

The four quadrants of the hexaxial reference figure

Figure 2-25. A, The hexaxial reference figure and, **B,** the four quadrants of the hexaxial reference figure.

The **perpendiculars of the lead axes** have the same attributes as those of the lead axes with which they coincide (Figure 2-26). For example, the perpendicular to the axis of lead II, which coincides with that of lead aVL, has one pole at $-30°$ and the other at $+150°$. **Table 2-1** summarizes the location of the negative and positive poles of the lead axes and their perpendiculars.

Table 2-1. The negative and positive poles of the lead axes and their perpendiculars

Lead	Location of lead axis poles		Location of the poles of the perpendicular (and its coincident lead axis)
	− Pole	+ Pole	
I	$\pm 180°$	$0°$	$-90°, +90°$ (aVF)
II	$-120°$	$+60°$	$+150°, -30°$ (aVL)
III	$-60°$	$+120°$	$+30°, -150°$ (aVR)
aVR	$+30°$	$-150°$	$-60°, +120°$ (III)
aVL	$+150°$	$-30°$	$-120°, +60°$ (II)
aVF	$-90°$	$+90°$	$\pm 180°, 0°$ (I)

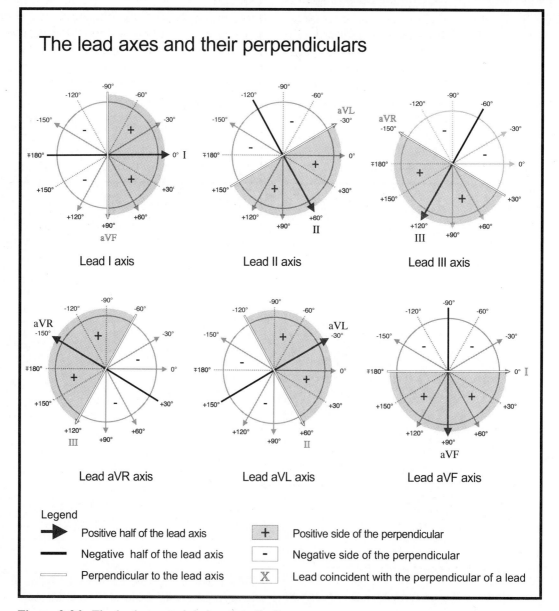

Figure 2-26. The lead axes and their perpendiculars.

The QRS Axis

The **normal QRS axis,** as determined using the hexaxial reference figure, lies between −**30° and** +**90°** in the frontal plane (Figure 2-27). A change or **"shift"** in the direction of the QRS axis from normal to one between −**30° and** −**90°** is considered **left axis deviation (LAD);** a shift of the QRS axis to one between +**90° and** +**180°, right axis deviation (RAD).** A QRS axis rarely falls between −**90° and** +**180°.** If it does, **extreme right axis deviation** or an **indeterminate axis** is present.

A QRS complex with **left axis deviation** (i.e., a QRS axis greater than −**30°**) is always abnormal. A QRS complex with **right axis deviation** (i.e., a QRS axis greater than +**90°**) may or may not be abnormal depending on the age and body build of the patient. Right axis deviation of up to +**120°** or more may be present in newborns and infants and up to about +**110°** in young adults with long, narrow chests and vertical hearts.

In the majority of adults, however, right axis deviation is seldom present without some cardiac or pulmonary disorder. For this reason, such a disorder should be suspected whenever right axis deviation is present in adults. In general, the causes of abnormal shift of the QRS axis to the left or right are **(1) ventricular enlargement** and **hypertrophy** and **(2) bundle branch** and **fascicular block** (See Chapters 10 and 12).

Left axis deviation (QRS axis greater than −**30°)** occurs in adults in the following cardiac disorders:

- **Left ventricular enlargement** and **hypertrophy.**
  - Hypertension
  - Aortic stenosis
  - Ischemic heart disease
  - Other disorders affecting the left ventricle
- **Left bundle branch block** and **left anterior fascicular block.**

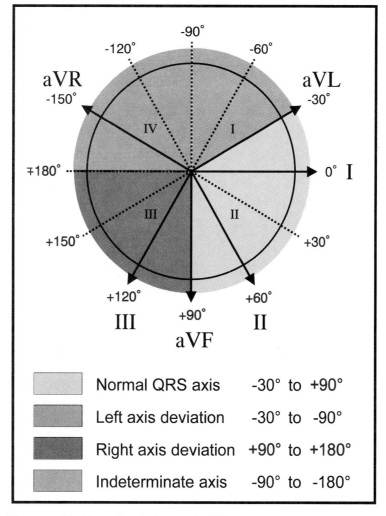

Normal QRS axis	-30° to	+90°
Left axis deviation	-30° to	-90°
Right axis deviation	+90° to	+180°
Indeterminate axis	-90° to	-180°

Figure 2-27. Normal and abnormal QRS axes.

Right axis deviation (QRS axis greater than +90°) occurs in adults with the following cardiac and pulmonary disorders:
- **Right ventricular enlargement** and **hypertrophy** secondary to:
  - Chronic obstructive pulmonary disease (COPD)
  - Pulmonary embolism
  - Congenital heart disease
  - Other disorders causing:
    - Severe pulmonary hypertension
    - Cor pulmonale
- **Right bundle branch block** and **left posterior fascicular block.**

The determination of the QRS axis may be useful in the following emergency situations:
- **In acute myocardial infarction** to determine if an acute left anterior or posterior fascicular block is present
- **In acute pulmonary embolism** to determine if right ventricular stretching and enlargement and subsequent acute right bundle branch block are present
- **In a tachycardia with wide QRS complexes** to differentiate between a tachycardia arising in the ventricles (**ventricular ectopy**) and one arising in the SA node, atria, or AV junction with wide QRS complexes caused by a **preexisting bundle branch block, aberrant ventricular conduction,** or **anomalous AV conduction** (see Chapter 3).

Determination of the QRS Axis

Several methods are used to determine the QRS axis. The most accurate method is by plotting **leads I and III** (or **leads I and II**) on a triaxial reference grid and calculating the axis by angulation. This method is somewhat time-consuming and not adaptable to emergency situations.

It is easier and quicker to approximate the QRS axes in the frontal plane using the hexaxial reference figure as follows:

- First, determine the net positivity or negativity of the **QRS complexes** in certain limb leads (i.e., whether the QRS complexes are **predominantly positive** or **negative**).
- Then, by using this information and knowing the perpendiculars to these leads, determine the approximate QRS axis on the hexaxial reference figure.

Lead I is usually evaluated first, then **lead II**. Between the two, it can be determined whether the QRS axis is normal or left or right axis deviation is present. Depending on the findings at this point, one or more of the other leads (i.e., **leads III, aVF, aVR,** and, rarely, **aVL**) are evaluated to determine the location of the QRS axis with greater accuracy if necessary. Figure 2-28 depicts the basics of determining the QRS axis using the hexaxial reference figure. Specific methods for determining the QRS axis are located in **Appendix A.**

Important points to remember in determining the QRS axis using the hexaxial reference figure are:

- A **predominantly positive QRS complex in both leads I and II** indicates a **normal QRS axis** (-30 to $+90$ degrees).
- A **predominantly positive QRS complex in lead I** and a **predominantly negative QRS complex in lead II** indicate a **left axis deviation** (-30 to -90 degrees).
- A **predominantly negative QRS complex in lead I** and a **predominantly positive QRS complex in lead aVR** indicate a **right axis deviation** ($> +120$ degrees).

Other important points to remember are:

- A **predominantly positive QRS complex in lead I** excludes **right axis deviation.**
- **Lead II** is the single lead that holds the clue in detecting left axis deviation since its perpendicular coincides with the positive pole of the axis of **lead aVL** ($-30°$).
- **Lead aVF,** in the presence of a predominantly positive QRS complex in **lead I,** helps to determine whether the QRS axis lies in quadrant I or II. A predominantly positive QRS complex in **lead aVF** indicates that the QRS axis is in quadrant II; a predominantly negative QRS complex in **lead aVF** indicates that the QRS axis is in quadrant I.
- A QRS axis between $-90°$ and $\pm 180°$ (quadrant IV) is rare except in ventricular ectopy.

Basic Steps in Determining the QRS Axis

There are three basic steps in determining the QRS axis:

Step One

■ **Determine the net positivity or negativity of the QRS complexes in lead I.**

A. **If the QRS complexes are predominantly positive in lead I,** the QRS axis lies between −90° and +90°, i.e., in **quadrant I** or **II.** The QRS axis may be between −30° and +90° (**normal QRS axis**) or between −30° and −90° (**left axis deviation**).

Step Two

If the QRS complexes are predominantly positive in lead I:

■ **Determine the net positivity or negativity of the QRS complexes in one or more of the following leads (i.e., leads II, aVF, and III):**

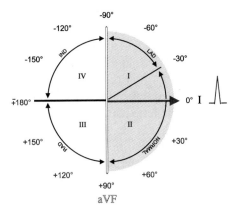

Lead II

A. **If the QRS complexes are predominantly positive in lead II,** the QRS axis is between −30° and +90° (**normal QRS axis**).

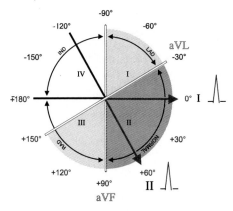

B. **If the QRS complexes are predominantly negative in lead II,** the QRS axis is between −30° and −90° (**left axis deviation**).

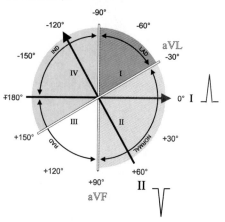

Note: The steps used in determining the QRS axis outlined here may be modified according to the specific method used in determining the QRS axis or to local protocol.

		Leads			Location of QRS Axis
I	II	aVF	III	aVR	
+	+	+	+		+30° to +90°
+	+	+	−		0° to +30°
+	+	−	−		0° to −30°
+	−	−	−		−30° to −90°
−	+	+	+	−	+90° to +120
−	+	+	+	+	+120° to +150
−	−	−	−		−90° to −150°

+ = Predominantly positive
− = Predominantly negative
± = Equiphasic

		Equiphasic Leads				Location of QRS Axis
I	II	aVF	III	aVR	aVL	
±	−	−	−	+		−90°
+	−	−	−	±		−60°
+	±	−	−	−		−30°
+	+	±	−	−		0°
+	+	+	±	−		+30°
+	+	+	+	−	±	+60°
±	+	+	+	−		+90°
−	+	+	+	±		+120°
−	±	+	+	+		+150°
−	−	±	+	+		±180°
−	−	−	±	+		−150°
−	−	−	−	+	±	−120°

Lead aVF

C. **If the QRS complexes are predominantly positive in lead aVF,** the QRS axis is between **0°** and **+90° (quadrant II).**

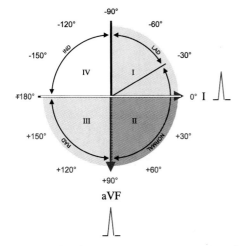

D. **If the QRS complexes are predominantly negative in lead aVF,** the QRS axis is between **0°** and **−90° (quadrant I).**

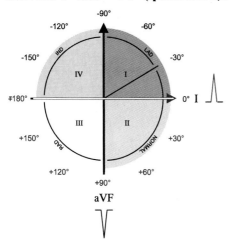

Lead III

E. **If the QRS complexes are predominantly positive in lead III,** the QRS axis is between **+30°** and **+90°.**

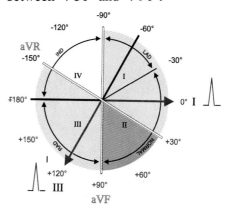

F. **If the QRS complexes are predominantly negative in lead III,** the QRS axis is between **+30°** and **−90°.**

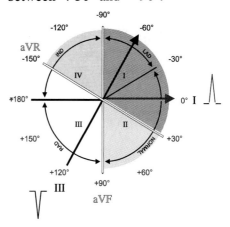

B. **If the QRS complexes are predominantly negative in lead I,** the QRS axis is greater than **+90°,** indicating **right axis deviation.** Most likely the QRS axis lies in **quadrant III** and, rarely, in **quadrant IV.**

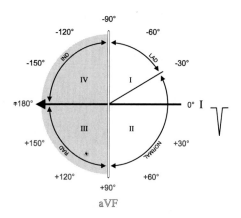

Step Three

If the QRS complexes are predominantly negative in lead I:

■ **Determine the net positivity or negativity of the QRS complexes in one or more of the following leads (i.e., leads II, aVF, III, and aVR).**

Lead II

A. **If the QRS complexes are predominantly positive in lead II,** the QRS axis is between **+90°** and **+150°.**

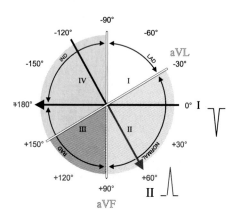

Lead aVF

C. **If the QRS complexes are predominantly positive in lead aVF,** the QRS axis is between **+90°** and **+180°** (quadrant III).

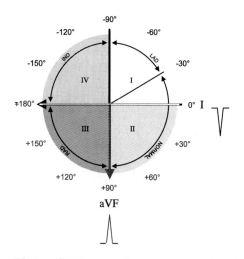

B. **If the QRS complexes are predominantly negative in lead II,** the QRS axis is greater than **+150°.**

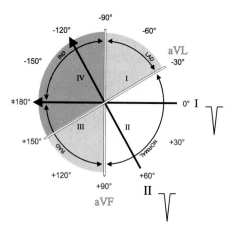

D. **If the QRS complexes are predominantly negative in lead aVF,** the QRS axis is between **−90°** and **−180°** (quadrant IV).

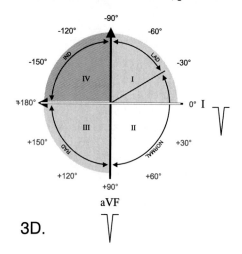

3D.

I	II	Leads aVF	III	aVR	Location of QRS Axis
+	+	+	+		+30° to +90°
+	+	+	−		0° to +30°
+	+	−	−		0° to −30°
+	−	−	−		−30° to −90°
−	+	+	+	−	+90° to +120
−	+	+	+	+	+120° to +150
−	−	−	−		−90° to −150°

+ = Predominantly positive
− = Predominantly negative
± = Equiphasic

I	II	Equiphasic Leads aVF	III	aVR	aVL	Location of QRS Axis
±	−	−	−	+		−90°
+	−	−	−	±		−60°
+	±	−	−	−		−30°
+	+	±	−	−		0°
+	+	+	±	−		+30°
+	+	+	+	−	±	+60°
±	+	+	+	−		+90°
−	+	+	+	±		+120°
−	±	+	+	+		+150°
−	−	±	+	+		±180°
−	−	−	±	+		−150°
−	−	−	−	+	±	−120°

Lead III

E. **If the QRS complexes are predominantly positive in lead III,** the QRS axis is between **+90°** and **−150°**.

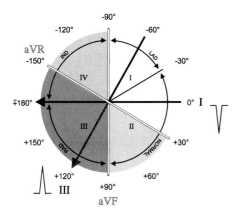

F. **If the QRS complexes are predominantly negative in lead III,** the QRS axis is between **−90°** and **−150°**.

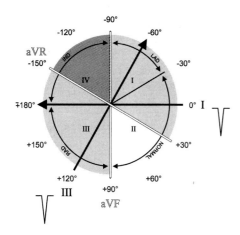

Lead aVR

G. **If the QRS complexes are predominantly positive in lead aVR,** the QRS axis is greater than **+120°** (**severe right axis deviation**).

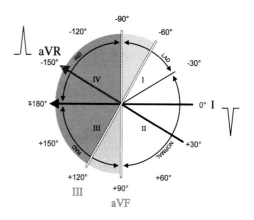

H. **If the QRS complexes are predominantly negative in lead aVR,** the QRS axis is between **+90°** and **+120°** (**mild to moderate right axis deviation**).

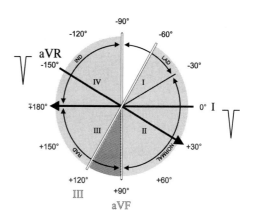

1. The part of the ECG when electrical activity of the heart is not being detected is:
   A. referred to as the isoelectric line
   B. referred to as the baseline
   C. a straight flat line
   D. all of the above

2. The sensitivity of the ECG machine is calibrated so that a _____ electrical signal produces a _____ deflection on the ECG.
   A. 0.5 millivolt: 1 mm
   B. 1 millivolt: 10 mm
   C. 5 millivolt: 10 mm
   D. 10 millivolt: 5 mm

3. An ECG lead composed of a single positive electrode and a zero reference point, the central terminal, is called a:
   A. unipolar lead
   B. multifocal lead
   C. bipolar lead
   D. MCL$_1$ lead

4. If the positive electrode is attached to the left leg or lower left anterior chest, all the electric currents generated in the heart that flow toward the positive electrode will be recorded as a _____ (_____) deflection.
   A. positive (inverted)
   B. negative (upright)
   C. positive (upright)
   D. negative (inverted)

5. An example of a unipolar lead would be:
   A. aVL
   B. V$_3$
   C. both of the above
   D. none of the above

6. The placement of the V$_4$ positive chest electrode is:
   A. left side of the sternum in the fourth intercostal space
   B. midclavicular line in the fifth intercostal space
   C. in the anterior axillary line at the fifth intercostal space
   D. in the midaxillary line at the sixth intercostal space

7. The placement of the V$_2$ positive chest electrode is:
   A. midway between V$_1$ and V$_3$
   B. right side of the sternum in the fourth intercostal space
   C. anterior axillary line at the same level as V$_1$
   D. left side of the sternum in the fourth intercostal space

8. The surface of the heart viewed on an ECG by the leads II, III, and aVF is the:
   A. lateral
   B. anterior
   C. inferior
   D. posterior

9. Left axis deviation with a QRS axis greater than $-30°$ occurs in adults with the following cardiac condition(s):
   A. hypertension
   B. aortic stenosis
   C. ischemic heart disease
   D. all of the above

10. Patients who have right ventricular enlargement and hypertrophy secondary to pulmonary embolism, COPD, or cor pulmonale may most likely have an axis deviation of:
    A. greater than $+90°$
    B. between 0 and $+90°$
    C. between 0 and $-60°$
    D. greater than $-60°$

Components of the Electrocardiogram

▼ OBJECTIVES

Upon completion of all or part of this chapter you should be able to complete the following objectives indicated by your instructor:

□ **1.** Define the following components of the electrocardiogram:
- □ P wave
- □ QRS complex
- □ T wave
- □ U wave
- □ PR interval
- □ QT interval
- □ R-R interval
- □ ST segment
- □ PR segment
- □ TP segment

□ **2.** Name and identify the components of the ECG, including the waves, complexes, segments, and intervals on an ECG.

□ **3.** Give the characteristics, description, and significance of the following waves and complexes:
- □ Normal P wave
- □ Abnormal P wave
- □ Ectopic P wave
- □ Normal QRS complex
- □ Abnormal QRS complex
- □ Normal T wave
- □ Abnormal T wave
- □ U wave

□ **4.** Give the characteristics, description, and significance of the following intervals and segments:
- □ Normal PR interval
- □ Abnormal PR interval
- □ QT interval
- □ R-R interval
- □ Normal ST segment
- □ Abnormal ST segment
- □ PR segment
- □ TP segment

□ **5.** Define the following:
- □ P pulmonale
- □ P mitrale
- □ Retrograde conduction
- □ J point
- □ Prime ('); double prime (")
- □ Notch in the R or S wave
- □ Ventricular activation time (VAT)
- □ Incomplete bundle branch block
- □ Complete bundle branch block
- □ Supraventricular arrhythmia
- □ Aberrant ventricular conduction (aberrancy)
- □ Anomalous AV conduction (preexcitation syndrome)
- □ Delta wave
- □ Ectopy
- □ QT_c
- □ Torsade de pointes

Waves

P Wave

Definition

A **P wave** represents **depolarization of the right and left atria.**

Normal Sinus P Wave

Characteristics

1. Pacemaker site: The pacemaker site is the SA node.

2. Relationship to cardiac anatomy and physiology: P wave (Figure 3-1) represents **normal depolarization of the atria.** Depolarization of the atria begins near the SA node and progresses across the atria from right to left and downward. The first part of the normal sinus P wave represents depolarization of the right atrium; the second part represents depolarization of the left atrium. During the P wave, the electrical impulse progresses from the SA node through the internodal atrial conduction tracts and most of the AV node. The P wave normally occurs during ventricular diastole.

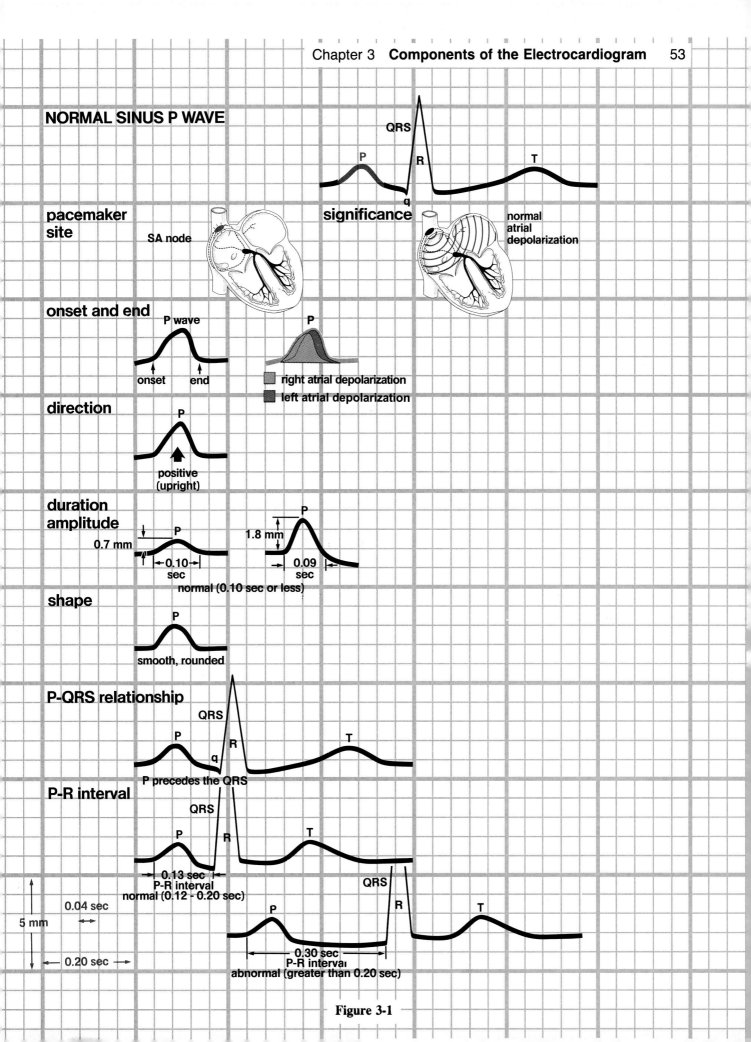

NORMAL SINUS P WAVE

QRS

P   R   T

q

pacemaker site

SA node

significance

normal atrial depolarization

onset and end

P wave

onset   end

P

right atrial depolarization

left atrial depolarization

direction

P

positive (upright)

duration amplitude

0.7 mm

P

|←0.10→|
sec

1.8 mm

P

0.09
sec

normal (0.10 sec or less)

shape

P

smooth, rounded

P-QRS relationship

QRS

P   R   T

q

P precedes the QRS

P-R interval

QRS

P   R   T

|← 0.13 sec →|
P-R interval
normal (0.12 - 0.20 sec)

0.04 sec

5 mm

|← 0.20 sec →|

QRS

P   R   T

|← 0.30 sec →|
P-R interval
abnormal (greater than 0.20 sec)

Figure 3-1

Description

1. Onset and end: The onset of the P wave is identified as the first abrupt or gradual deviation from the baseline. The point where the wave flattens out to return to the baseline, joining with the PR segment, marks the end of the P wave.

2. Direction: The direction is positive (upright) in lead II.

3. Duration: The duration is 0.10 second or less.

4. Amplitude: The amplitude is 0.5 to 2.5 mm in lead II. The normal P wave is rarely over 2 mm high.

5. Shape: The shape is smooth and rounded.

6. P Wave-QRS complex relationship: A QRS complex normally follows each sinus P wave, but in certain arrhythmias, such as AV blocks (see Chapter 9), a QRS complex may not follow each sinus P wave.

7. PR interval: The PR interval may be normal (0.12 to 0.20 second) or abnormal (greater than 0.20 second or less than 0.12 second).

Significance

A normal sinus P wave indicates that the electrical impulse responsible for the P wave originated in the SA node and that normal depolarization of the right and left atria has occurred.

Notes

Abnormal Sinus P Wave

Characteristics

1. Pacemaker site: The pacemaker site is the SA node.

2. Relationship to cardiac anatomy and physiology: An **abnormal sinus P wave** (Figure 3-2) represents **depolarization of altered, damaged, or abnormal atria.** Increased right atrial pressure and right atrial dilatation and hypertrophy (right atrial overload)—as found in chronic obstructive pulmonary disease, status asthmaticus, acute pulmonary embolism, and acute pulmonary edema—may result in tall and symmetrically peaked P waves (**P pulmonale**). Abnormally tall P waves may also occur in sinus tachycardia (see Chapter 5).

Increased left atrial pressure and left atrial dilatation and hypertrophy (left atrial overload)—as found in hypertension, mitral and aortic valvular disease, acute myocardial infarction, and pulmonary edema secondary to left heart failure—may cause wide, notched P waves (**P mitrale**). Such P waves may also result from a delay or block of the progression of electrical impulses through the interatrial conduction tract between the right and left atria.

Description

1. Onset and end: The onset and end of the abnormal sinus P wave are the same as those of a normal P wave.

2. Direction: The direction is positive (upright) in lead II.

3. Duration: The duration may be normal (0.10 second or less) or greater than 0.10 second.

4. Amplitude: The amplitude may be normal (0.5 to 2.5 mm) or greater than 2.5 mm in lead II. By definition, a P pulmonale is 2.5 mm or greater in amplitude.

5. Shape: The abnormal sinus P wave may be tall and symmetrically peaked or may be wide and notched.

6. P wave-QRS complex relationship: The P wave-QRS complex relationship is the same as that of a normal sinus P wave.

7. PR interval: The PR interval may be normal (0.12 to 0.20 second) or abnormal (greater than 0.20 second).

Significance

An abnormal sinus P wave indicates that the electrical impulse responsible for the P wave originated in the SA node and that depolarization of altered, damaged, or abnormal atria has occurred.

Notes

ABNORMAL SINUS P WAVE

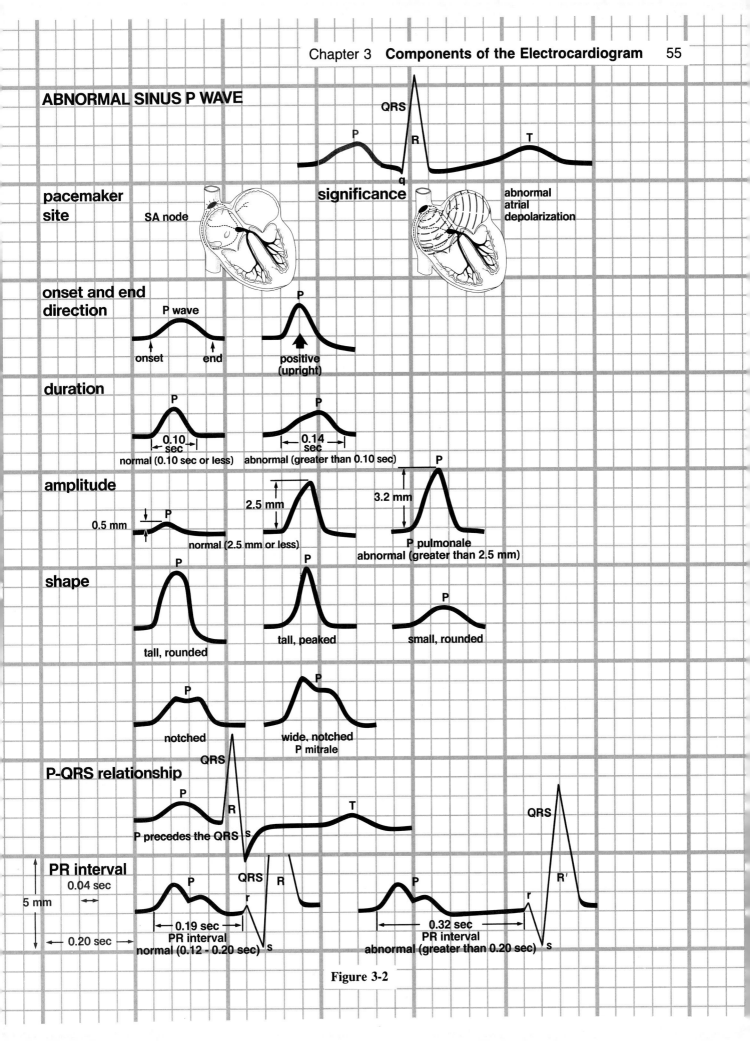

pacemaker site — SA node

significance — abnormal atrial depolarization

onset and end direction

P wave

onset   end

positive (upright)

duration

P

0.10 sec

normal (0.10 sec or less)

P

0.14 sec

abnormal (greater than 0.10 sec)

amplitude

0.5 mm   P

2.5 mm

normal (2.5 mm or less)

3.2 mm   P

P pulmonale
abnormal (greater than 2.5 mm)

shape

P

tall, rounded

P

tall, peaked

P

small, rounded

P

notched

P

wide, notched
P mitrale

P-QRS relationship

QRS

P   R

T

P precedes the QRS   S

QRS

PR interval

0.04 sec

5 mm

0.20 sec

P   QRS   R

r

S

0.19 sec
PR interval
normal (0.12 - 0.20 sec)

P

r   R'

S

0.32 sec
PR interval
abnormal (greater than 0.20 sec)

Figure 3-2

Ectopic P Wave (P Prime or P′)

Characteristics

1. Pacemaker site: The pacemaker site is an ectopic pacemaker in the atria outside of the SA node or in the AV junction or ventricles.

2. Relationship to cardiac anatomy and physiology: An **ectopic P wave (P′)** (Figure 3-3) represents **atrial depolarization occurring in an abnormal direction or sequence or both.** If the ectopic pacemaker is in the atria, depolarization of the atria may occur in a normal direction (right to left and downward) or in a retrograde direction (left to right and upward), depending on the ectopic pacemaker's location. If the ectopic pacemaker is in the AV junction or ventricles, the electrical impulse travels upward through the AV junction into the atria **(retrograde conduction),** causing retrograde atrial depolarization.

Ectopic P waves occur in various atrial, junctional, and ventricular arrhythmias, including:

- Wandering atrial pacemaker
- Premature atrial contractions
- Nonparoxysmal atrial tachycardia
- Paroxysmal atrial tachycardia
- Premature junctional contractions
- Junctional escape rhythm
- Nonparoxysmal junctional tachycardia
- Paroxysmal junctional tachycardia
- Premature ventricular contractions (occasionally)

See Chapter 6, 7, or 8, as appropriate, for details.

Description

1. Onset and end: The onset and end of the abnormal ectopic P wave are the same as those of a normal P wave.

2. Direction: The ectopic P wave may be either positive (upright) or negative (inverted) in lead II if the ectopic pacemaker is in the atria. It is always negative (inverted) in lead II if the ectopic pacemaker is in the AV junction or ventricles.

Generally, if the ectopic pacemaker is in the left atrium or in the lower right atrium near the AV node, the ectopic P wave is negative (inverted). If the ectopic pacemaker is in any other part of the right atrium, the ectopic P wave is positive (upright) and may resemble a normal sinus P wave.

3. Duration: The duration is 0.10 second or less.

4. Amplitude: The amplitude is usually less than 2.5 mm in lead II, but it may be greater.

5. Shape: The ectopic P wave may be smooth and rounded, peaked, or dimple-shaped.

6. P′ wave-QRS complex relationship: The ectopic P wave may precede, be buried in, or follow the QRS complex with which it is associated. If the ectopic P wave is buried in the QRS complex, it is not seen and is said to be hidden or invisible. The ectopic P wave may also be superimposed on the preceding T wave, resulting in a T wave that differs in amplitude and shape from the other T waves not so affected.

7. P′R interval: Generally, the **P′R interval** is normal (0.12 to 0.20 second) if the ectopic pacemaker is in the upper or middle part of the atria. It is slightly less than 0.12 second if the ectopic pacemaker is in the lower part of the atria, close to the AV node. If the ectopic pacemaker is in the upper part of the AV junction, the ectopic P wave usually precedes the QRS complex, and the P′R interval is less than 0.12 second. If the ectopic pacemaker is in the lower part of the AV junction or in the ventricles, the ectopic P wave usually follows the QRS complex. In this case, the interval between the end of the QRS complex and the onset of the P′ is called the **R-P′ interval.** It is usually less than 0.21 second.

Significance

An ectopic P wave indicates that the electrical impulse responsible for the ectopic P wave originated in part of the atria outside the SA node or in the AV junction or ventricles and that depolarization of the right and left atria has occurred in an abnormal direction or sequence, or both.

Notes

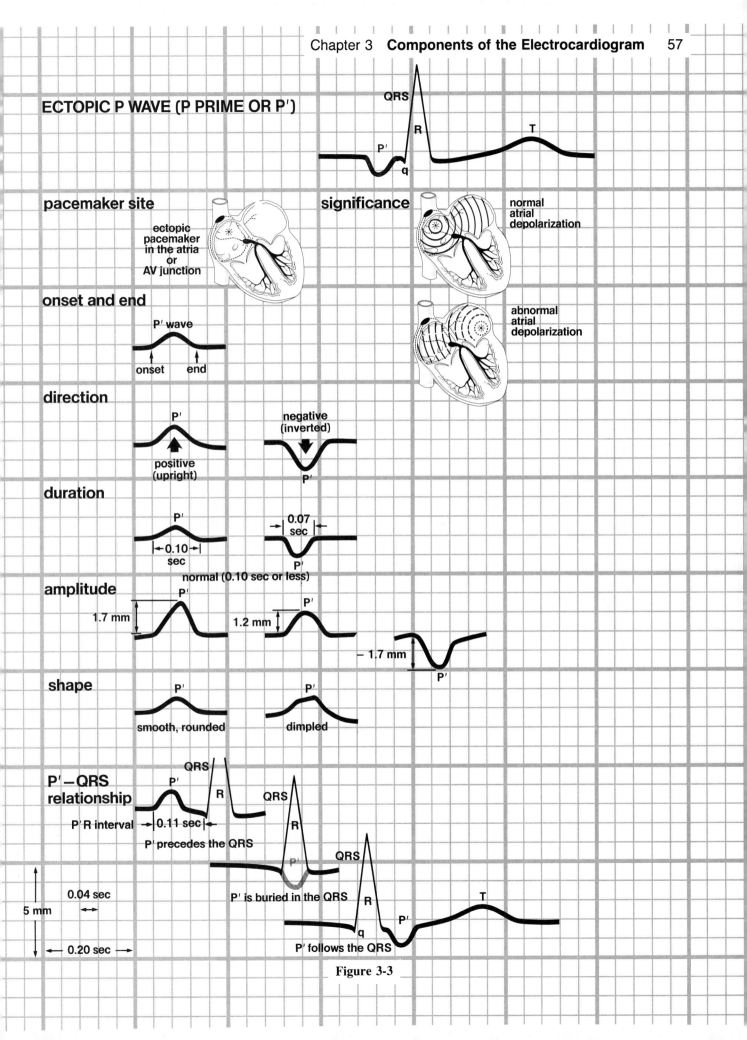

ECTOPIC P WAVE (P PRIME OR P')

QRS

R

P'

q

T

pacemaker site

ectopic
pacemaker
in the atria
or
AV junction

significance

normal
atrial
depolarization

abnormal
atrial
depolarization

onset and end

P' wave

onset   end

direction

P'

positive
(upright)

negative
(inverted)

P'

duration

P'

←0.10→
sec

0.07
sec

P'

normal (0.10 sec or less)

amplitude

P'

1.7 mm

P'

1.2 mm

− 1.7 mm

P'

shape

P'

smooth, rounded

P'

dimpled

**P'−QRS
relationship**

QRS

P'

R

P'R interval →|0.11 sec|←

P' precedes the QRS

QRS

R

P'

QRS

P' is buried in the QRS

R

q

P'

T

P' follows the QRS

0.04 sec

5 mm

0.20 sec

Figure 3-3

QRS Complex

Definition

A **QRS complex** represents **depolarization of the right and left ventricles.**

Normal QRS Complex

Characteristics

1. Pacemaker site: The pacemaker site of the electrical impulse responsible for a normal QRS complex is the SA node or an ectopic or escape pacemaker in the atria or AV junction.

2. Relationship to cardiac anatomy and physiology: A normal QRS complex (Figure 3-4) represents **normal depolarization of the ventricles.** Depolarization begins in the left side of the interventricular septum near the AV junction and progresses across the interventricular septum from left to right. Then, beginning at the endocardial surface of the ventricles, depolarization progresses through the ventricular walls to the epicardial surface. The first short part of the QRS complex, usually the Q wave, represents depolarization of the interventricular septum; the rest of the QRS complex represents the simultaneous depolarization of the right and left ventricles. Because the left ventricle is larger than the right ventricle and has more muscle mass, the QRS complex represents, for the most part, depolarization of the left ventricle.

The electrical impulse that causes normal ventricular depolarization originates above the ventricles in the SA node or in an ectopic or escape pacemaker in the atria or AV junction and has normal conduction down the right and left bundle branches to the Purkinje network. The QRS complex precedes ventricular systole.

Description

1. Onset and end: The onset of the QRS complex is identified as the point where the first wave of the complex just begins to deviate, abruptly or gradually, from the baseline. The end of the QRS complex is the point where the last wave of the complex begins to flatten out (sharply or gradually) at, above, or below the baseline. This point, the junction between the QRS complex and the ST segment, is called the **"junction"** or **"J" point.**

2. Components: The QRS complex consists of one or more of the following: positive (upright) deflections called R waves and negative (inverted) deflections called Q, S, and QS waves.

- *R wave* The R wave is the first positive deflection in the QRS complex. Subsequent positive deflections that extend above the baseline are called **R prime (R′), R double prime (R″),** and so forth.

- *Q wave* The Q wave is the first negative deflection in the QRS complex not preceded by an R wave.

- *S wave* The S wave is the first negative deflection that extends below the baseline in the QRS complex following an R wave. Subsequent negative deflections are called **S prime (S′), S double prime (S″),** and so forth.

- *QS wave* A QS wave is a QRS complex that consists entirely of a single, large negative deflection.

    Note: *Although there may be only one Q wave, there can be more than one R and S wave in the QRS complex.*

- *Notch* A notch in the R wave is a negative deflection that does not extend below the baseline; a notch in the S wave is a positive deflection that does not extend above the baseline.

The waves composing the QRS complex are usually identified by upper or lower case letters depending on the relative size of the waves. The **large waves** that form the major deflections are identified by **upper case letters (QS, R, S).** The **smaller waves** that are less than one-half the amplitude of the major deflections are identified by **lower case letters (q, r, s).** Thus, the ventricular depolarization complex can be described more accurately by using upper and lower case letters assigned to the waves (for example, **qR, Rs, qRs**).

NORMAL QRS COMPLEX

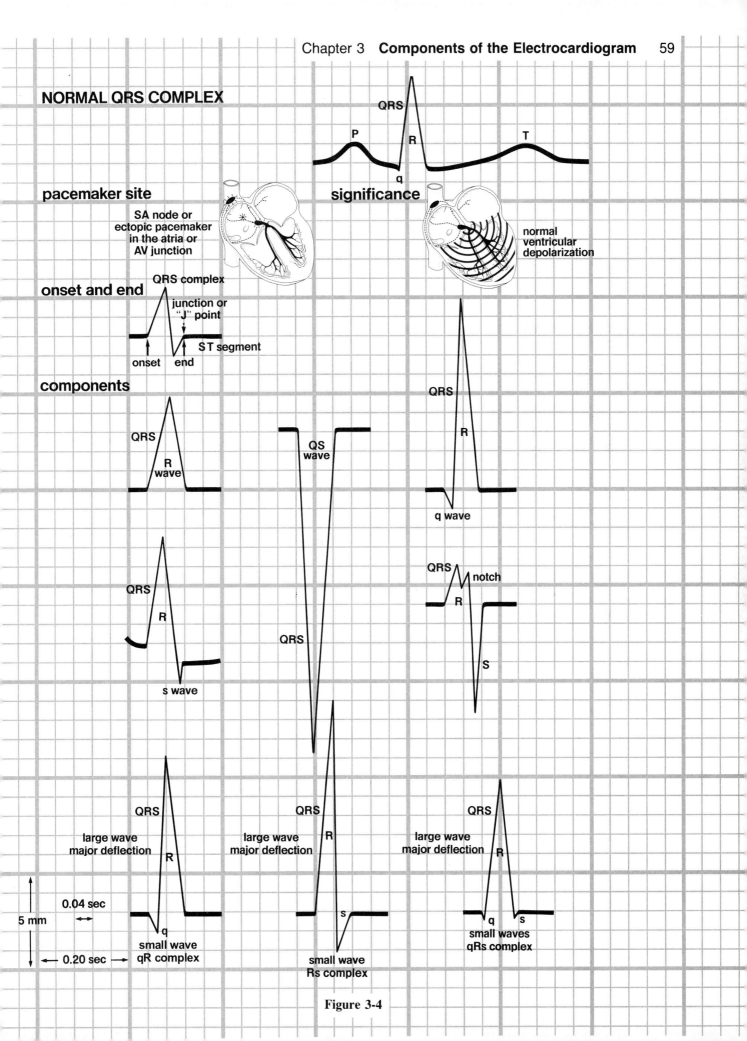

pacemaker site

SA node or ectopic pacemaker in the atria or AV junction

significance

normal ventricular depolarization

onset and end

QRS complex

junction or "J" point

ST segment

onset   end

components

QRS
R wave

QS wave

QRS
R
q wave

QRS
R
s wave

QRS

QRS
R   notch
S

large wave major deflection

QRS
R

q
small wave
qR complex

large wave major deflection

QRS
R
s
small wave
Rs complex

large wave major deflection

QRS
R
q   s
small waves
qRs complex

0.04 sec

5 mm

0.20 sec

Figure 3-4

3. Direction: The direction of the QRS complex may be predominantly positive (upright), predominantly negative (inverted), or equiphasic (partly positive, partly negative). A predominantly positive QRS complex, for example, has more area encompassed by the R wave, the major deflection, than is encompassed by the Q and S waves.

4. Duration: The duration of the normal QRS complex is 0.10 second or less (0.06 to 0.10 second) in adults and 0.08 second or less in children. The QRS complex is measured from the onset of the Q or R wave to the end of the last wave of the complex or the J point. The duration of the Q wave does not normally exceed 0.04 second.

The time from the onset of the QRS complex to the peak of the R wave is the **ventricular activation time (VAT).** The VAT represents the time taken for the depolarization of the interventricular septum plus depolarization of the ventricle from the endocardium to the epicardium under the facing lead. The upper limit of the normal VAT is 0.05 second.

5. Amplitude: The amplitude of the R or S wave in the QRS complex in lead II may vary from 1 to 2 mm to 15 mm or more. The normal Q wave is less than 25% of the height of the succeeding R wave.

6. Shape: The waves in the QRS complex are generally narrow and sharply pointed.

Significance

A normal QRS complex indicates that the electrical impulse has progressed normally from the bundle of His to the Purkinje network through the right and left bundle branches and that normal depolarization of the right and left ventricles has occurred.

Notes

NORMAL QRS COMPLEX—CONT.

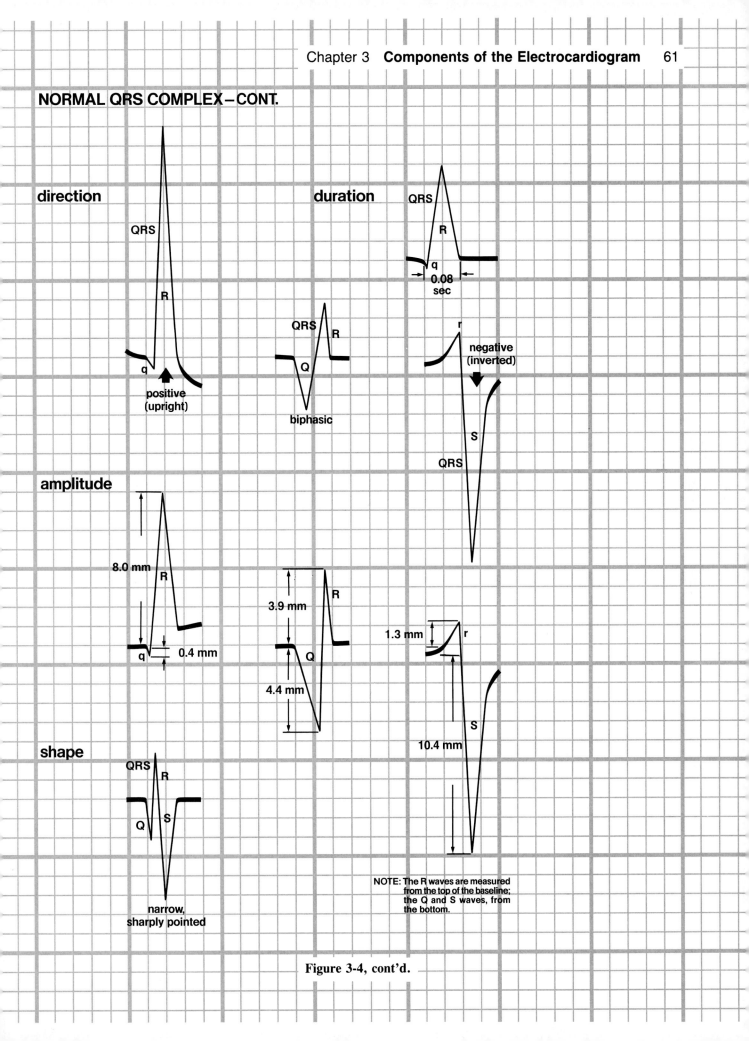

Figure 3-4, cont'd.

Abnormal QRS Complex

Characteristics

1. Pacemaker site: The pacemaker site of the electrical impulse responsible for an abnormal QRS complex is the SA node or an ectopic or escape pacemaker in the atria, AV junction, bundle branches, Purkinje network, or ventricular myocardium.

2. Relationship to cardiac anatomy and physiology: An **abnormal QRS complex** (Figure 3-5) represents **abnormal depolarization of the ventricles.** This may result from **(a)** a partial or complete block in the conduction of electrical impulses through a bundle branch (**bundle branch block** and **aberrant ventricular conduction**), **(b)** abnormal conduction of electrical impulses from the atria to the ventricles through abnormal anatomical pathways bypassing both the AV node and bundle of His (**anomalous AV conduction** or **preexcitation syndrome**), or **(c)** an electrical impulse originating in a **ventricular ectopic or escape pacemaker.**

(a) Bundle branch block results from partial or complete block in conduction of the electrical impulse from the bundle of His to the Purkinje network through the right or left bundle branch while conduction continues uninterrupted through the unaffected bundle branch. A block in one bundle branch causes the ventricle on that side to be depolarized later than the other.

For example, in **complete left bundle branch block,** because of a block in conduction through the left bundle branch, depolarization of the left ventricle is delayed, resulting in an abnormal QRS complex—one that is greater than 0.12 second in duration and appears bizarre, that is, abnormal in size and shape. On the other hand, in **complete right bundle branch block,** the block is in the right bundle branch and, therefore, depolarization of the right ventricle is delayed, also resulting in an abnormal QRS complex.

In **partial** or **incomplete bundle branch block,** conduction of the electrical impulse is only partially blocked, resulting in less of a delay in depolarization of the ventricle on the side of the block than in complete bundle branch block. Consequently, the QRS complex is greater than 0.10 second but less than 0.12 second in duration and often appears normal.

Complete and incomplete bundle branch block may be present in any **supraventricular arrhythmia,** that is, any arrhythmia arising above the ventricles in the SA node, atria, or AV junction, including normal sinus rhythm. Certain supraventricular arrhythmias with bundle branch block may mimic ventricular arrhythmias (see Chapter 8).

Aberrant ventricular conduction (or, simply, **aberrancy**) is a transient inability of the right or left bundle branch to conduct an electrical impulse normally. This may occur when an electrical impulse arrives at the bundle branch while it is still refractory after conducting a previous electrical impulse. This results in an abnormal QRS complex often resembling an incomplete or complete bundle branch block.

Aberrant ventricular conduction may occur in the following supraventricular arrhythmias:
- Premature atrial contractions
- Premature junctional contractions
- Nonparoxysmal atrial tachycardia
- Paroxysmal atrial tachycardia
- Atrial flutter
- Atrial fibrillation
- Nonparoxysmal junctional tachycardia
- Paroxysmal junctional tachycardia

These supraventricular arrhythmias with aberrant ventricular conduction may mimic ventricular arrhythmias (see Chapter 8).

(b) Anomalous AV conduction or **preexcitation syndrome** is a clinical condition associated with abnormal conduction pathways between the atria and ventricles that bypass the AV node and bundle of His and allow the electrical impulses to initiate depolarization of the ventricles earlier than usual. This results in a PR interval of less than 0.12 second, a QRS complex greater than 0.10 second, and an abnormal slurring of the onset of the QRS complex—the **delta wave.** The delta wave represents the early, abnormal depolarization of the ventricles, which begins at the point where the abnormal conduction pathway enters the ventricles.

Supraventricular tachycardia and atrial flutter and fibrillation with anomalous AV conduction may resemble ventricular tachycardia (see Chapter 8).

(c) An electrical impulse originating in an **ectopic or escape pacemaker** in the bundle branches, Purkinje network, or myocardium of one of the ventricles depolarizes that ventricle earlier than the other. The result is an abnormal QRS complex that is greater than 0.12 second in duration and appears bizarre. Such QRS complexes typically occur in ventricular arrhythmias such as accelerated idioventricular rhythm, ventricular escape rhythm, ventricular tachycardia, and premature ventricular contractions (see Chapter 8). The occurrence of ventricular ectopic beats or rhythms is often referred to as **"ventricular ectopy."**

ABNORMAL QRS COMPLEX

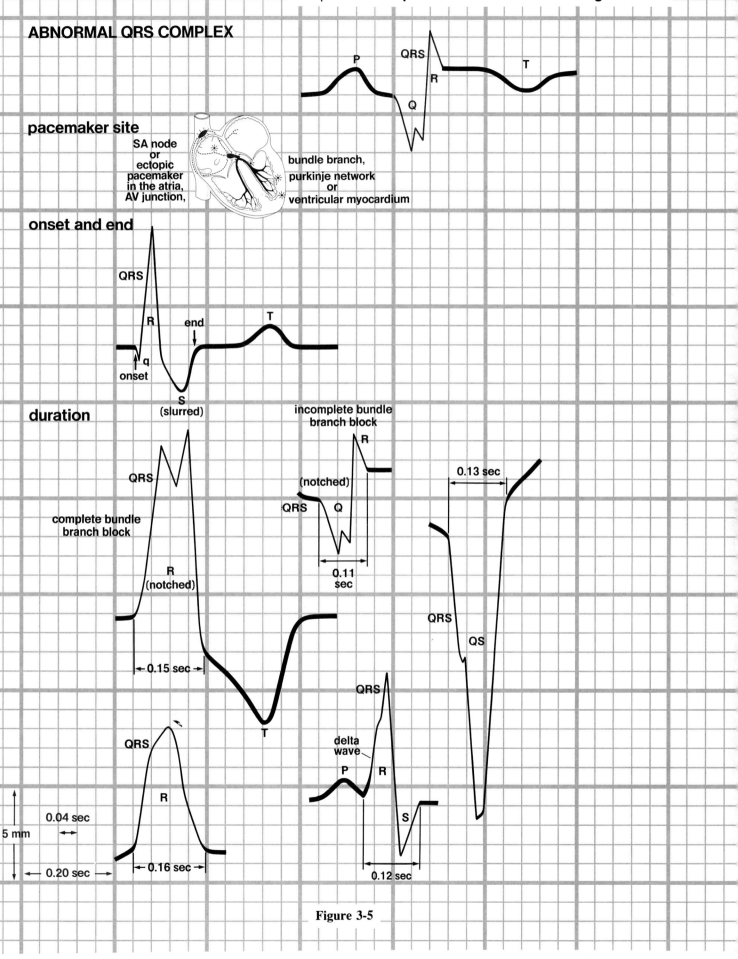

pacemaker site

SA node
or
ectopic
pacemaker
in the atria,
AV junction,

bundle branch,
purkinje network
or
ventricular myocardium

onset and end

QRS

R

↑ q
onset

end

T

S
(slurred)

duration

QRS

complete bundle
branch block

R
(notched)

←0.15 sec→

T

QRS

R

0.04 sec

5 mm

←0.20 sec→   ←0.16 sec→

incomplete bundle
branch block

R

(notched)

QRS   Q

0.11
sec

0.13 sec

QRS

QS

QRS

delta
wave

P   R

S

0.12 sec

Figure 3-5

Description

1. Onset and end: The onset and end of the abnormal QRS complex are the same as those of a normal QRS complex.

2. Duration: The duration of the abnormal QRS complex is greater than 0.10 second. If a bundle branch block is present and the duration of the QRS complex is between 0.10 and 0.12 second, the bundle branch block is called **"incomplete."** If the duration of the QRS complex is greater than 0.12 second, the bundle branch block is called **"complete."**

The duration of a QRS complex caused by an electrical impulse originating in an ectopic or escape pacemaker in the Purkinje network or ventricular myocardium is always greater than 0.12 second; typically, it is 0.16 second or greater. However, if the electrical impulse originates in a bundle branch, the duration of the QRS complex may be only slightly greater than 0.10 second and appear normal.

3. Direction: The direction of the abnormal QRS complex may be predominantly positive (upright), predominantly negative (inverted), or equiphasic (partly positive, partly negative).

ABNORMAL QRS COMPLEX – CONT.

direction

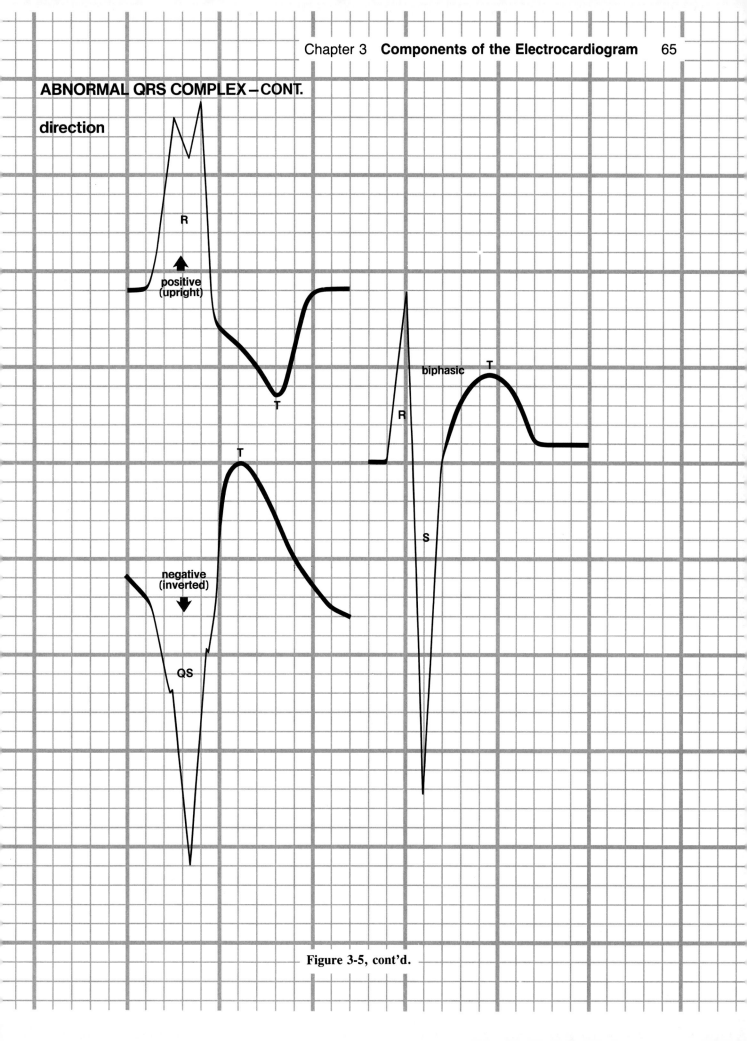

R

positive
(upright)

T

biphasic

R

T

T

S

negative
(inverted)

QS

Figure 3-5, cont'd.

4. Amplitude: The amplitude of the waves in the abnormal QRS complex varies from 1 to 2 mm to 20 mm or more.

5. Shape: An abnormal QRS complex varies widely in shape, from one that appears quite normal—narrow and sharply pointed (as in incomplete bundle branch block)—to one that is wide and bizarre, slurred and notched (as in complete bundle branch block and ventricular arrhythmias).

Significance

An abnormal QRS complex indicates that abnormal depolarization of the ventricles has occurred because of (1) a block in the progression of the electrical impulse from the bundle of His to the Purkinje network through the right or left bundle branch (bundle branch block, aberrant ventricular conduction); (2) the progression of the electrical impulse from the atria to the ventricles through an abnormal conduction pathway (anomalous AV conduction or preexcitation syndrome); or (3) the origination of the electrical impulse responsible for the ventricular depolarization in a ventricular ectopic or escape pacemaker (see below).

Notes

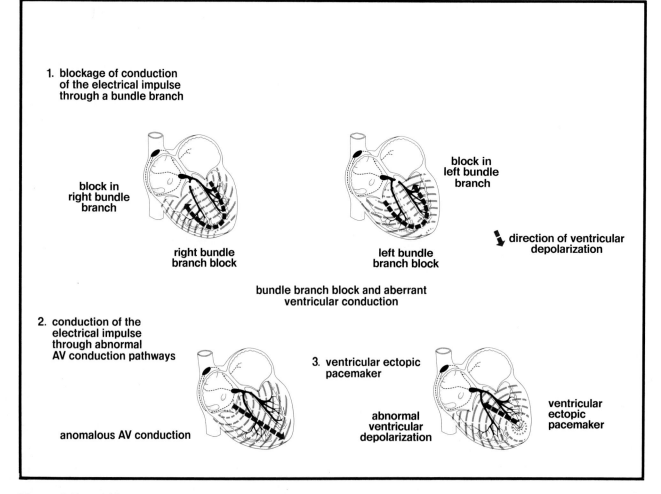

1. blockage of conduction of the electrical impulse through a bundle branch

block in right bundle branch

right bundle branch block

block in left bundle branch

left bundle branch block

direction of ventricular depolarization

bundle branch block and aberrant ventricular conduction

2. conduction of the electrical impulse through abnormal AV conduction pathways

anomalous AV conduction

3. ventricular ectopic pacemaker

abnormal ventricular depolarization

ventricular ectopic pacemaker

Figure 3-5, cont'd.

ABNORMAL QRS COMPLEX – CONT.

amplitude

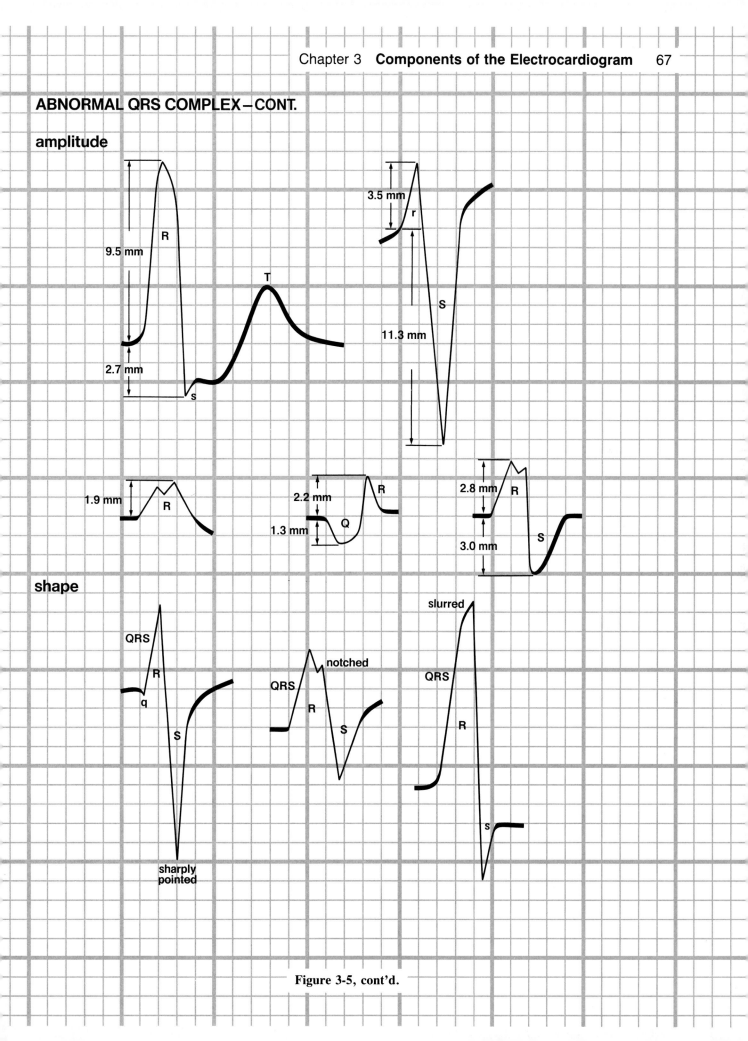

shape

Figure 3-5, cont'd.

T Wave

Definition

A **T wave** represents **ventricular repolarization.**

Normal T Wave

Characteristics

1. Relationship to cardiac anatomy and physiology: A **normal T wave** (Figure 3-6) represents **normal repolarization of the ventricles.** Normal repolarization begins at the epicardial surface of the ventricles and progresses inwardly through the ventricular walls to the endocardial surface. The T wave occurs during the last part of ventricular systole.

Description

1. Onset and end: The onset of the T wave is identified as the first abrupt or gradual deviation from the ST segment (or the point where the slope of the ST segment appears to become abruptly or gradually steeper). If the ST segment is absent, the T wave begins at the end of the QRS complex (or the **J point**). The point where the T wave returns to the baseline marks the end of the T wave. In the absence of an ST segment, the T wave is sometimes called the **ST-T** wave. Often the onset and end of the T wave are difficult to determine with certainty.

2. Direction: The direction of the normal T wave is positive (upright) in lead II.

3. Duration: The duration is 0.10 to 0.25 second or greater.

4. Amplitude: The amplitude is less than 5 mm.

5. Shape: The normal T wave is sharply or bluntly rounded and slightly asymmetrical. Ordinarily, the first, upward part of the T wave is longer than the second, downward part.

6. T wave-QRS complex relationship: The T wave always follows the QRS complex.

Significance

A normal T wave preceded by a normal ST segment indicates that normal repolarization of the right and left ventricles has occurred.

Notes

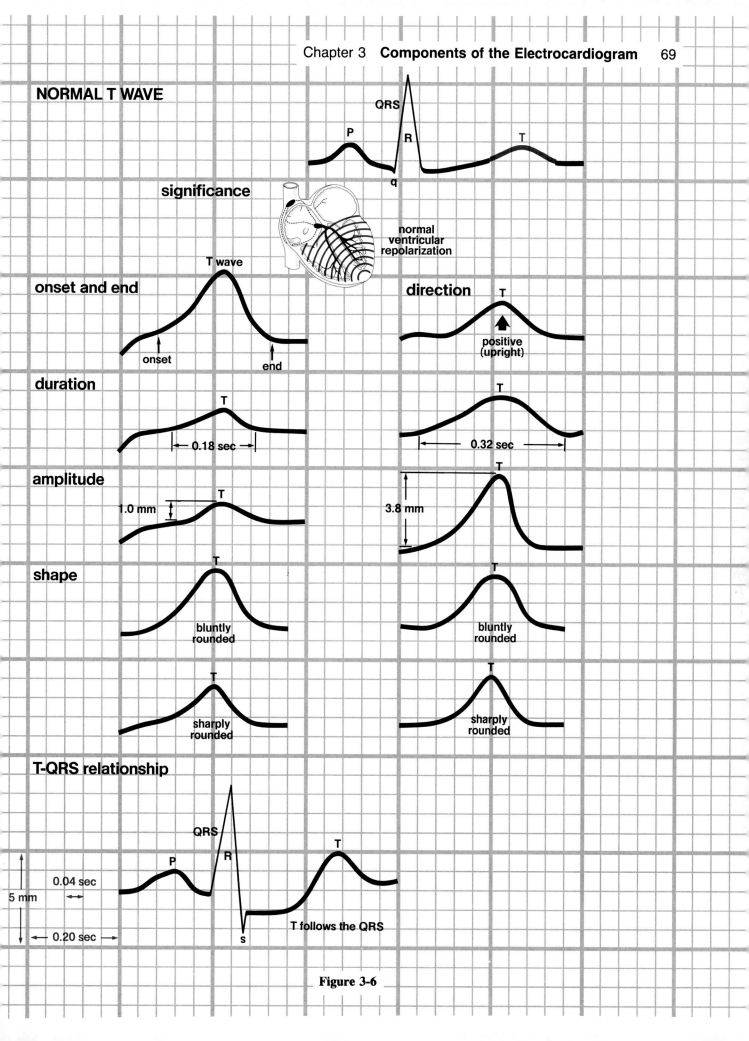

NORMAL T WAVE

QRS

P R T

q

significance

normal
ventricular
repolarization

onset and end

T wave

onset end

direction

T

positive
(upright)

duration

T

0.18 sec

T

0.32 sec

amplitude

T

1.0 mm

3.8 mm

T

shape

T

bluntly
rounded

T

bluntly
rounded

T

sharply
rounded

T

sharply
rounded

T-QRS relationship

QRS

P R T

0.04 sec

5 mm

0.20 sec

s

T follows the QRS

Figure 3-6

Abnormal T Wave

Characteristics

1. Relationship to cardiac anatomy and physiology: An **abnormal T wave** (Figure 3-7) represents **abnormal ventricular repolarization.** Abnormal repolarization may begin at either the epicardial or endocardial surface of the ventricles. When abnormal repolarization begins at the epicardial surface of the ventricles, it progresses inwardly through the ventricular walls to the endocardial surface, as it normally does, but at a slower rate, producing an abnormally tall, upright T wave in lead II. When it begins at the endocardial surface of the ventricles, it progresses outwardly through the ventricular walls to the epicardial surface, producing a negative T wave in lead II. Abnormal ventricular repolarization may result from myocardial ischemia, acute myocardial infarction, myocarditis, pericarditis, ventricular enlargement (hypertrophy), electrolyte imbalance (e.g., excess serum potassium), or administration of certain cardiac drugs (e.g., quinidine, procainamide); it also commonly occurs where there is abnormal depolarization of the ventricles (as in bundle branch block and ectopic ventricular arrhythmias). Abnormal ventricular repolarization may also occur in athletes and in persons who are hyperventilating.

Description

1. Onset and end: The onset and end of an abnormal T wave are the same as those of a normal T wave.

2. Direction: The abnormal T wave may be positive (upright) and abnormally tall or low, negative (inverted), or biphasic (partially positive and partially negative) in lead II. The abnormal T wave may or may not be in the same direction as that of the QRS complex. The T wave following an abnormal QRS complex is almost always opposite in direction to it; it is abnormally wide and tall or deeply inverted.

3. Amplitude: The amplitude varies.

ABNORMAL T WAVE

significance

onset and end

direction

amplitude

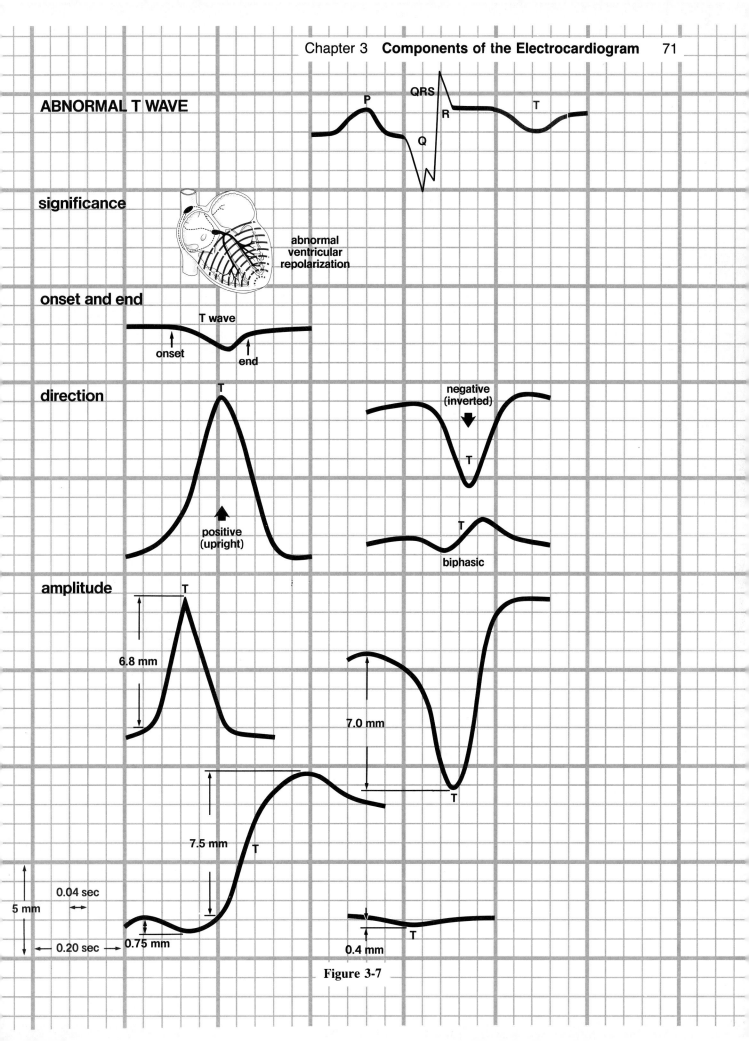

Figure 3-7

4. Duration: The duration is 0.10 to 0.25 second or greater.

5. Shape: The abnormal T wave may be rounded, blunt, sharply peaked, wide, or notched.

6. T wave-QRS complex relationship: The abnormal T wave always follows the QRS complex.

Significance

An abnormal T wave indicates that abnormal repolarization of the ventricles has occurred.

Notes

ABNORMAL T WAVE—CONT.

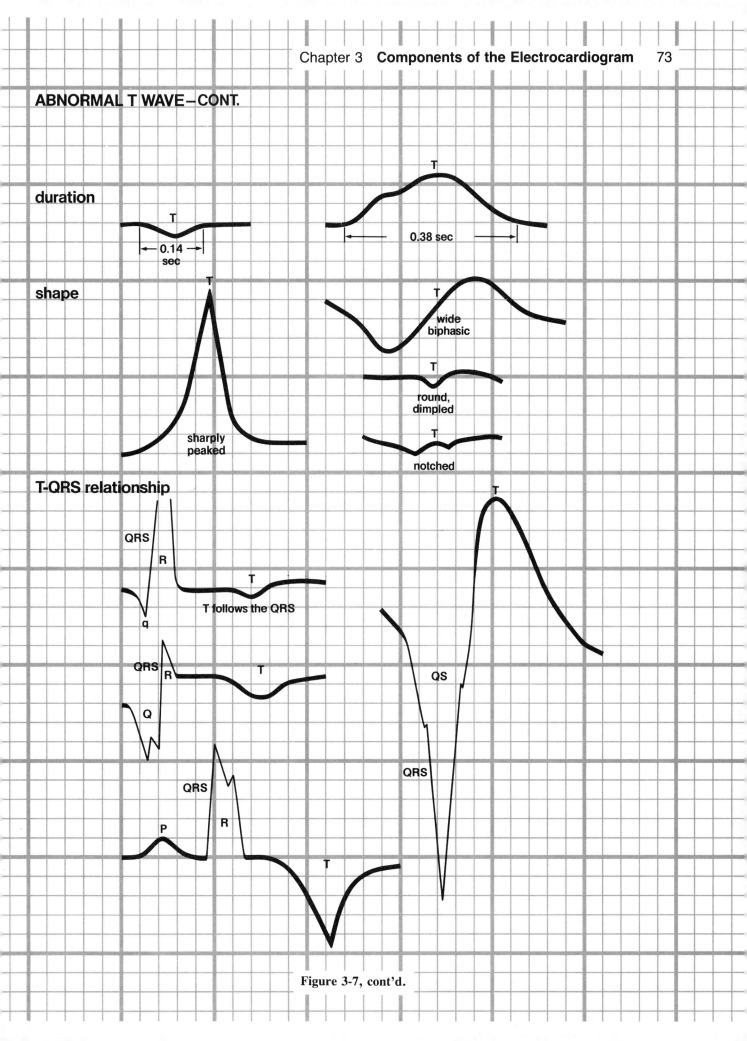

duration

0.14 sec

0.38 sec

shape

sharply peaked

wide biphasic

round, dimpled

notched

T-QRS relationship

QRS

R

q

T follows the QRS

QRS

R

Q

T

QRS

P

R

T

QS

QRS

Figure 3-7, cont'd.

U Wave

Definition

A **U wave** probably represents the **final stage of repolarization of the ventricles.**

Characteristics

1. Relationship to cardiac anatomy and physiology: A **U wave** (Figure 3-8) probably represents **repolarization of a small segment of the ventricles** (such as the papillary muscles or ventricular septum) after most of the right and left ventricles have been repolarized. Although uncommon and not easily identified, the U wave can best be seen when the heart rate is slow.

Description

1. Onset and end: The onset of the U wave is identified as the first abrupt or gradual deviation from the baseline or the downward slope of the T wave. The point where the U wave returns to the baseline or downward slope of the T wave marks the end of the U wave.

2. Direction: The direction of a normal U wave is positive (upright), the same as that of the preceding normal T wave in lead II. An abnormal U wave may be flat or negative (inverted).

3. Duration: The duration is not determined routinely.

4. Amplitude: The amplitude of a normal U wave is usually less than 2 mm and always smaller than that of the preceding T wave in lead II. A U wave taller than 2 mm is considered to be abnormal.

5. Shape: The U wave is rounded and symmetrical.

6. U wave relationship to other waves: The U wave always follows the peak of the T wave and occurs before the next P wave.

Significance

A U wave indicates that repolarization of the ventricles has occurred. An abnormally tall U wave may be present in hypokalemia, cardiomyopathy, left ventricular hypertrophy, and diabetes and may follow administration of digitalis, quinidine, and procainamide.

Notes

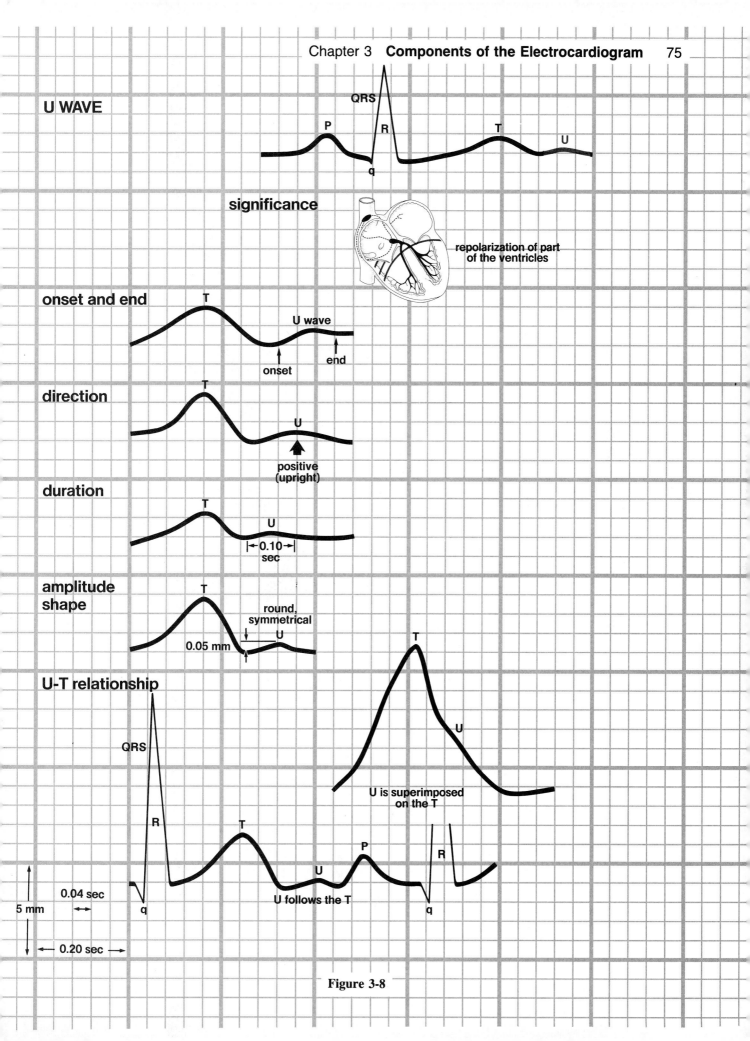

U WAVE

significance

repolarization of part
of the ventricles

onset and end

U wave

onset   end

direction

U

positive
(upright)

duration

U

|← 0.10 →|
sec

amplitude
shape

round,
symmetrical

U

0.05 mm

U-T relationship

QRS

R

T

U

U is superimposed
on the T

P

R

T

U

q

q

U follows the T

0.04 sec

5 mm

← 0.20 sec →

Figure 3-8

Intervals

PR Interval

Definition

A **PR interval** represents the **time of progression of the electrical impulse from the SA node through the entire electrical conduction system of the heart to the ventricular myocardium, including the depolarization of the atria.**

Normal PR Interval

Characteristics

1. Relationship to cardiac anatomy and physiology: A **normal PR interval** (Figure 3-9) represents the **time from the onset of atrial depolarization to the onset of ventricular depolarization** during which the electrical impulse progresses normally from the SA node through the internodal atrial conduction tracts, AV junction, bundle branches, and Purkinje network to the ventricular myocardium. The PR interval includes a P wave and the short, usually flat (isoelectric) segment, the **PR segment** that follows it.

Description

1. Onset and end: The PR interval begins with the onset of the P wave and ends with the onset of the QRS complex.

2. Duration: The duration of the normal PR interval is 0.12 to 0.20 second and is dependent on the heart rate. When the heart rate is fast, the PR interval is normally shorter than when the heart rate is slow (Example: heart rate 120, PR interval 0.16 second; heart rate 60, PR interval 0.20 second).

Significance

A normal PR interval indicates that the electrical impulse originated in the SA node or an ectopic pacemaker in the adjacent atria and has progressed normally through the electrical conduction system of the heart to the ventricular myocardium. The major significance of a normal PR interval is that the electrical impulse has been conducted through the AV node and bundle of His normally and without delay.

Notes

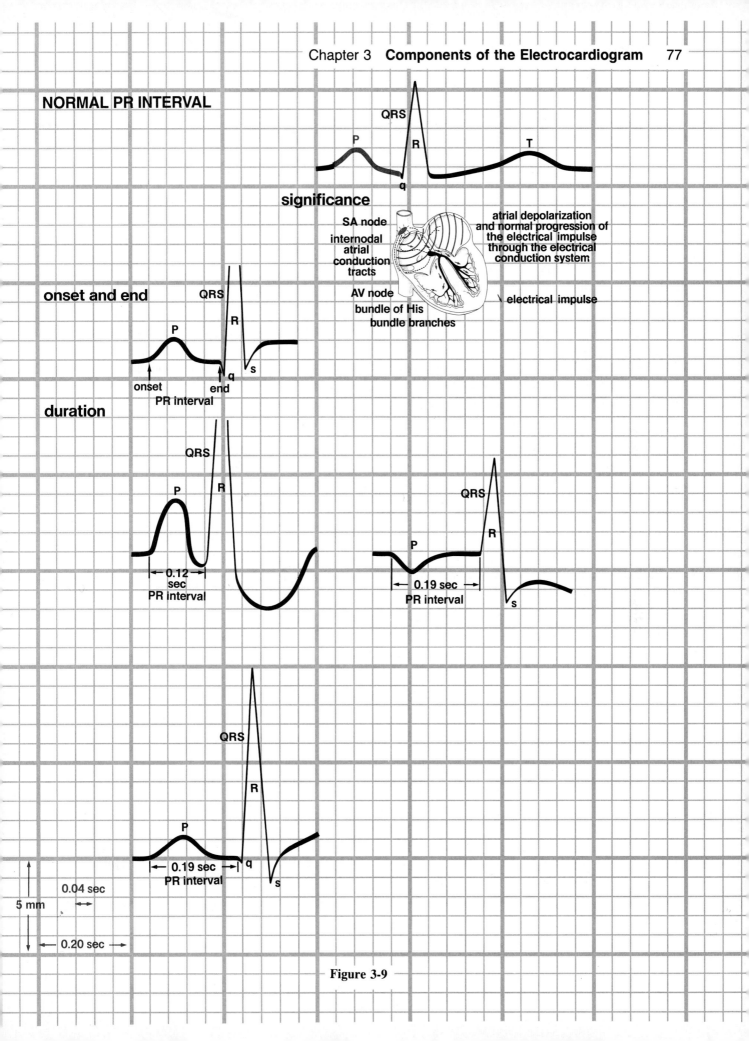

NORMAL PR INTERVAL

QRS

P   R   q   T

significance

SA node
internodal atrial conduction tracts
AV node
bundle of His
bundle branches

atrial depolarization and normal progression of the electrical impulse through the electrical conduction system

electrical impulse

onset and end

QRS   R   P   q   s

onset   end
PR interval

duration

QRS   P   R
← 0.12 → sec
PR interval

QRS   P   R
← 0.19 sec →
PR interval   s

QRS   P   R
← 0.19 sec → q
PR interval   s

0.04 sec
5 mm
← 0.20 sec →

Figure 3-9

Abnormal PR Interval

Characteristics

1. Relationship to cardiac anatomy and physiology: A **PR interval greater than 0.20 second** represents **delayed progression of the electrical impulse through the AV node, bundle of His, or, rarely, the bundle branches.** The P wave of a prolonged PR interval may be normal or abnormal.

A **PR interval less than 0.12 second** is commonly present when the **electrical impulse originates in an ectopic pacemaker in the atria close to the AV node or in an ectopic or escape pacemaker in the AV junction.** Negative (inverted) P waves in lead II are commonly associated with abnormally short PR intervals.

A **PR interval less than 0.12 second** also occurs if the **electrical impulse progresses from the atria to the ventricles through abnormal conduction pathways, which bypass the AV node and bundle of His, depolarizing the ventricles earlier than usual.** In this AV conduction abnormality—the **anomalous AV conduction** or **preexcitation syndrome**—the short PR interval is commonly followed by a wide, abnormally shaped QRS complex with a **delta wave,** the slurring of the onset of the QRS complex. The P waves in this condition may be positive (upright) or negative (inverted) in lead II.

Description

1. Onset and end: The onset and end of the **abnormal PR interval** (Figure 3-10) are the same as those of a normal PR interval.

2. Duration: The duration of the abnormal PR interval may be greater than 0.20 second or less than 0.12 second.

Significance

An abnormally long PR interval indicates that a delay of progression of the electrical impulse through the AV node, bundle of His, or, rarely, the bundle branches is present. An abnormally short PR interval indicates (1) that the electrical impulse originated in an ectopic pacemaker in the atria near the AV node or in an ectopic or escape pacemaker in the AV junction or (2) that the electrical impulse progressed from the atria to the ventricles through atrioventricular conduction pathways other than the AV node and bundle of His (see below).

Notes

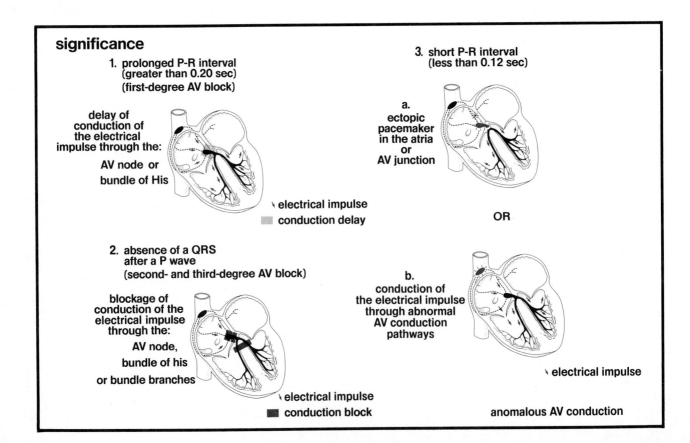

significance

1. prolonged P-R interval
   (greater than 0.20 sec)
   (first-degree AV block)

delay of
conduction of
the electrical
impulse through the:

AV node or
bundle of His

⬈ electrical impulse
▨ conduction delay

2. absence of a QRS
   after a P wave
   (second- and third-degree AV block)

blockage of
conduction of the
electrical impulse
through the:

AV node,
bundle of his
or bundle branches

⬈ electrical impulse
◼ conduction block

3. short P-R interval
   (less than 0.12 sec)

a.
ectopic
pacemaker
in the atria
or
AV junction

OR

b.
conduction of
the electrical impulse
through abnormal
AV conduction
pathways

⬈ electrical impulse

anomalous AV conduction

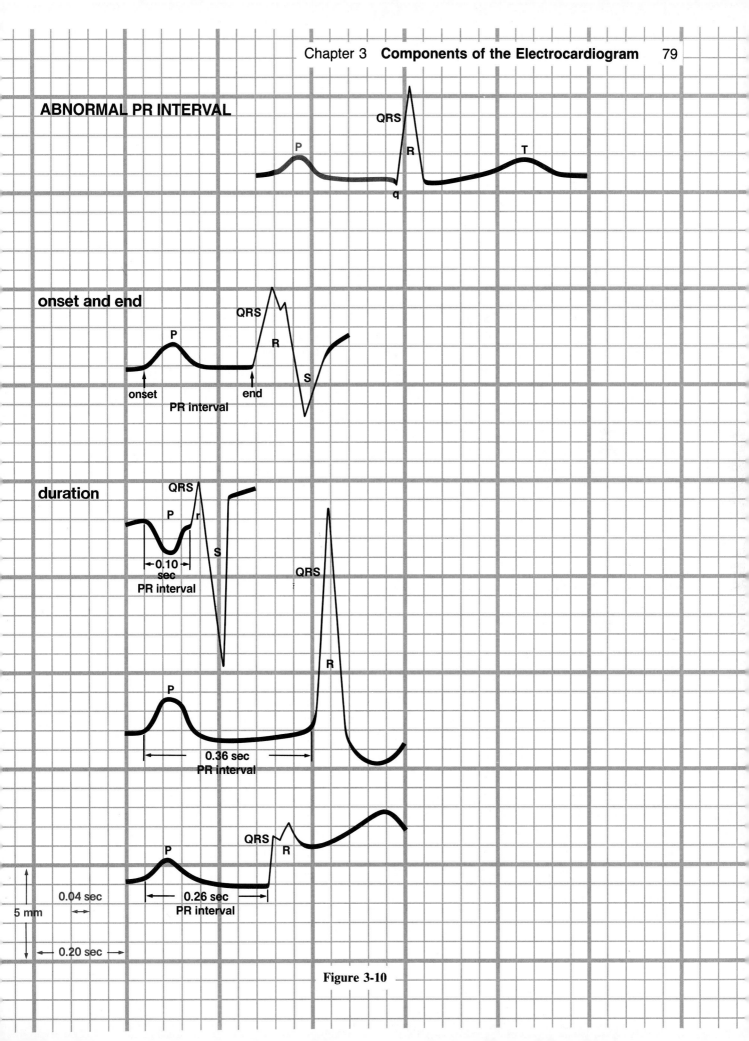

ABNORMAL PR INTERVAL

onset and end

duration

Figure 3-10

QT Interval

Definition

A **QT interval** represents the **time between the onset of depolarization and the termination of repolarization of the ventricles.**

Characteristics

1. Relationship to cardiac anatomy and physiology: The **QT interval** (Figure 3-11) represents **the refractory period of the ventricles during which they depolarize and repolarize.**

An abnormally prolonged QT interval, one that exceeds the average QT interval for any given heart rate by 10%, represents a slowing in the repolarization of the ventricles. This occurs in electrolyte imbalance (hypokalemia and hypocalcemia), excess of certain drugs (quinidine, procainamide, disopyramide, amiodarone, phenothiazines, and tricyclic antidepressants), liquid protein diets, pericarditis, acute myocarditis, acute myocardial infarction, left ventricular hypertrophy, hypothermia, and central nervous system disorders (e.g., subarachnoid hemorrhage, intracranial trauma) or it can occur without a known cause (idiopathic). The QT interval is also prolonged in bradyarrhythmias (e.g., marked sinus bradycardia, third-degree AV block with slow ventricular escape rhythm).

An abnormally short QT interval, one that is less than the average QT interval for any given heart rate by 10%, represents an increase in the rate of repolarization of the ventricles. This occurs in digitalis therapy and hypercalcemia.

Description

1. Onset and end: The onset of the QT interval is identified as the point where the first wave of the QRS complex just begins to deviate, abruptly or gradually, from the baseline. The end of the QT interval is the point where the T wave returns to the baseline.

2. Duration: The duration of the QT interval is dependent on the heart rate, being somewhat less then half of the preceding R-R interval. In general, a QT interval less than half the R-R interval is normal, one that is greater than half is abnormal, and one

that is about half is "borderline." When the heart rate is fast, the QT interval is shorter than when the heart rate is slow (Example: heart rate 120, QT interval about 0.29 second; heart rate 60, QT interval about 0.39 second). The QT intervals may be equal or unequal in duration depending on the underlying rhythm. The average duration of the QT interval normally expected at a given heart rate, the **corrected QT interval** (or **QTc**), and the normal range of 10% above and 10% below the average value are shown in **Table 3-1** on the page to the right.

Note: The determination of the QT interval should be made in the lead where the T wave is most prominent and not deformed by a U wave and should not include the U wave. Furthermore, the measurement of the QT interval assumes that the duration of the QRS complex is normal with an average value of 0.08 second. If the QRS is widened beyond 0.08 second for any reason, the excess widening beyond 0.08 second must be subtracted from the actual measurement to obtain the correct QT interval.

Significance

A QT interval represents the time between the onset of ventricular depolarization and the end of ventricular repolarization, the refractory period of the ventricles. A prolonged QT interval indicates slowing of ventricular repolarization. The most common causes of this are electrolyte imbalance (hypokalemia and hypocalcemia), drug therapy (quinidine, procainamide, disopyramide, and amiodarone), pericarditis, acute myocarditis, acute myocardial infarction, left ventricular hypertrophy, and hypothermia. The prolongation of the QT interval following administration of excessive amounts of such antiarrhythmic agents as quinidine, procainamide, and disopyramide may provoke the appearance of **torsade de pointes,** an ominous form of ventricular tachycardia.

A decrease in the QT interval indicates an increase in the rate of repolarization of the ventricles. The most common causes of this are digitalis therapy and hypercalcemia.

Notes

QT INTERVAL

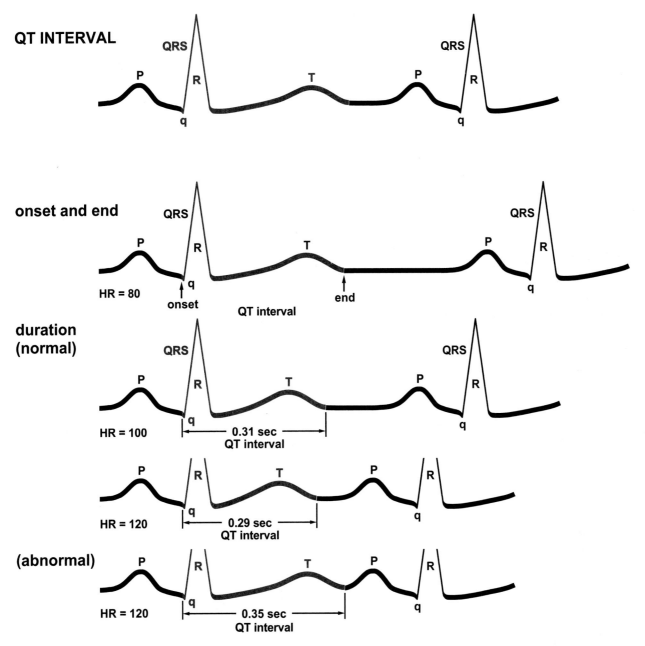

Figure 3-11

Table 3-1. QT$_c$ intervals

Heart rate/min	R-R interval (sec)	QT$_c$ (sec) and normal range
40	1.5	0.46 (0.41-0.51)
50	1.2	0.42 (0.38-0.46)
60	1.0	0.39 (0.35-0.43)
70	0.86	0.37 (0.33-0.41)
80	0.75	0.35 (0.32-0.39)
90	0.67	0.33 (0.30-0.36)
100	0.60	0.31 (0.28-0.34)
120	0.50	0.29 (0.26-0.32)
150	0.40	0.25 (0.23-0.28)
180	0.33	0.23 (0.21-0.25)
200	0.30	0.22 (0.20-0.24)

R-R Interval

Definition

An **R-R interval** represents the **time between two successive ventricular depolarizations.**

Characteristics

1. Relationship to cardiac anatomy and physiology: An **R-R interval** (Figure 3-12) normally represents **one cardiac cycle** during which the atria and ventricles contract and relax once.

Description

1. Onset and end: The onset of the R-R interval is generally considered to be the peak of one R wave; the end, the peak of the succeeding R wave.

2. Duration: The duration is dependent on the heart rate. When the heart rate is fast, the R-R interval is shorter than when the heart rate is slow (example: heart rate 120, R-R interval 0.50 second; heart rate 60, R-R interval 1.0 second). The R-R intervals may be equal or unequal in duration depending on the underlying rhythm.

Significance

An R-R interval represents the time between two successive ventricular depolarizations.

Notes

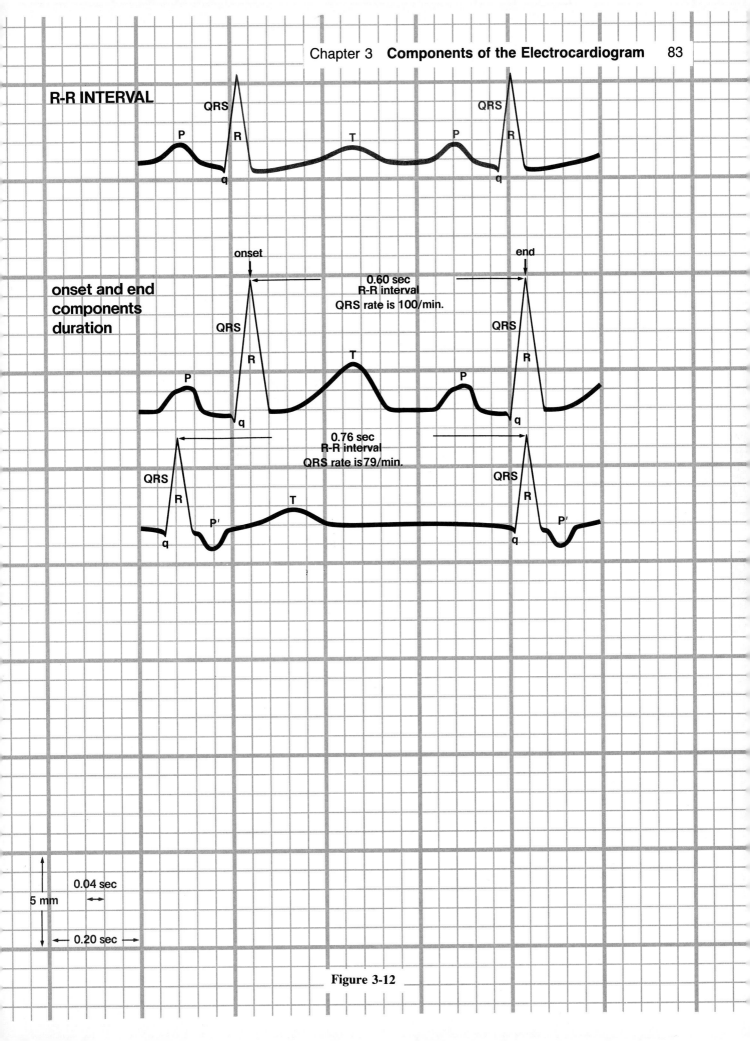

R-R INTERVAL

**onset and end
components
duration**

Figure 3-12

Segments

ST Segment

Definition

An **ST segment** represents the **early part of re-polarization of the right and left ventricles.**

Normal ST Segment

Characteristics

1. Relationship to cardiac anatomy and physiology: The **ST segment** (Figure 3-13) represents the **early part of ventricular repolarization.**

Description

1. Onset and end: The ST segment begins with the end of the QRS complex and ends with the onset of the T wave. The junction between the QRS complex and the ST segment is called the **"junction"** or **"J" point.**

2. Duration: The duration is 0.20 second or less and is dependent on the heart rate. When the heart rate is fast, the ST segment is shorter than when the heart rate is slow.

3. Amplitude: Normally, the ST segment is flat (isoelectric). However, it may be slightly elevated or depressed and still be normal if it is elevated or depressed by **less than 1.0 mm, 0.08 second (2 small squares)** after the **J point** of the QRS complex. The TP segment is normally used as a baseline reference for the determination of the amplitude of the ST segment. However, if the TP segment is absent because of a very rapid heart rate, the PR segment is used instead.

4. Appearance: If slightly elevated, the ST segment may be flat, concave, or arched. If slightly depressed, the ST segment may be flat, sagging, or downsloping.

Significance

A normal ST segment followed by a normal T wave indicates that normal repolarization of the right and left ventricles has occurred.

Notes

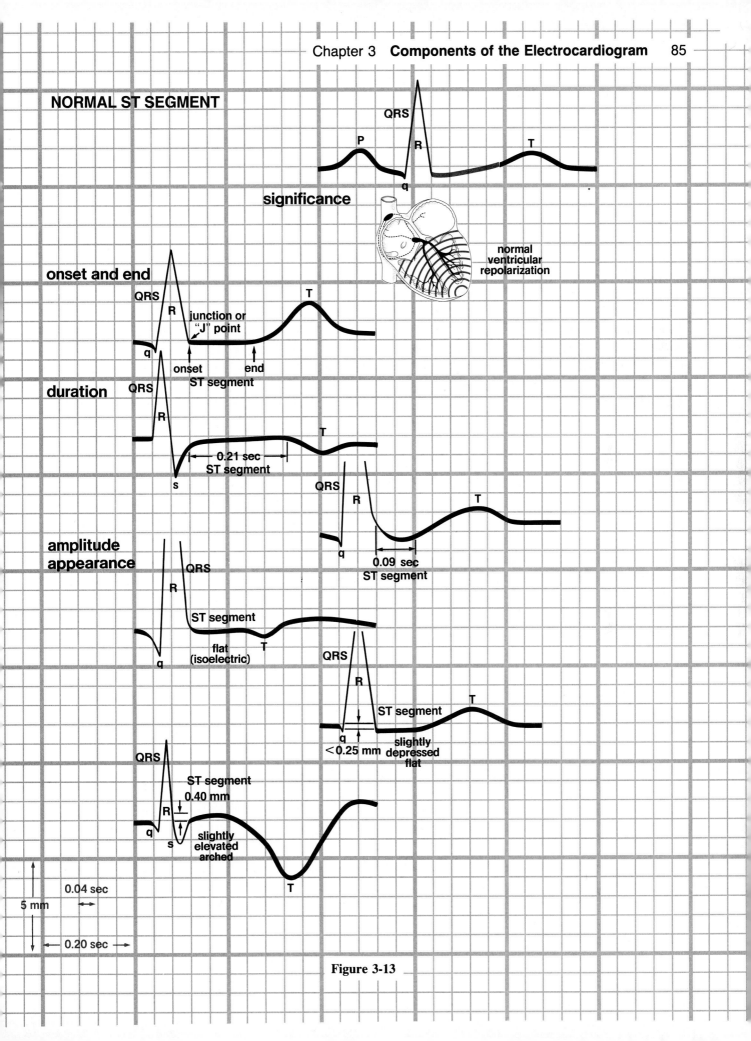

NORMAL ST SEGMENT

significance

normal
ventricular
repolarization

onset and end

junction or
"J" point

onset
ST segment

end

duration

0.21 sec
ST segment

0.09 sec
ST segment

amplitude
appearance

ST segment

flat
(isoelectric)

ST segment
<0.25 mm

slightly
depressed
flat

ST segment
0.40 mm

slightly
elevated
arched

0.04 sec

5 mm

0.20 sec

Figure 3-13

Abnormal ST Segment

Characteristics

1. Relationship to cardiac anatomy and physiology: An **abnormal ST segment** (Figure 3-14) signifies **abnormal ventricular repolarization,** a common consequence of myocardial ischemia and acute myocardial infarction. It is also present in ventricular fibrosis or aneurysm, pericarditis, left ventricular enlargement (hypertrophy), and administration of digitalis.

Description

1. Onset and end: The onset and end of the abnormal ST segment are the same as those of a normal ST segment.

2. Duration: The duration is 0.20 second or less.

ABNORMAL ST SEGMENT

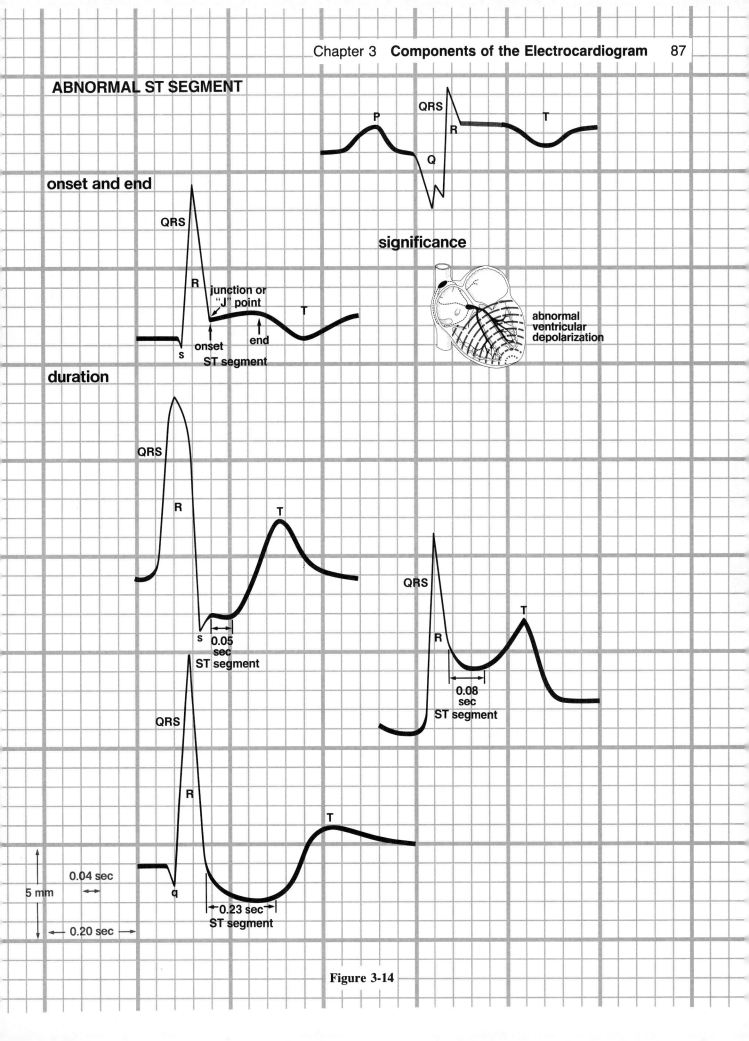

onset and end

QRS

R

junction or
"J" point

T

onset
ST segment

end

s

significance

abnormal
ventricular
depolarization

duration

QRS

R

T

s 0.05
sec
ST segment

QRS

R

T

0.08
sec
ST segment

QRS

R

T

q

0.23 sec
ST segment

0.04 sec

5 mm

0.20 sec

P

QRS

R

Q

T

Figure 3-14

3. Amplitude: An ST segment is abnormal when it is elevated or depressed **1.0 mm or more, 0.08 second (2 small squares)** after the **J point** of the QRS complex.

4. Appearance: If elevated, the ST segment may be flat, concave, or arched. If depressed, the ST segment may be flat, sagging, or downsloping.

Significance

An abnormal ST segment indicates that abnormal ventricular repolarization has occurred. The most common causes of an abnormal ST segment are coronary artery disease (coronary insufficiency, myocardial infarction), left ventricular hypertrophy, digitalis effect, and pericarditis.

Notes

ABNORMAL ST SEGMENT — CONT.

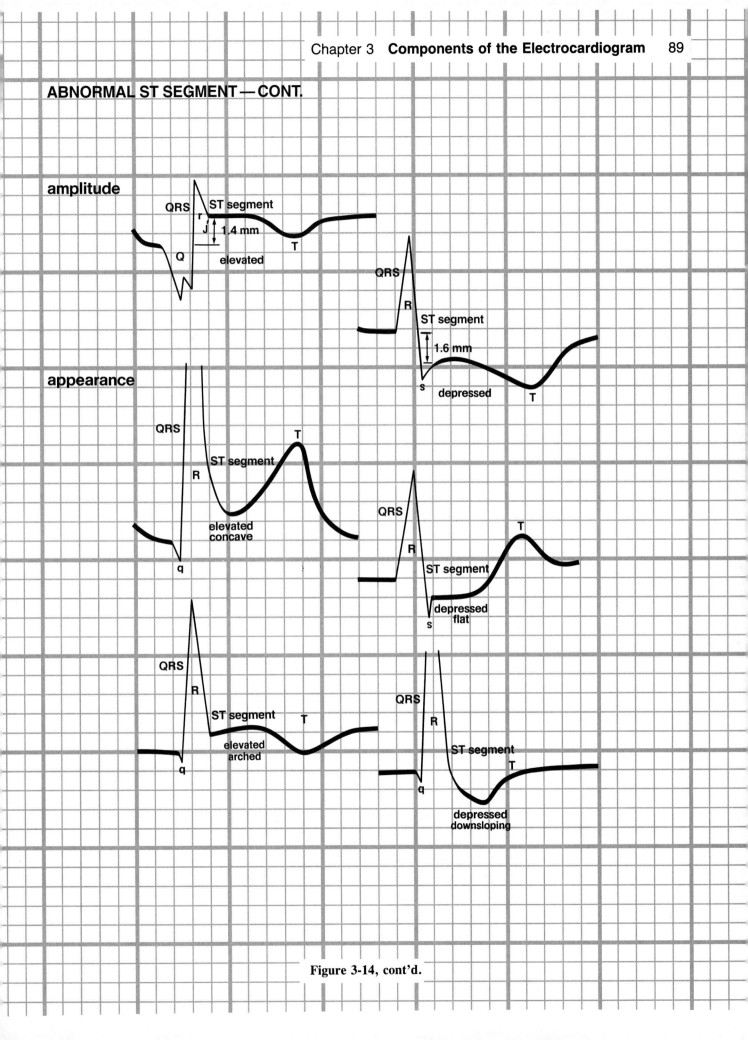

Figure 3-14, cont'd.

PR Segment

Definition

A **PR segment** represents the **time of progression of the electrical impulse from the AV node through the bundle of His, bundle branches, and Purkinje network to the ventricular myocardium.**

Characteristics

1. Relationship to cardiac anatomy and physiology: The **PR segment** (Figure 3-15) represents the **time from the end of atrial depolarization to the onset of ventricular depolarization** during which the electrical impulse progresses from the AV node through the bundle of His, bundle branches, and Purkinje network to the ventricular myocardium.

Description

1. Onset and end: The onset of the PR segment begins with the end of the P wave and ends with the onset of the QRS complex.

2. Duration: The duration normally varies from about 0.02 to 0.10 second. It may be greater than 0.10 second if there is a delay in the progression of the electrical impulse through the AV node or bundle of His, or, rarely, the bundle branches.

3. Amplitude: Normally, the PR segment is flat (isoelectric).

Significance

A PR segment of 0.10-second duration or less indicates that the electrical impulse has been conducted through the AV junction and bundle branches normally and without delay. A PR segment exceeding 0.10 second in duration indicates a delay in the conduction of the electrical impulse through the AV junction or, rarely, the bundle branches.

Notes

PR SEGMENT

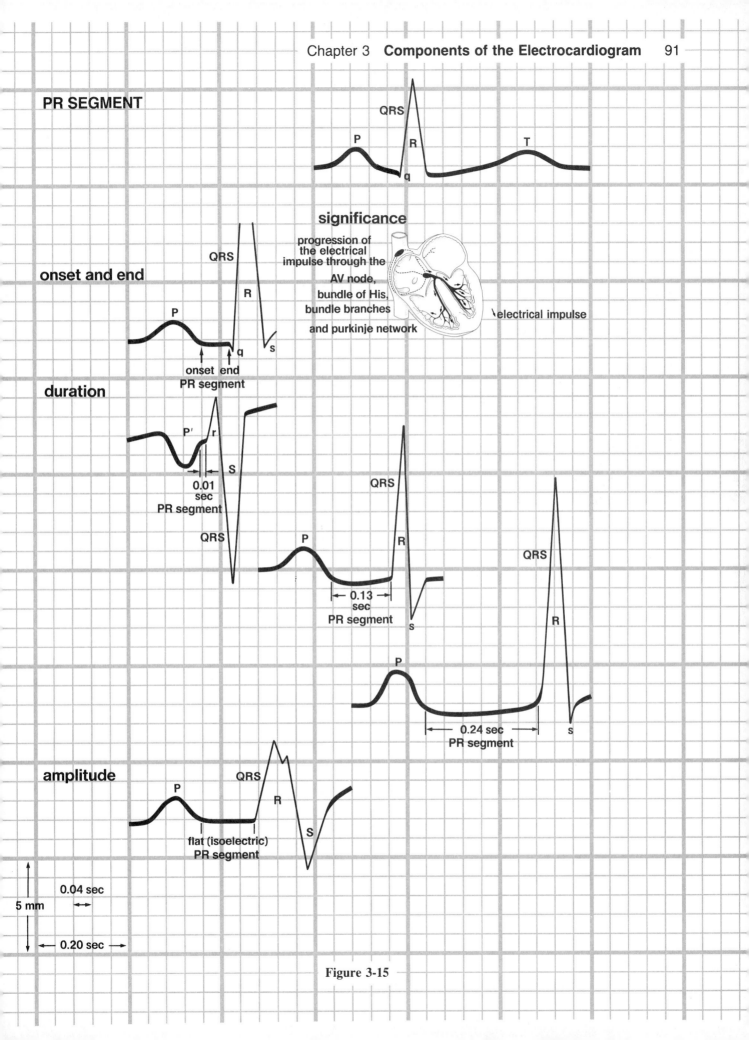

QRS
P
R
q
T

significance

progression of
the electrical
impulse through the

AV node,
bundle of His,
bundle branches

and purkinje network

electrical impulse

onset and end

QRS
R
P
q
s
onset end
PR segment

duration

P' r
S
0.01
sec
PR segment

QRS

QRS

P
R
s
0.13
sec
PR segment

QRS

P
R
s
0.24 sec
PR segment

amplitude

P
QRS
R
S
flat (isoelectric)
PR segment

0.04 sec

5 mm

0.20 sec

Figure 3-15

TP Segment

Definition

A **TP segment** is the interval **between two successive P-QRST complexes** during which electrical activity of the heart is absent.

Characteristics

1. Relationship to cardiac anatomy and physiology: A **TP segment** (Figure 3-16) represents the **time from the end of ventricular repolarization to the onset of atrial depolarization** during which electrical activity of the heart is absent.

Description

1. Onset and end: The TP segment begins with the end of the T wave and ends with the onset of the following P wave.

2. Duration: The duration is 0.0 to 0.40 second or greater and is dependent on the heart rate. When the heart rate is fast, the TP segment is shorter than when the heart rate is slow (example: heart rate about 120 or greater, TP segment 0 second; heart rate about 60 or less, TP segment 0.04 second or greater).

3. Amplitude: Usually, the TP segment is flat (isoelectric).

Significance

A TP segment indicates the absence of any electrical activity of the heart. The TP segment is used as the baseline reference for the determination of ST segment elevation or depression.

Notes

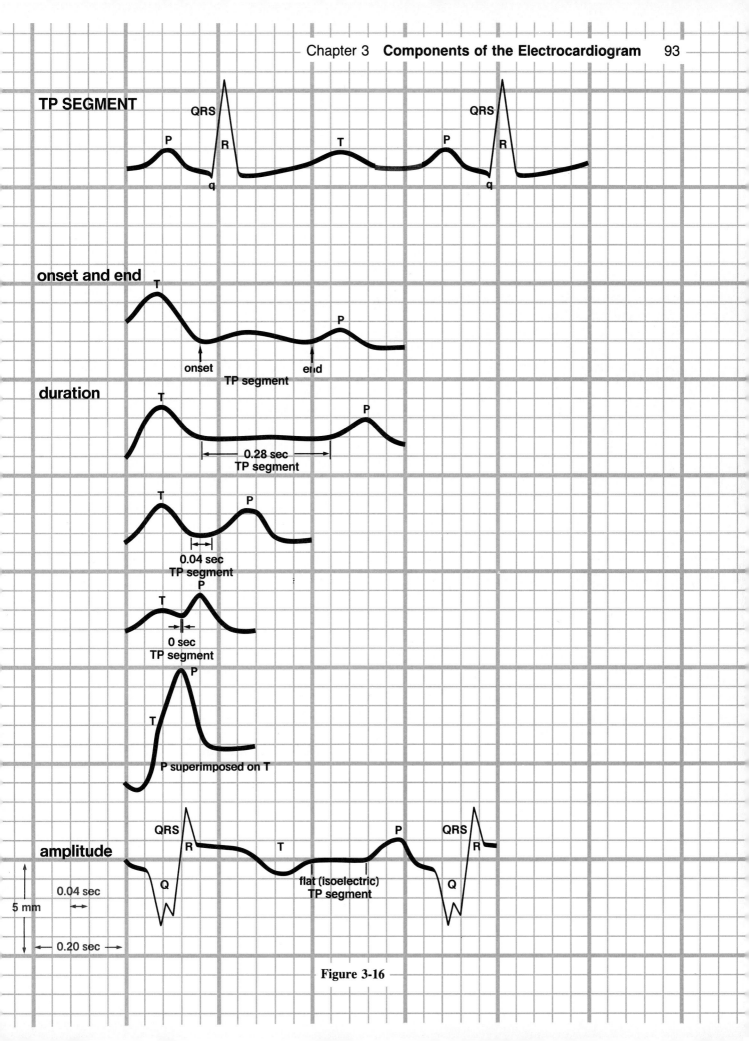

Figure 3-16

1. Wide, notched P waves may be caused by:
   A. hypertension
   B. mitral and aortic valvular disease
   C. acute MI
   D. all of the above

2. The normal PR interval is between:
   A. 0.8 and 0.24 second
   B. 0.8 and 0.16 second
   C. 0.12 and 0.20 second
   D. 0.10 and 0.24 second

3. An ectopic P wave represents atrial depolarization occurring in:
   A. an abnormal sequence
   B. an abnormal direction
   C. all of the above
   D. none of the above

4. A normal QRS complex represents normal:
   A. repolarization of the atria
   B. depolarization of the ventricles
   C. repolarization of the ventricles
   D. depolarization of the atria

5. The time taken for the depolarization of the interventricular septum plus depolarization of the ventricle from the endocardium to the epicardium under the facing lead is called the:
   A. ventricular activation time
   B. septal excitation time
   C. atrial repolarization phase
   D. none of the above

6. Aberrant ventricular conduction may occur in:
   A. sinus bradycardia with PVCs
   B. paroxysmal atrial tachycardia and PACs
   C. PVCs
   D. all of the above

7. Myocardial ischemia, acute MI, excess serum potassium, and administration of procainamide can cause an abnormal _____ on the ECG.
   A. P wave
   B. QRS complex
   C. T wave
   D. U wave

8. A U wave indicates that repolarization of the ventricles has occurred. An abnormally tall U wave may be present in:
   A. hypothermia, vertigo
   B. hypokalemia, cardiomyopathy
   C. cardiac tamponade, diabetes
   D. CVA, syncope

9. A delay of progression of the electrical impulse through the AV node or bundle of His would show on an ECG as a(n):
   A. prolonged QRS complex
   B. peaked T wave
   C. elevated ST segment
   D. prolonged PR interval

10. An abnormal ST segment indicates:
    A. abnormal ventricular repolarization
    B. abnormal atrial repolarization
    C. abnormal ventricular depolarization
    D. none of the above

CHAPTER
4

ECG Interpretation

Arrhythmia Determination

Step One: Identify and Analyze the QRS Complexes

Step Two: Determine the Heart Rate

Step Three: Determine the Ventricular Rhythm

Step Four: Identify and Analyze the P, P′, F, or f Waves

Step Five: Determine the PR or RP′ Intervals and AV Conduction Ratio

Step Six: Determine the Site of Origin of the Arrhythmia

Step Seven: Identify the Arrhythmia

Step Eight: Evaluate the Significance of the Arrhythmia

BASIC DYSRHYTHMIAS

Upon completion of all or part of this chapter you should be able to complete the following objectives indicated by your instructor:

☐ 1. List the seven steps in determining an arrhythmia.

☐ 2. List and describe the three steps in identifying and analyzing the QRS complexes.

☐ 3. Define heart rate and describe the following methods of determining it:
  ☐ Six-second count method
  ☐ Heart rate calculator ruler method
  ☐ Triplicate method
  ☐ R-R interval method
    ☐ Seconds method
    ☐ Small square method
    ☐ Large square method
    ☐ Conversion table method

☐ 4. List and describe two methods of determining the ventricular rhythm.

☐ 5. Define the following terms as they apply to ventricular rhythm:
  Essentially regular ☐ Irregular

☐ 6. List and describe the three steps in identifying and analyzing the P, P′, F, and f waves.

☐ 7. Define the basic differences between the following components of the ECG, including shape, width, height, relationship to the QRS complexes, and rate and rhythm:
  ☐ Normal P wave
  ☐ Abnormal P wave
  ☐ Atrial flutter waves
  ☐ Atrial fibrillation waves
  ☐ "Coarse"
  ☐ "Fine"

☐ 8. List and describe the three steps in determining the PR and RP′ intervals and the AV conduction ratio.

☐ 9. Define normal and abnormal PR intervals.

☐ 10. Give the causes of a PR interval less than 0.12 second in duration and one greater than 0.20 second.

☐ 11. Define the following terms:
  ☐ Atrioventricular (AV) block
  ☐ Variable AV block
  ☐ Isoelectric line
  ☐ Incomplete AV block
  ☐ Complete AV block
  ☐ First-degree AV block
  ☐ Second-degree AV block
  ☐ Third-degree AV block
  ☐ Dropped beat
  ☐ Wenckebach phenomenon
  ☐ AV dissociation
  ☐ AV conduction ratio
  ☐ Anomalous AV conduction

☐ 12. List the most likely site or sites of origin (or pacemaker sites) of arrhythmias under the following circumstances:
  ☐ Upright P waves preceding each QRS complex in lead II
  ☐ Negative P waves preceding each QRS complex in lead II
  ☐ Negative P waves following each QRS complex in lead II
  ☐ QRS complexes occurring alone without P waves
  ☐ Atrial flutter waves
  ☐ Atrial fibrillation waves
  ☐ Normal QRS complexes with no set relationship to the P waves
  ☐ Slightly widened QRS complexes (0.10 to 0.12 second in duration) with no set relationship to the P waves
  ☐ Widened QRS complexes (greater than 0.12 second in duration and bizarre) with no set relationship to the P waves

Arrhythmia Determination

Step One

Identify and Analyze the QRS Complexes

- **Identify the QRS complexes** (Figure 4-1).
- **Note the duration and shape of the QRS com-** plexes. The QRS complexes may be normal (0.10 second or less wide) or abnormal (greater than 0.10 second wide and bizarre-appearing).
- **Compare the QRS complexes** to determine if all QRS complexes are equal in duration and shape or if one or more of the QRS complexes differ from the others, indicating **ectopy** or **aberrancy**.

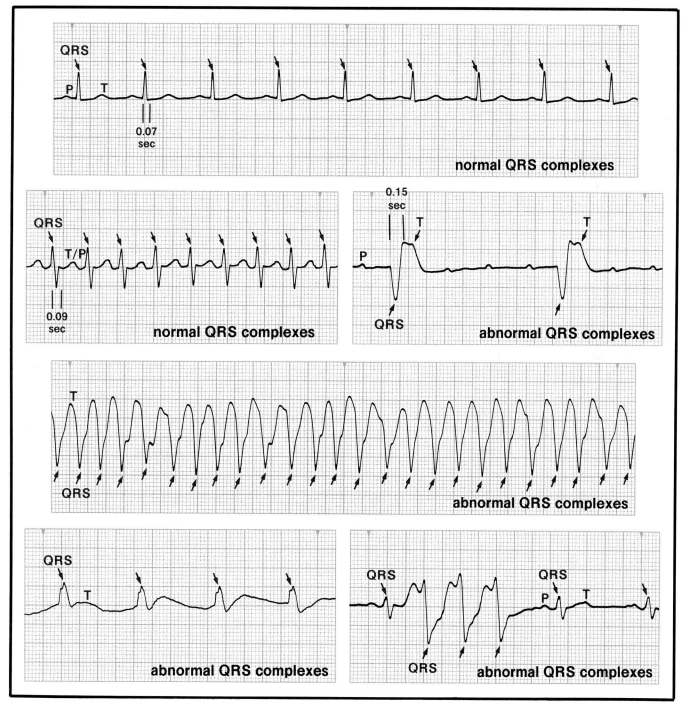

Figure 4-1. Identifying the QRS complexes.

The QRS complexes of **ventricular arrhythmias (ectopy)** are typically wide and bizarre. The QRS complexes may also be wide and bizarre in a **supraventricular arrhythmia** (i.e., one that originates in the SA node or in the atria or AV junction) if a **bundle branch block** or **aberrant ventricular conduction (aberrancy)** is present. Less commonly, **anomalous AV conduction** is the cause of abnormal QRS complexes in arrhythmias originating in the SA node or atria.

Step Two

Determine the Heart Rate

* **Calculate the heart rate** by determining the number of ventricular depolarizations (QRS complexes) or beats that occur in the ECG in 1 minute.

The heart rate can be determined by using the six-second count method, a heart rate calculator ruler, the R-R interval method, or the triplicate method.

The Six-Second Count Method

The **six-second count method** is the simplest way of determining the heart rate and is generally considered the fastest, with the exception of the heart rate calculator ruler method. The six-second count method, however, is the least accurate. This method can be used when the rhythm is either regular or irregular.

The short, vertical lines (or some other similar marking) at the top of most ECG papers divide the ECG paper strip into **three-second intervals** (Figure 4-2) when the paper is run at a standard speed of 25 mm per second. Two of these intervals are equal to a **six-second interval** (Figure 4-3).

The heart rate is calculated by determining the number of QRS complexes in a six-second interval and multiplying this number by 10. The result is the heart rate in beats per minute. The heart rate calculated by this method is almost always an approximation of the actual heart rate.

> **Example.** If there are **eight QRS complexes** in a six-second interval, the heart rate is:
>
> $8 \times 10 = 80$ beats per minute.

To obtain a more accurate heart rate when the rate is extremely slow and/or the rhythm is grossly irregular, the number of QRS complexes should be determined in a longer interval, such as a **twelve-second interval,** and the multiplier should be adjusted accordingly.

> **Example.** If there are **six QRS complexes** in a twelve-second interval, the heart rate is:
>
> $6 \times 5 = 30$ **beats per minute.**

In adults, a heart rate less than 60 beats per minute indicates **bradycardia;** a heart rate above 100 per minute indicates **tachycardia.**

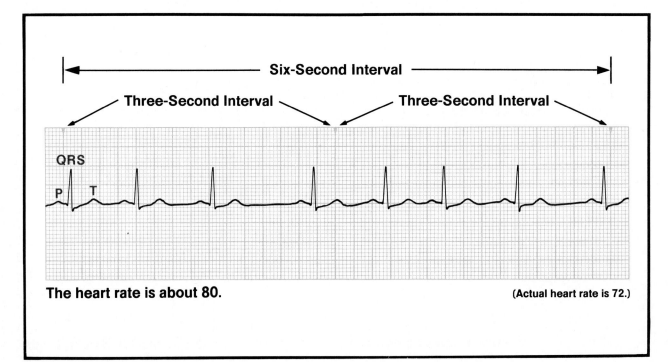

The heart rate is about 80.   (Actual heart rate is 72.)

Figure 4-2. Three- and six-second intervals.

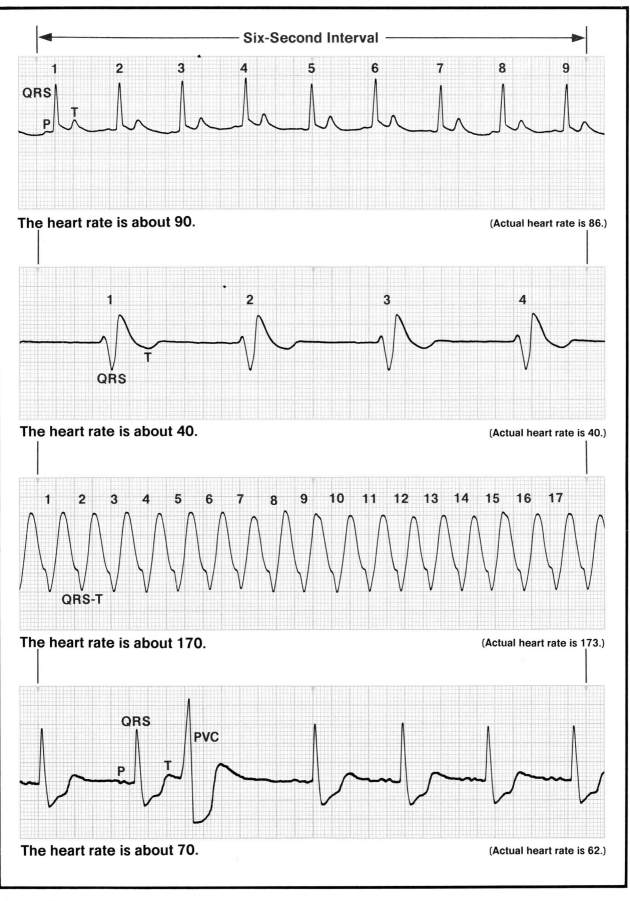

Figure 4-3. Six-second count method.

Heart Rate Calculator Ruler Method

A **heart rate calculator ruler** such as the one supplied with this book, shown in **Figure 4-4,** is a device that can be used to determine the heart rate rapidly and accurately. This method is most accurate if the rhythm is regular. The directions printed on the ruler should be followed (e.g., "Third complex from arrow is rate/min").

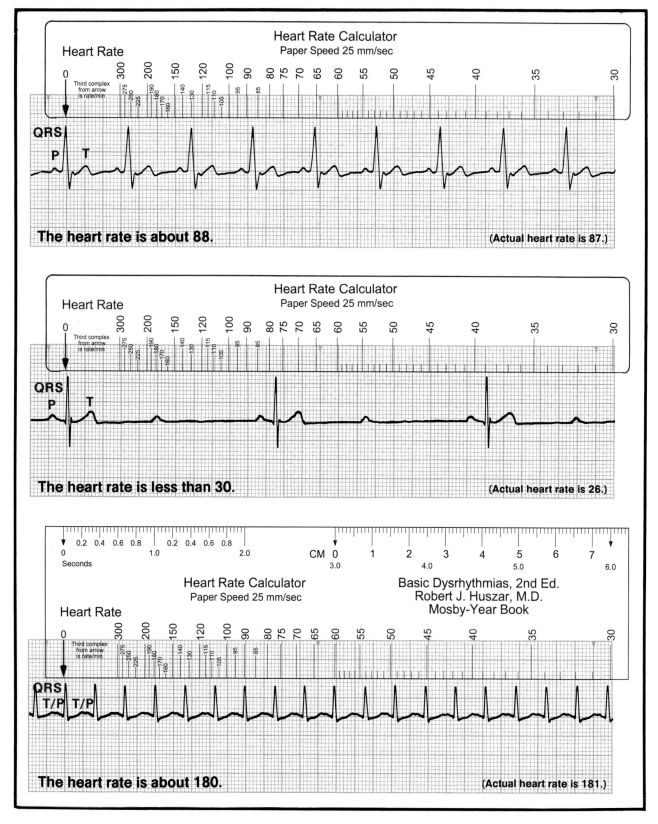

Figure 4-4. Heart rate calculator ruler method.

R-R Interval Method

The **R-R interval** may be used four different ways to determine the heart rate. The rhythm must be regular if the calculation of the heart rate is to be accurate. The four ways are as follows:

1. Measure the distance in seconds between the peaks of 2 consecutive R waves, and divide this number into 60 to obtain the heart rate (Figure 4-5).

Example.   If the distance between the **peaks of 2 consecutive R waves** is 0.56 second, the heart rate is:

60/0.56 = 107 beats per minute.

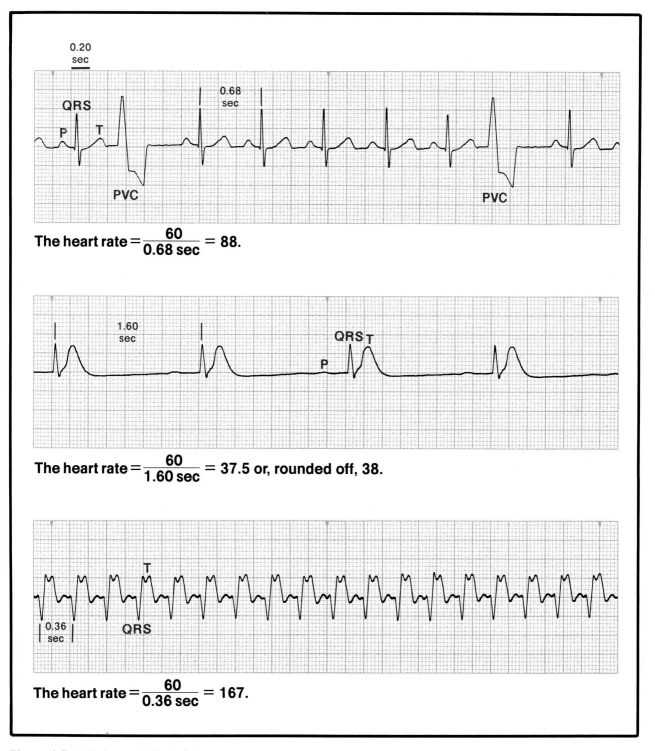

The heart rate $= \dfrac{60}{0.68 \text{ sec}} = 88.$

The heart rate $= \dfrac{60}{1.60 \text{ sec}} = 37.5$ or, rounded off, 38.

The heart rate $= \dfrac{60}{0.36 \text{ sec}} = 167.$

Figure 4-5. R-R interval Method 1.

2. Count the large squares (0.20-second spaces) between the peaks of 2 consecutive R waves, and divide this number into 300 to obtain the heart rate (Figure 4-6).

Example.   If there are 2.5 large squares between the **peaks of 2 consecutive R waves,** the heart rate is:

300/2.5 = 120 beats per minute.

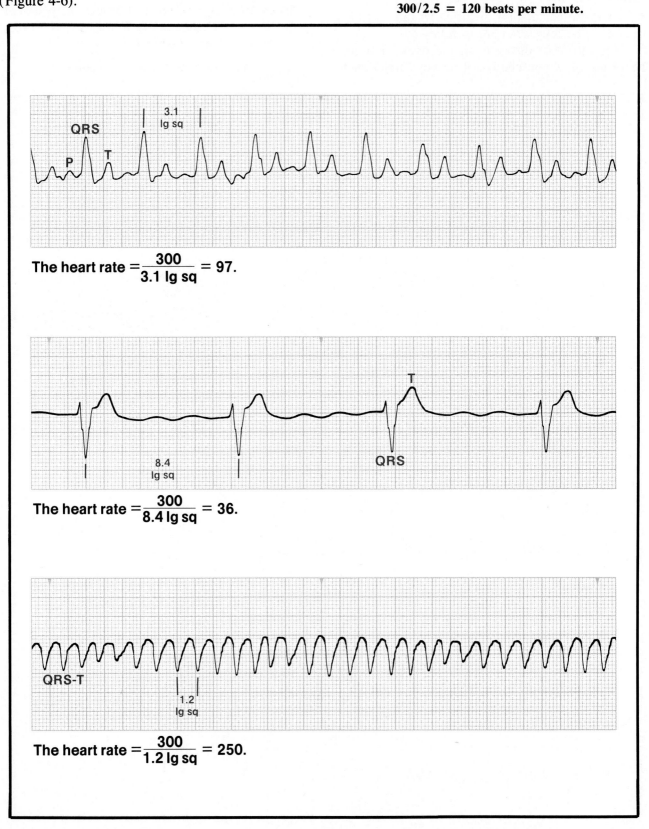

The heart rate $= \dfrac{300}{3.1 \text{ lg sq}} = 97.$

The heart rate $= \dfrac{300}{8.4 \text{ lg sq}} = 36.$

The heart rate $= \dfrac{300}{1.2 \text{ lg sq}} = 250.$

Figure 4-6. R-R interval Method 2.

3. Count the small squares (0.04-second spaces) between the peaks of 2 consecutive R waves, and divide this number into 1,500 to obtain the heart rate (Figure 4-7).

Example. If there are 19 small squares between the **peaks of 2 consecutive R waves,** the heart rate is:

1500/19 = 78.9 or, rounded off, 80 beats per minute.

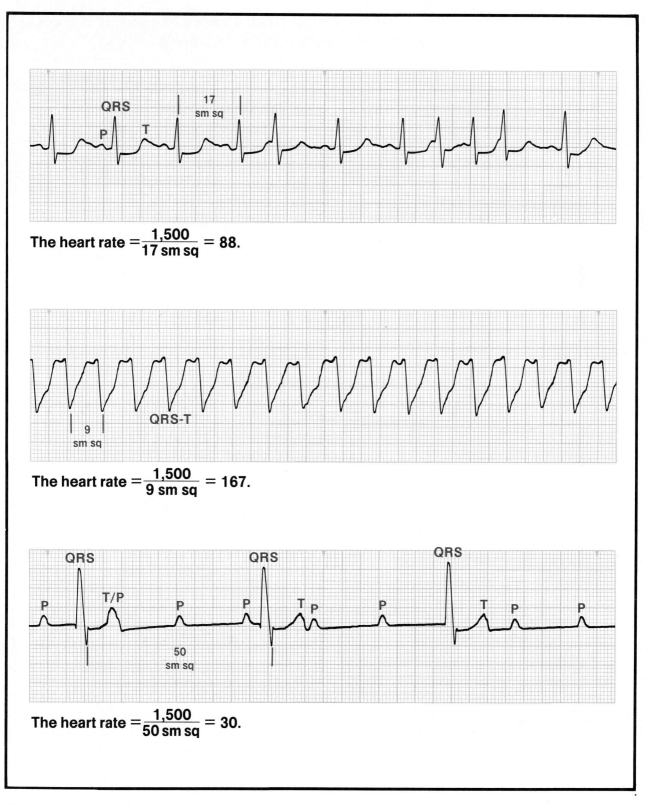

Figure 4-7. R-R interval Method 3.

4. Count the small squares (0.04-second spaces) between the peaks of two consecutive R waves, and, using a **rate conversion table (Table 4-1),** convert the number of small squares into the heart rate (Figure 4-8).

Example.   If there are 17 small squares between the **peaks of 2 consecutive R waves,** the heart rate is:

88 beats per minute.

Table 4-1. Table for conversion of the number of small squares (0.04-second spaces) between the peaks of two consecutive R waves into the heart rate

0.04-sec spaces	Heart rate/min	0.04-sec spaces	Heart rate/min	0.04-sec spaces	Heart rate/min	0.04-sec spaces	Heart rate/min
5	300	16	94	27	56	38	40
6	250	17	88	28	54	39	39
7	214	18	84	29	52	40	38
8	188	19	79	30	50	41	37
9	167	20	75	31	48	42	36
10	150	21	72	32	47	43	35
11	136	22	68	33	45	44	34
12	125	23	65	34	44	45	33
13	115	24	63	35	43	47	32
14	107	25	60	36	42	48	31
15	100	26	58	37	41	50	30

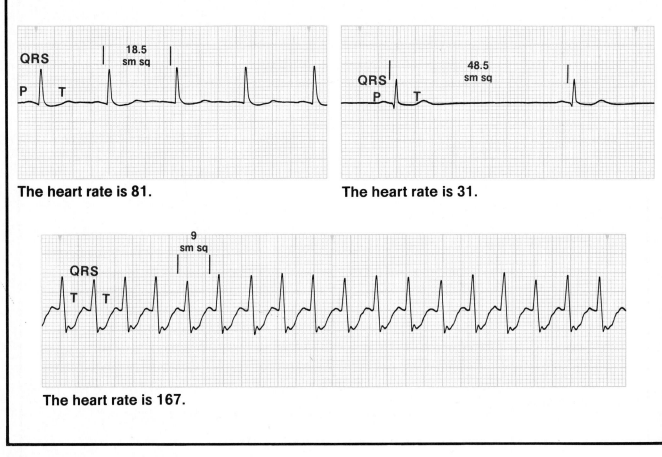

Figure 4-8. R-R interval Method 4.

Triplicate Method

The **triplicate method** of determining the heart rate will be accurate only if the rhythm is regular (Figure 4-9).

The heart rate per minute is determined as follows:

1. Select an R wave that lines up with a dark vertical line, and label it **"A."**
2. Number the next six dark vertical lines consecutively from left to right: **"300," "150," "100," "75," "60,"** and **"50."** These numbers represent heart rate in beats per minute.
3. Identify the first R wave to the right of the R wave labeled **"A,"** and label this R wave **"B."**
4. Identify the numbered dark vertical lines on either side of the R wave labeled **"B."**
5. Estimate the distance of the R wave labeled **"B"** from the nearest of the two adjacent numbered dark vertical lines with respect to the total distance between them, for example, one quarter, one third, or one half of the total distance.
6. Estimate the heart rate by equating the estimated distance of the R wave labeled **"B"** from the nearest adjacent numbered, dark vertical line to beats per minute.

    Examples. If the **R wave labeled "B"** is halfway between the **"150"** dark vertical line and the **"100"** dark vertical line, the heart rate is **about 125 beats per minute.**

                 If the **R wave labeled "B"** is a third of the way between the **"75"** dark vertical line and the **"60"** dark vertical line, the heart rate is **about 70 beats per minute.**

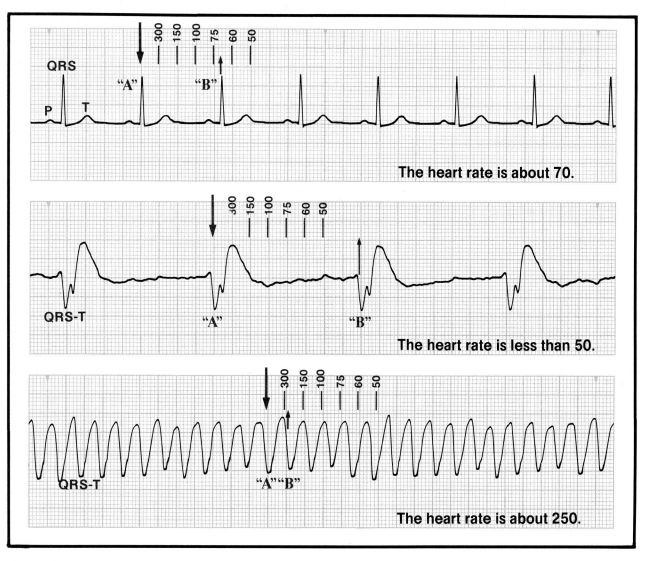

Figure 4-9. Triplicate method.

Step Three

Determine the Ventricular Rhythm

- **Determine the ventricular rhythm** by estimating the R-R intervals, measuring them using **ECG calipers** or, if calipers are not available, a **pencil and paper,** or counting the small squares between the R waves and then by comparing the R-R intervals to each other (Figure 4-10).

For example, an R-R interval (preferably one located on the left side of the ECG strip for the sake of convenience) is measured first. Second, the R-R intervals in the rest of the strip are compared to the one first measured, in a systematic way from left to right.

If ECG calipers are used, one tip of the calipers is placed on the peak of one R wave; the other is adjusted so that it rests on the peak of the adjacent R wave. Without changing the distance between the tips of the calipers, the other R-R intervals are compared to the R-R interval first measured. If a pencil and paper are used, the straight edge of the paper is placed near the peaks of the R waves and the distance between two consecutive R waves (the R-R interval) is marked off. This R-R interval is then compared to the other R-R intervals in the ECG strip.

If the shortest and longest R-R intervals vary by

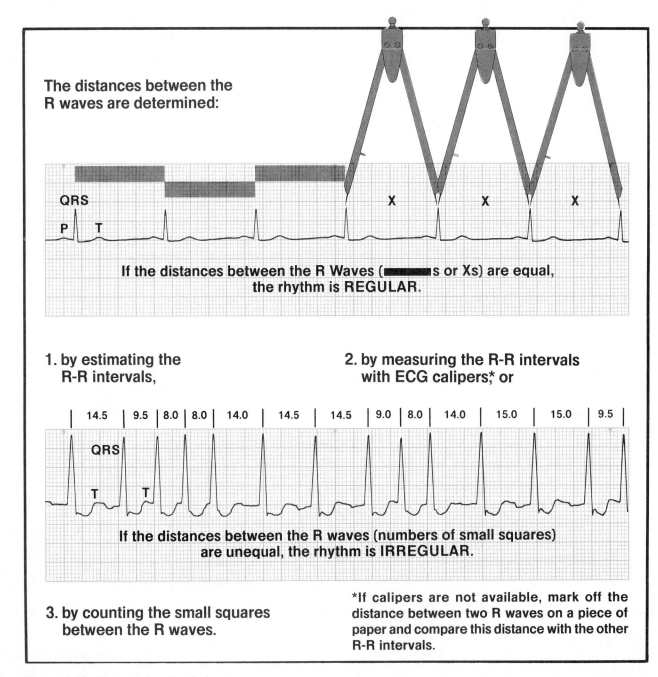

Figure 4-10. Determining the rhythm.

less than 0.16 second (four small squares) in a given ECG strip, the rhythm is considered to be **"essentially regular"** (Figure 4-11). (Thus, the R-R intervals of an "essentially regular" rhythm may be precisely equal or slightly unequal.) If the shortest and longest R-R intervals vary by more than 0.16 second, the rhythm is considered to be **irregular.**

The rhythm may be **slightly irregular, occasionally irregular, regularly irregular,** or **irregularly irregular.** Other terms used interchangeably to describe an irregularly irregular rhythm are **grossly** and **totally irregular** (Figure 4-12). These terms apply to atrial as well as ventricular rhythms.

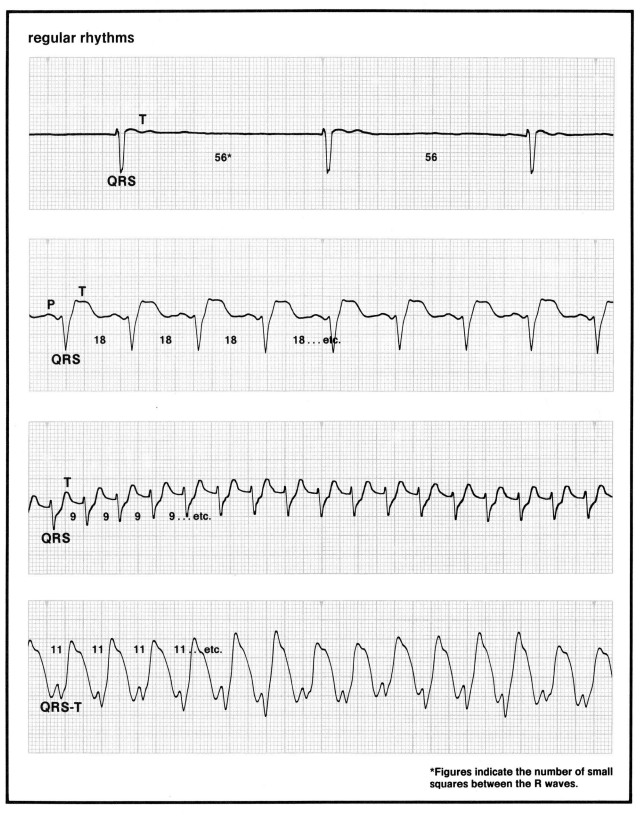

regular rhythms

*Figures indicate the number of small squares between the R waves.

Figure 4-11. Regular rhythms.

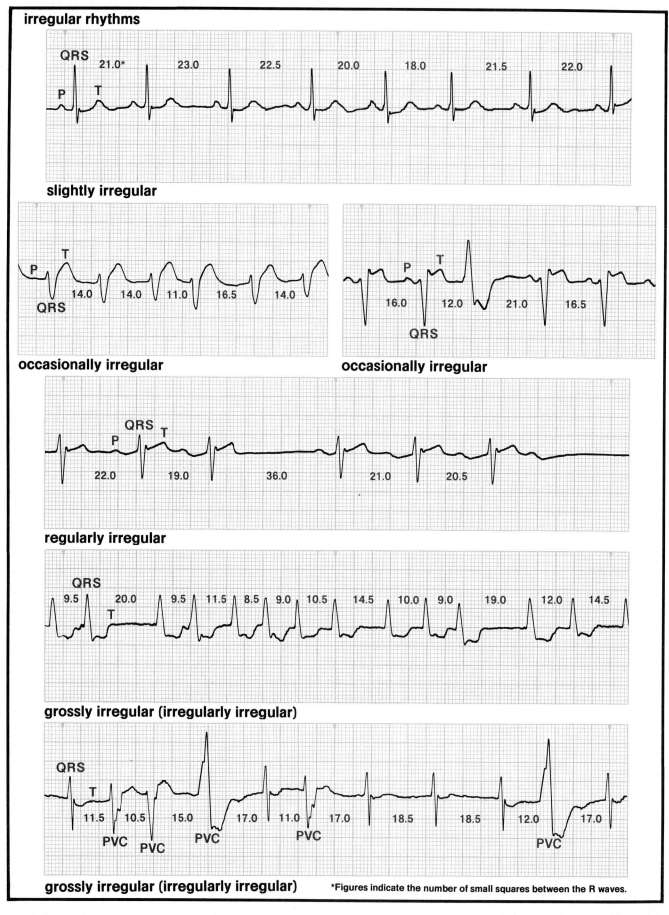

Figure 4-12. Irregular rhythms.

Step Four

Identify and Analyze the P, P′, F, or f Waves

- **Identify the P, P′, F, or f waves.**
- **Determine the atrial rate and rhythm.**

- **Note the association of the P, P′, F, or f waves to the QRS complexes.**

A **normal P wave** is a positive, smoothly rounded wave in lead II (Figure 4-13). It is 0.5 to 2.5 mm high and 0.10 second or less wide. It typically appears before each QRS complex, but it may occur

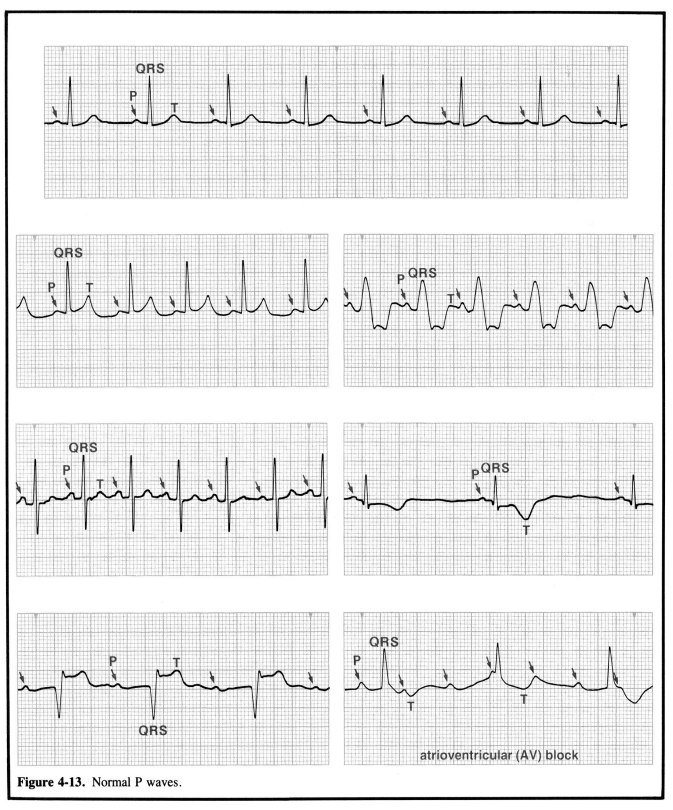

Figure 4-13. Normal P waves.

singly without a QRS complex following it, as in **atrioventricular (AV) block.** An atrioventricular (AV) block is a condition where there is a complete or incomplete (partial) block in the conduction of electrical impulses from the atria to the ventricles through the atrioventricular (AV) junction or the bundle branches. (See Chapter 9.)

An **abnormal P wave** may be positive, negative, or flat (isoelectric) in lead II (Figure 4-14). It may be smoothly rounded, peaked, or deformed. Its height may be normal (0.5 to 2.5 mm) or abnormal (less than 0.5 mm or greater than 2.5 mm). Its duration may be normal (0.10 second or less) or abnormal (greater than 0.10 second). Like a normal P

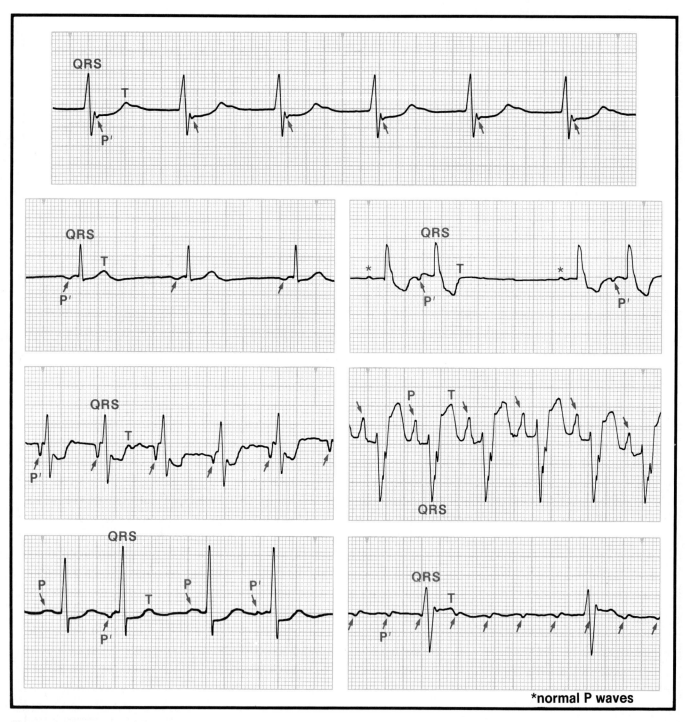

Figure 4-14. Abnormal P waves.

wave, it may appear before the QRS complex or occur alone without a QRS complex following it. Unlike a normal P wave, however, an abnormal P wave may regularly appear after each QRS complex or be buried (or "hidden") in the QRS complex.

Next, determine the atrial rate and rhythm and whether each QRS complex is regularly accompa-

nied by a P wave. The rate of the P waves is usually that of the QRS complexes, but it may be less; if an **AV block** is present, it may be greater.

If P waves are absent, determine if **atrial flutter (F)** or **fibrillation (f) waves** are present (Figure 4-15).

Atrial flutter waves are typically negative,

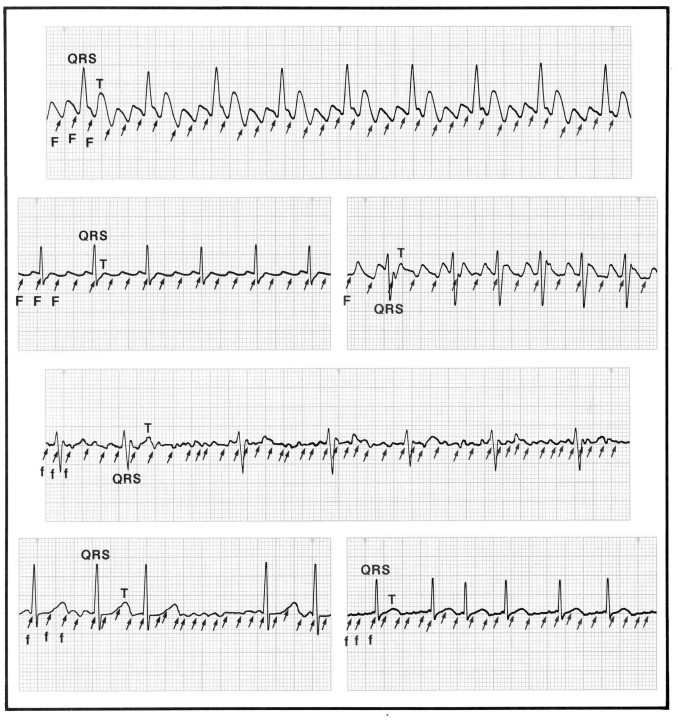

Figure 4-15. F and f waves.

V-shaped waves followed by positive, sharply pointed atrial T waves in lead II. The rate of the F waves is usually between 240 and 350 per minute. Their rhythm is typically regular. QRS complexes commonly occur regularly after every other or every fourth F wave, but they may occur irregularly at varying F wave-to-QRS complex ratios if a **variable AV block** is present.

Atrial fibrillation waves are irregularly shaped, rounded waves, each dissimilar in configuration and amplitude to the other. If the f waves are less than 1 mm high, they are called **"fine" fibrillatory waves;** if greater than 1 mm high, **"coarse" fibrillatory waves.** If the f waves are extremely fine, they may not be identified as such, and the sections of the ECG between the T waves and QRS complexes may appear only slightly wavy or even flat **(isoelectric).** The rate of the f waves is usually between 350 and 600 (average 400) per minute, and their rhythm extremely irregular. Typically, in atrial fibrillation, the QRS complexes occur irregularly with no set pattern, reflecting the extremely irregular atrial rhythm.

Step Five

Determine the PR or RP' Intervals and AV Conduction Ratio

- **Determine the PR intervals** by measuring the distance in seconds between the onset of the P wave and the onset of the first wave of the QRS complex, be it a Q, R, or QS wave.
- **Compare the PR intervals** to determine if all PR intervals are equal in duration.
- **Determine the AV conduction ratio** by noting the number of P (or F) waves followed by QRS complexes in a given set of P (or F) waves.

A **normal PR interval** is 0.12 to 0.20 second in duration (Figure 4-16). It indicates that the electrical impulse causing the P wave originated in the SA node or upper or middle part of the atria. It also indicates that the conduction of the electrical impulse through the AV node, bundle of His, and bundle branches is normal. When the heart rate is fast, the PR interval is shorter than when the heart rate is slow.

A PR interval **less than 0.12 second** or one **greater than 0.20 second** is abnormal (Figure 4-17). A PR interval less than 0.12 second indicates (1) that the electrical impulse originated in the lower part of the atria or in the AV junction or (2) that the electrical impulse progressed from the atria to the

ventricles through atrioventricular (AV) conduction pathways other than the AV node and bundle of His **(anomalous AV conduction).**

An abnormally prolonged PR interval of greater than 0.20 second indicates a delay in the conduction of the electrical impulse through the AV node, bundle of His, or, rarely, the bundle branches. When this occurs, a **first-degree AV block** is present.

If a QRS complex does not follow a P wave, a PR interval is absent. This indicates a blockage of the conduction of the electrical impulse through the AV node, bundle of His, or bundle branches into the ventricles. If QRS complexes follow some P waves and not others, an **incomplete AV block (second-degree AV block)** is present.

Determine the equality of the PR intervals at this point. When unequal PR intervals are present, there is usually an increase in their duration until a P wave is not followed by a QRS complex **(nonconducted P wave** or **dropped beat).** This indicates that there is, typically, a progressive delay in the conduction of the electrical impulse through the AV node (or, less commonly, the bundle of His or bundle branches) into the ventricles until conduction is completely blocked. This kind of second-degree AV block, which occurs cyclically, is called a **Wenckebach block.**

When second-degree AV block is present, an **AV conduction ratio** is commonly determined. This is the number of P waves followed by QRS complexes in a given set of P waves. The following are examples of AV conduction ratios.

- If all P waves are followed by QRS complexes, the AV conduction ratio is **1:1.**
- If, for every two P waves, one is followed by a QRS complex, the AV conduction ratio is **2:1.**
- If, for every three P waves, two are followed by QRS complexes, the AV conduction ratio is **3:2.**
- If, for every five P waves, one is followed by a QRS complex, the AV conduction ratio is **5:1.**

If QRS complexes are present but do not regularly precede or follow the P waves, a **complete AV block (third-degree AV block)** is present. Another term used to describe the condition when QRS complexes occur totally unrelated to the P, P', or F waves is **AV dissociation.**

If a P wave follows the QRS complex, an **RP' interval** is present, indicating that the electrical impulse responsible for the P' wave and QRS complex has originated in the AV junction or ventricles. An RP' interval is usually 0.20 second or less.

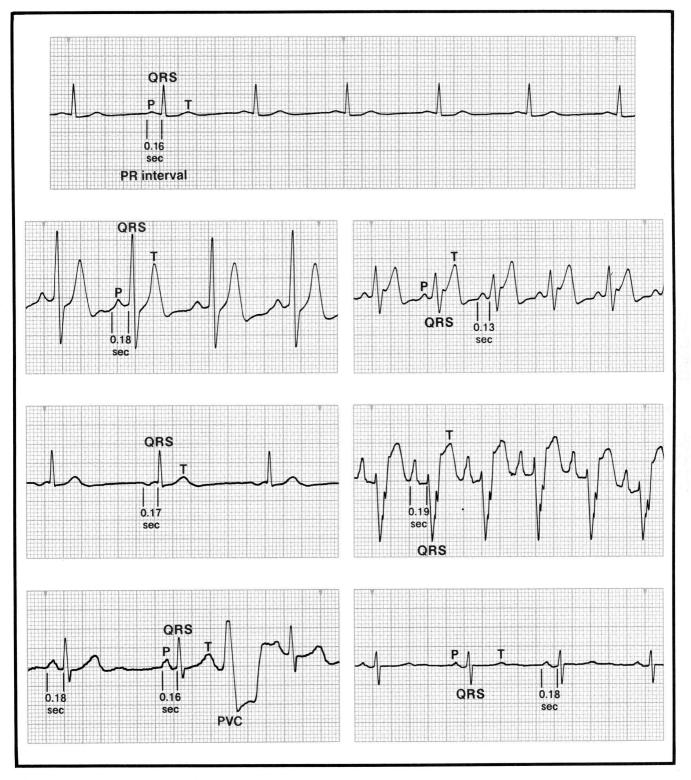

Figure 4-16. Normal PR intervals.

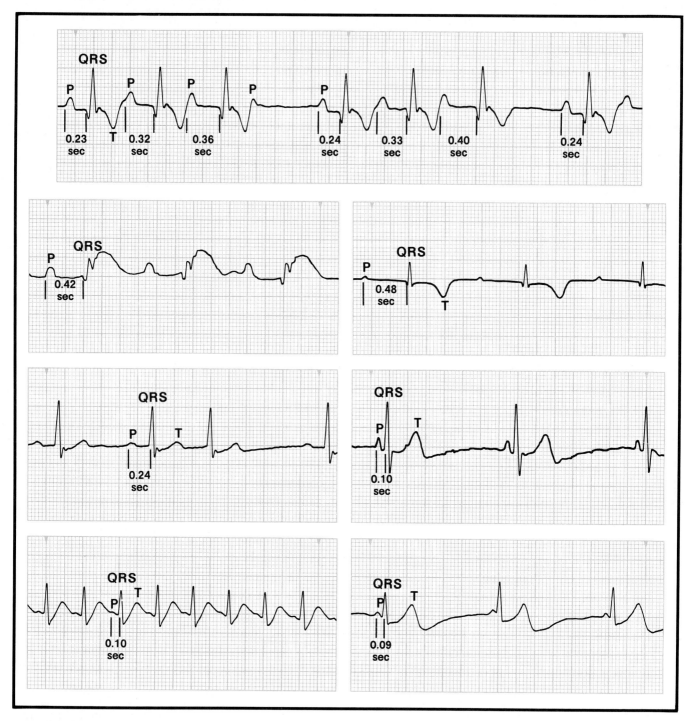

Figure 4-17. Abnormal PR intervals.

Step Six

Determine the Site of Origin of the Arrhythmia

- **Determine the site of origin of the arrhythmia** by analyzing the P waves, the QRS complexes, and their association to each other.

If P waves are associated with the QRS complexes (i.e., the P waves regularly precede or follow the QRS complexes), the **site of origin** (or **pacemaker site**) of the arrhythmia is that of the P waves (Figure 4-18). Conversely, if the P waves are not associated with the QRS complexes, that is, the P waves and the QRS complexes occur independently of each other (i.e., **atrioventricular [AV] dissociation**), or if the P waves are absent, the **site of origin** of the arrhythmia is that of the QRS complexes (Figure 4-19).

The electrical impulses causing the P waves may have originated in the **SA node** or an ectopic or escape pacemaker in the **atria, AV junction,** or **ventricles.** The site of origin of the electrical impulses responsible for the P waves can usually be deduced by noting the direction of the P waves in lead II and their relationship to the QRS complexes. **Table 4-2** summarizes the determination of the pacemaker site of arrhythmias with P waves associated with the QRS complexes.

- **If the P waves are upright (positive) in lead II,** the electrical impulses responsible for them may have originated either in the **SA node** or in the **atria.** When upright P waves have a set relationship to the QRS complexes, they always precede the QRS complexes. The PR interval may be **normal** (0.12 to 0.20 second), **prolonged** (greater than 0.20 second—indicating first-degree AV block), or **short** (less than 0.12 second—indicating anomalous AV conduction).

- **If the P waves are negative (inverted) in lead II (P'),** the electrical impulses responsible for them may have originated in the **lower part of the atria near the AV junction,** in the **AV junction** itself, or in the **ventricles.** The exact location of the site of origin of negative P' waves can be deduced by analyzing their relationship to the QRS complexes in lead II as follows:

    If the negative P' waves regularly precede the QRS complexes, the electrical impulses responsible

for the P' waves may have originated either in the **lower part of the atria near the AV junction** or in the **proximal part of the AV junction** itself. Typically, the P'R interval is less than 0.12 second, but it may be greater if first-degree AV block is present.

    If the negative P' waves regularly follow the QRS complexes, the electrical impulses responsible for the P' waves may have originated either in the **distal part of the AV junction** or in the **ventricles.** If the QRS complexes are greater than 0.12 second in duration and appear bizarre, it is more likely that the P' waves originated in the ventricles. The RP' intervals are usually less than 0.20 second.

    If the negative P' waves have no set relationship to the QRS complexes, occurring at a rate different from that of the QRS complexes (i.e., AV dissociation), the electrical impulses responsible for the P' waves may have originated either in the **lower part of the atria near the AV junction** or in the **AV junction.** The electrical impulses responsible for the QRS complexes may have originated in the **AV junction** or the **ventricles.**

- If **atrial flutter or fibrillation waves** are present, the electrical impulses responsible for them have originated in the **atria.**

If the QRS complexes have no set relationship to the P waves, occurring at a rate different from that of the P waves, or if P waves are absent, the electrical impulses causing the QRS complexes may have originated in an ectopic or escape pacemaker in the **AV junction** or **ventricles** (i.e., **bundle branch, Purkinje network,** or **ventricular myocardium**). The site of origin of the electrical impulses responsible for such QRS complexes can be deduced by noting the duration and shape of the QRS complex and whether or not a preexisting bundle branch block or aberrant ventricular conduction

Table 4-2. Determination of the pacemaker site of arrhythmias with P waves associated with the QRS complexes

Pacemaker site	Direction of the P wave in lead II	P/QRS relationship	P-R interval
SA node **OR** Atria	Positive (upright)	P precedes QRS complex	0.12-0.20 sec or greater **OR** less than 0.12 sec*
Lower atria **OR** Proximal AV junction	Negative (inverted)	P precedes QRS complex	Less than 0.12 sec
Distal AV junction **OR** Ventricles	Negative (inverted)	P follows QRS complex	None

*In association with anomalous AV conduction

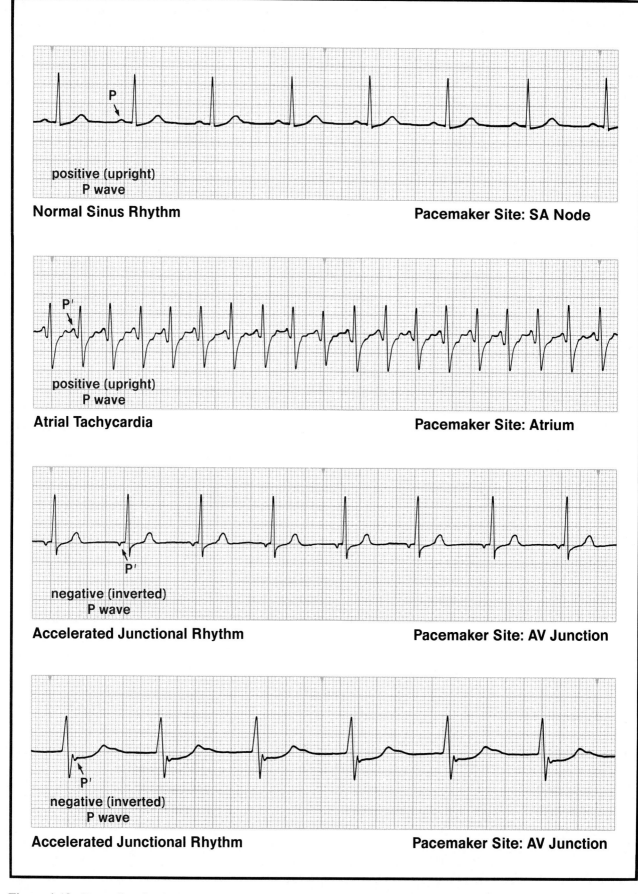

Figure 4-18. Examples of arrhythmias with P waves associated with the QRS complexes and their pacemaker sites.

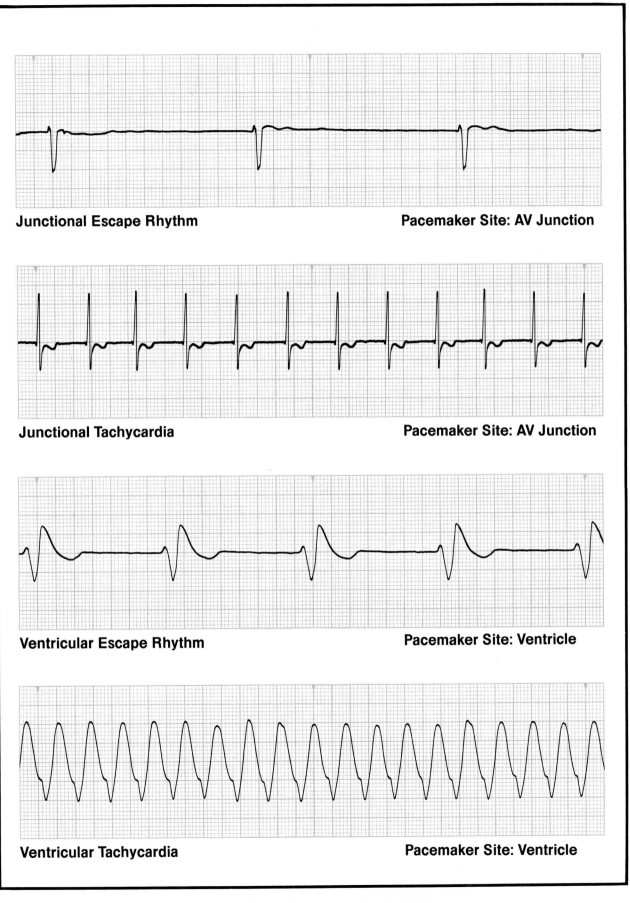

Junctional Escape Rhythm   Pacemaker Site: AV Junction

Junctional Tachycardia   Pacemaker Site: AV Junction

Ventricular Escape Rhythm   Pacemaker Site: Ventricle

Ventricular Tachycardia   Pacemaker Site: Ventricle

Figure 4-19. Examples of arrhythmias with QRS complexes not associated with P waves and their pacemaker sites.

is present. Often, the pacemaker site of wide and bizarre QRS complexes, occurring independently of the P waves or in their absence, cannot be determined with accuracy based on an ECG obtained from a single monitoring lead II. In such instances, a **12-lead ECG** or **lead MCL₁** is extremely helpful. **Table 4-3** summarizes the determination of the pacemaker site of arrhythmias with QRS complexes not associated with P waves.

- If the QRS complexes are 0.10 second or less in duration, the electrical impulses responsible for the QRS complexes most likely have originated in the **AV junction.**
- If the QRS complexes are between 0.10 and 0.12 second in duration, the electrical impulses responsible for the QRS complexes may have originated in the **AV junction** (in which case a preexisting incomplete bundle branch block or aberrant ventricular conduction has to be present) or in the **proximal part of a bundle branch in the ventricles near the bundle of His.**
- If the QRS complexes are greater than 0.12 second in duration and appear bizarre, the electrical impulses responsible for the QRS complexes may have originated in the **AV junction** (in which case a preexisting complete bundle branch block or aberrant ventricular conduction has to be present) or in the **distal part of a bundle branch, the Purkinje network,** or **ventricular myocardium.**

Table 4-3. Determination of the pacemaker site of arrhythmias with QRS complexes not associated with P waves

| Pacemaker site | QRS complex | |
	Duration	Appearance
AV junction	0.10 sec or less	Normal
AV junction* **OR** Proximal bundle branch	0.10-0.12 sec	Normal
AV junction† **OR** Distal bundle branch, Purkinje network, or ventricular myocardium	Greater than 0.12 sec	Bizarre

*In association with a preexisting incomplete bundle branch block or aberrant ventricular conduction.

†In association with a preexisting complete bundle branch block or aberrant ventricular conduction.

Step Seven

Identify the Arrhythmia

The identification of arrhythmias is presented in detail in Chapters 5 through 9.

Step Eight

Evaluate the Significance of the Arrhythmia

The evaluation of the significance of arrhythmias is presented in detail in Chapters 5 through 9.

ECG Interpretation

The following is an outline of the steps in interpreting an ECG to determine the presence of an **arrhythmia** and its identity. The ECG interpretation may be performed in the order shown or in accordance with local prehospital or hospital protocols.

A. **Step One:** Identify and analyze the QRS complexes
1. Identify the QRS complexes
2. Note the duration and shape of the QRS complexes
3. Assess the equality of the QRS complexes
B. **Step Two:** Determine the heart rate
C. **Step Three:** Determine the ventricular rhythm
D. **Step Four:** Identify and analyze the P, P′, F, or f waves
1. Identify the P, P′, F, or f waves
2. Determine the atrial rate and rhythm
3. Note the association of the P, P′, F, or f waves to the QRS complexes
E. **Step Five:** Determine the PR or RP′ intervals and AV conduction ratio
1. Determine the PR intervals
2. Assess the equality of the PR intervals
3. Determine the AV conduction ratio
F. **Step Six:** Determine the site of origin of the arrhythmia
G. **Step Seven:** Identify the arrhythmia
H. **Step Eight:** Evaluate the significance of the arrhythmia

1. The heart rate can be determined by:
   A. the six-second count method
   B. a heart rate calculator ruler
   C. the R-R interval method
   D. all of the above

2. In adults, a heart rate less than _____ beats per minute indicates _____ and a heart rate greater than _____ per minute indicates _____ .
   A. 60, bradycardia: 120, tachycardia
   B. 50, tachycardia: 120, bradycardia
   C. 60, bradycardia: 100, tachycardia
   D. 50, tachycardia: 100, bradycardia

3. The rhythm must be regular if the calculation of the heart rate is to be accurate using the _____ method.
   A. triplicate
   B. R-R interval
   C. both of the above
   D. none of the above

4. If there are four large squares between the peaks of two consecutive R waves, the heart rate is _____ beats per minute.
   A. 50
   B. 75
   C. 100
   D. 150

5. The rate of the P waves is:
   A. the same as that of the QRS complexes
   B. sometimes less than the rate of QRS complexes
   C. greater than the QRS rate in AV block
   D. all of the above

6. If QRS complexes are present but do not regularly precede or follow the P waves:
   A. a complete AV block is present
   B. the AV conduction ratio should be calculated
   C. an incomplete AV block is present
   D. none of the above

7. If atrial flutter or fibrillation waves are present, the electrical impulses responsible for them have originated in the:
   A. ventricle
   B. atria
   C. septum
   D. bundle of His

8. The pacemaker site of inverted P waves in lead II is in the:
   A. ventricles
   B. lower atria
   C. AV junction
   D. all of the above

9. If the QRS complexes are 0.10 second or less in duration, the electrical impulses responsible for the QRS complexes most likely have originated in the:
   A. SA node
   B. Purkinje network
   C. AV junction in the presence of a right bundle branch block
   D. interventricular septum

10. A QRS which has a bizarre appearance and a duration greater than 0.12 second most likely has a pacemaker site in (the):
    A. AV junction in the presence of aberrant ventricular conduction
    B. Purkinje network
    C. ventricular myocardium
    D. all of the above

Sinus Node Arrhythmias

Normal Sinus Rhythm (NSR)

Sinus Arrhythmia

Sinus Bradycardia

Sinus Arrest and Sinoatrial (SA) Exit Block

Sinus Tachycardia

OBJECTIVES

Upon completion of all or part of this chapter you should be able to complete the following objectives indicated by your instructor:

☐ **1.** Define and give the diagnostic characteristics, cause, and clinical significance of the following arrhythmias:

☐ Normal sinus   ☐ Sinus arrest
   rhythm (NSR)   ☐ Sinoatrial (SA) exit
☐ Sinus arrhythmia   block
☐ Sinus bradycardia   ☐ Sinus tachycardia

Normal Sinus Rhythm (NSR)

Definition

Normal sinus rhythm (NSR) (Figure 5-1) is the normal rhythm of the heart, originating in the SA node, and characterized by a heart rate of 60 to 100 beats per minute.

Diagnostic Characteristics

Heart rate: The heart rate is 60 to 100 beats per minute.

Rhythm: The atrial and ventricular rhythms are essentially regular.

Pacemaker site: The pacemaker site is the SA node.

P waves: The sinus P waves are identical and precede each QRS complex. They are positive (upright) in lead II.

PR intervals: The PR intervals are normal (0.12 to 0.20 second) and generally constant but may vary slightly with the heart rate.

R-R and P-P intervals: The R-R intervals may be equal or vary slightly. The difference between the longest and shortest R-R (or P-P) interval is less than 0.16 second in normal sinus rhythm.

QRS complexes: A QRS complex typically follows each P wave. The QRS complexes are normal (0.10 second or less) unless a preexisting bundle branch block or anomalous AV conduction is present, in which case the QRS complexes are abnormal (greater than 0.10 second).

Clinical Significance

Normal sinus rhythm is of no clinical significance. No treatment is indicated.

Notes

Normal Sinus Rhythm (NSR)

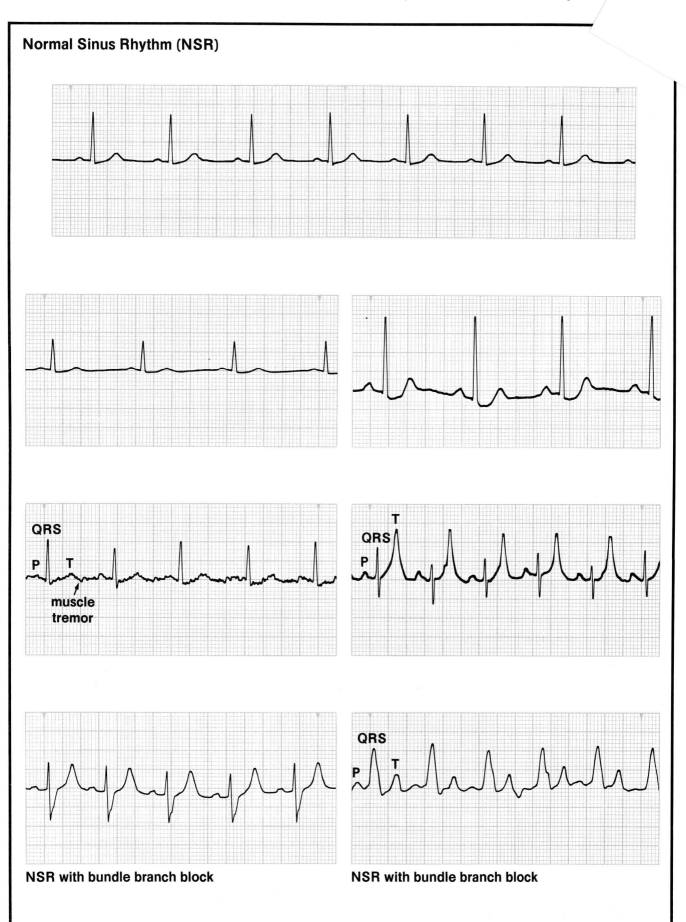

NSR with bundle branch block   NSR with bundle branch block

Figure 5-1

Sinus Arrhythmia

Definition

Sinus arrhythmia (Figure 5-2) is an irregularity of the heart beat caused by a cyclic increase and decrease in the rate of a sinus rhythm.

Diagnostic Characteristics

Heart rate: The heart rate is 60 to 100 beats per minute. Occasionally, the heart rate may slow to less than 60 and increase to over 100 beats per minute. Typically, the heart rate *increases* during inspiration and *decreases* during expiration.

Rhythm: The atrial and ventricular rhythms are regularly irregular as the heart rate gradually increases and slows; the changes in rate occur in cycles.

Pacemaker site: The pacemaker site is the SA node.

P waves: The sinus P waves are identical and precede each QRS complex. They are positive (upright) in lead II. **Sinus arrhythmia** is considered to be present when the difference between the longest and shortest P-P (or R-R) interval is greater than 0.16 second.

PR intervals: The PR intervals are normal and constant.

R-R intervals: The R-R intervals are unequal. The most common type of sinus arrhythmia is related to respiration in which the R-R intervals become shorter during inspiration as the heart rate increases and longer during expiration as the heart rate decreases. In another, less common type of sinus arrhythmia, the R-R intervals become shorter and longer without any relation to respiration. The difference between the longest and shortest R-R interval is greater than 0.16 second in sinus arrhythmia.

QRS complexes: A QRS complex normally follows each P wave. The QRS complexes are normal unless a preexisting bundle branch block or anomalous AV conduction is present.

Cause of Arrhythmia

The most common type of sinus arrhythmia, the one related to respiration, is a normal phenomenon commonly seen in children, young adults, and elderly individuals. It is caused by the inhibitory vagal (parasympathetic) effect of respiration on the SA node. The other, less common type of sinus arrhythmia is not related to respiration. It may occur in healthy individuals, but it is more commonly found in adult patients with heart disease, especially following acute inferior myocardial infarction, or in patients receiving certain drugs such as digitalis and morphine.

Clinical Significance

Usually, sinus arrhythmia is of no clinical significance per se and generally does not require treatment. Marked sinus arrhythmia may cause palpitations, dizziness, and even syncope.

Notes

Sinus Arrhythmia

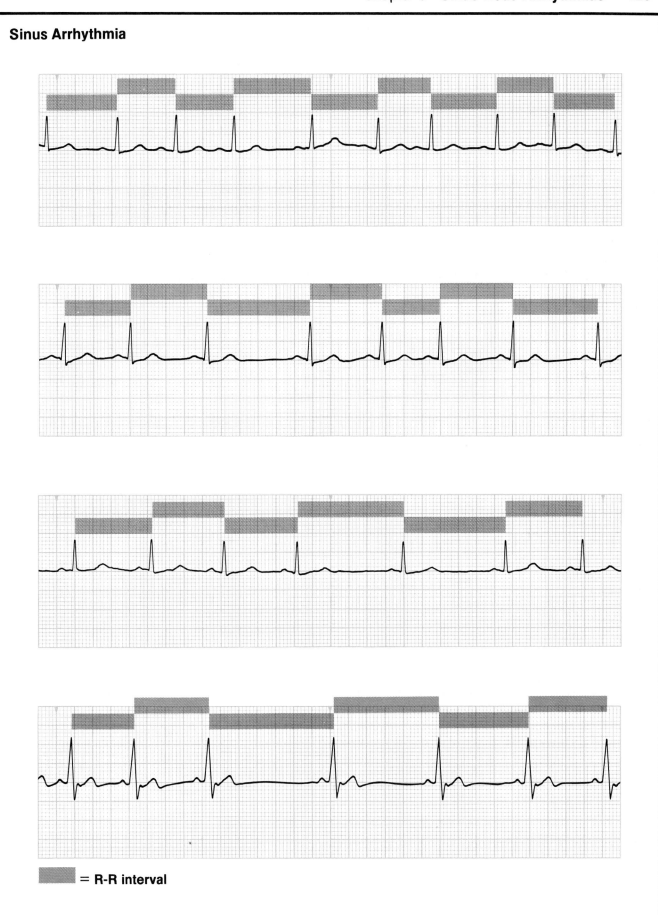

= R-R interval

Figure 5-2

Sinus Bradycardia

Definition

Sinus bradycardia (Figure 5-3) is an arrhythmia originating in the SA node, characterized by a rate of less than 60 beats per minute.

Diagnostic Characteristics

Heart rate: The heart rate is less than 60 beats per minute.

Rhythm: The rhythm is essentially regular, but it may be irregular if sinus arrhythmia is also present.

Pacemaker site: The pacemaker site is the SA node.

P waves: The sinus P waves are identical and precede each QRS complex. They are positive (upright) in lead II.

PR intervals: The PR intervals are normal and constant. However, they tend to be at the upper limits of normal.

R-R intervals: The R-R intervals are usually equal but may vary.

QRS complexes: A QRS complex normally follows each P wave. The QRS complexes are normal unless a preexisting bundle branch block or anomalous AV conduction is present.

Cause of Arrhythmia

Sinus bradycardia may be caused by either an excessive inhibitory vagal (parasympathetic) tone or a decrease in sympathetic tone on the SA node, disease in the SA node, myxedema, hypothermia, hypoxia, or administration of digitalis, propranolol, or diltiazem or verapamil. Sinus bradycardia is common in acute inferior myocardial infarction. Sinus bradycardia may be associated with vomiting and vasovagal syncope and follow carotid sinus stimulation. It is common during sleep and in trained athletes.

Clinical Significance

Sinus bradycardia with a heart rate between 50 and 59 beats per minute (**mild sinus bradycardia**) usually does not produce symptoms by itself. Such a bradycardia without symptoms is an **asymptomatic bradycardia.** If the heart rate is 30 to 45 beats per minute or less (**marked sinus bradycardia**), hypotension with reduction in cardiac output and decreased perfusion of the brain and other vital organs may occur. This may result in dizziness, lightheadedness, or syncope. When symptoms occur, the bradycardia is called a **symptomatic bradycardia** regardless of the heart rate.

In the presence of acute myocardial infarction, mild sinus bradycardia may actually be beneficial in some patients because of the decrease in the workload of the heart, which reduces the oxygen requirements of the myocardium, minimizes the extension of the infarction, and lessens the predisposition to certain arrhythmias. Marked sinus bradycardia, however, may result in hypotension with a marked reduction of cardiac output and lead to congestive heart failure, syncope, and shock and predispose the patient to more serious arrhythmias (i.e., premature ventricular contractions, ventricular tachycardia or fibrillation, or ventricular asystole).

Symptomatic sinus bradycardia, whatever the heart rate, must be treated promptly with atropine or a transcutaneous pacemaker to reverse the consequences of reduced cardiac output and to prevent the occurrence of serious ventricular arrhythmias.

Notes

Sinus Bradycardia

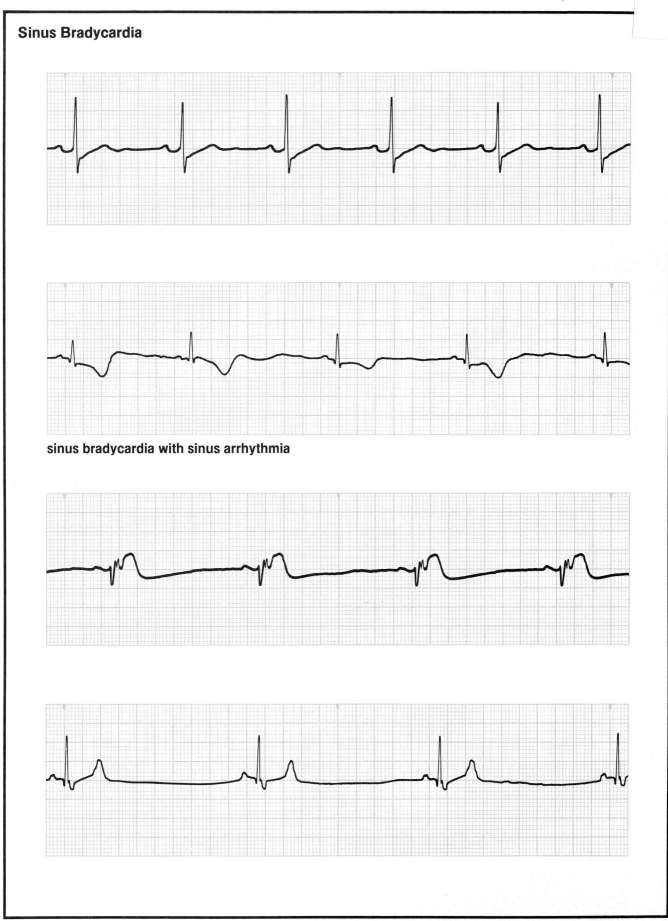

sinus bradycardia with sinus arrhythmia

Figure 5-3

Sinus Arrest and Sinoatrial (SA) Exit Block

Definition

Sinus arrest (Figure 5-4) is an arrhythmia caused by episodes of failure in the automaticity of the SA node, resulting in bradycardia, asystole, or both.

Sinoatrial (SA) exit block (Figure 5-4) is an arrhythmia caused by a block in the conduction of the electrical impulse from the SA node to the atria, resulting, like sinus arrest, in bradycardia, asystole, or both.

Diagnostic Characteristics

Heart rate: The heart rate is usually 60 to 100 beats per minute but may be less.

Rhythm: The rhythm is irregular when sinus arrest or SA exit block is present.

Pacemaker site: The pacemaker site is the SA node.

P waves: The sinus P waves of the underlying rhythm are identical and precede each QRS complex. If an electrical impulse is not generated by the SA node **(sinus arrest)** or if it is generated by the SA node but blocked from entering the atria **(sinoatrial [SA] exit block),** atrial depolarization does not occur and, consequently, neither does a P wave **(dropped P wave).** Often, it is difficult to distinguish sinus arrest from SA exit block when a P wave does not occur. Typically, an SA exit block is indicated by the absence of the normally expected sinus P wave(s) on the ECG. In addition, the long P-P interval caused by SA exit block is twice (or a multiple of) the P-P interval of the underlying rhythm since the underlying rhythm remains undisturbed. The long P-P interval caused by sinus arrest is, typically, not a multiple of the P-P interval of the underlying rhythm since the timing of the SA node is reset by the arrest.

PR intervals: The PR intervals are those of the underlying rhythm and may be normal or abnormal.

R-R intervals: The R-R intervals are unequal when sinus arrest or SA exit block is present.

QRS complexes: A QRS complex normally follows each P wave. The QRS complexes are normal unless a preexisting bundle branch block or anomalous AV conduction is present. A QRS complex is absent when a P wave does not occur.

Cause of Arrhythmia

Sinus arrest results from a marked depression in the automaticity of the SA node. SA exit block results from a block in the conduction of the electrical impulse from the SA node into the atria.

Sinus arrest or SA exit block may be precipitated by an increase in vagal (parasympathetic) tone on the SA node, hypoxia, hyperkalemia, or an excessive dose of digitalis or propranolol. The arrhythmias may also be caused by damage to the SA node or adjacent atrium from acute inferior myocardial infarction, acute myocarditis, or degenerative forms of fibrosis. SA exit block may also result from quinidine toxicity.

Clinical Significance

Transient sinus arrest and SA exit block may have no clinical significance per se if an AV junctional escape pacemaker takes over promptly. If a ventricular escape pacemaker takes over with a slow heart rate or if an escape pacemaker does not take over at all, resulting in transient ventricular asystole, lightheadedness may occur, followed by syncope. The signs and symptoms, clinical significance, and management of sinus arrest and SA exit block with excessively slow heart rates are the same as those in symptomatic sinus bradycardia.

Intermittent sinus arrest or SA exit block can, however, progress to prolonged sinus arrest **(atrial standstill).** If a junctional or ventricular escape pacemaker does not take over, ventricular asystole occurs, requiring immediate treatment.

Notes

**Sinus Arrest and
Sinoatrial (SA) Exit Block**

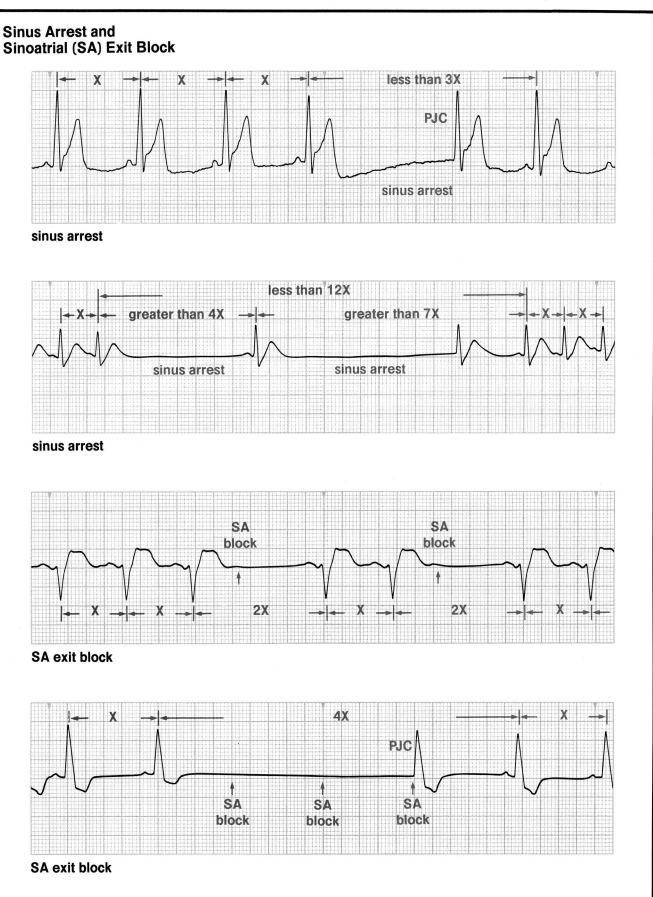

Figure 5-4

Sinus Tachycardia

Definition

Sinus tachycardia (Figure 5-5) is an arrhythmia originating in the SA node, characterized by a rate of over 100 beats per minute.

Diagnostic Characteristics

Heart rate: The heart rate is over 100 beats per minute and may be as high as 180 beats per minute or greater with extreme exertion. The onset and termination of **sinus tachycardia** are typically gradual. Vagal maneuvers, such as carotid sinus massage, may cause transient slowing of the heart rate, with a gradual return to the prestimulation rate following the carotid massage.

Rhythm: The rhythm is essentially regular.

Pacemaker site: The pacemaker site is the SA node.

P waves: The sinus P waves are usually normal but may be slightly taller and more peaked than usual. The sinus P waves are identical and precede each QRS complex. They are positive (upright) in lead II. When the heart rate is very rapid, the sinus P waves may be buried in the preceding T waves (**buried P waves**) and not be easily identified.

PR intervals: The PR intervals are normal and constant. They are shorter when the heart rate is fast than when the rate is slow.

R-R intervals: The R-R intervals may be equal but may vary slightly.

QRS complexes: The QRS complexes are normal unless a preexisting bundle branch block, aberrant ventricular conduction, or anomalous AV conduction is present. A QRS complex normally follows each P wave. Sinus tachycardia with abnormal QRS complexes may resemble ventricular tachycardia (see Ventricular Tachycardia, page 172).

Cause of Arrhythmia

Sinus tachycardia in adults is a normal response of the heart to the demand for increased blood flow, as in exercise and exertion. It may also be caused by the ingestion of stimulants (coffee, tea, and alcohol) or smoking or by an increase in catecholamines and sympathetic tone resulting from anxiety, pain, or stress. Sinus tachycardia may also be caused by pathophysiologic conditions (fever, thyrotoxicosis, anemia, hypovolemia, hypoxia, congestive heart failure, pulmonary embolism, myocardial ischemia, acute myocardial infarction, and hypotension or shock) or an excessive dose of atropine or a sympathomimetic drug, such as epinephrine, isoproterenol, and norepinephrine.

Clinical Significance

Sinus tachycardia per se in healthy individuals is a benign arrhythmia and does not require treatment. When its cause is removed or treated, sinus tachycardia resolves gradually and spontaneously. Because a rapid heart rate increases the workload of the heart, the oxygen requirements of the heart are increased. For this reason, sinus tachycardia in acute myocardial infarction may increase myocardial ischemia and the frequency and severity of chest pain, cause an extension of the infarct or even pump failure (e.g., congestive heart failure, hypotension, and cardiogenic shock), or predispose the patient to more serious arrhythmias.

Treatment of sinus tachycardia should be directed to correcting the underlying cause of the arrhythmia.

Notes

Sinus Tachycardia

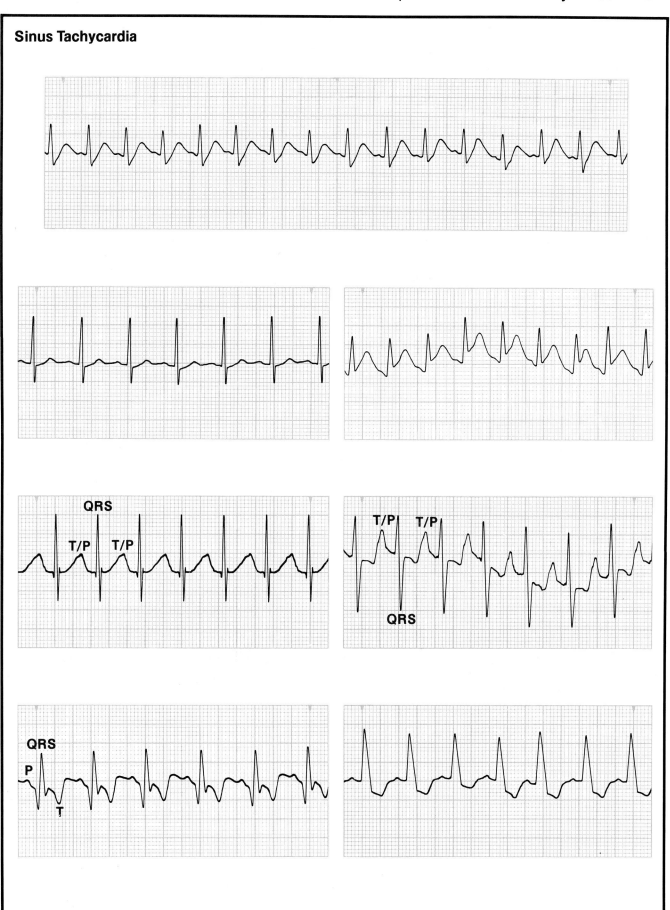

Figure 5-5

1. Typically, the heart rate _____ during inspiration and _____ during expiration.
   A. increases: increases
   B. increases: decreases
   C. decreases: increases
   D. decreases: decreases

2. The most common type of sinus arrhythmia, the one related to respiration, is:
   A. caused by the sympathetic effect on the SA node
   B. extremely rare in children
   C. a normal phenomenon commonly seen in young adults
   D. all of the above

3. Another less common type of sinus arrhythmia is not related to respiration. It may occur in healthy individuals but is more commonly found in adult patients:
   A. with heart disease
   B. with an acute MI
   C. on digitalis
   D. all of the above

4. An arrhythmia originating in the SA node with a regular rate of less than 60 beats per minutes is called:
   A. sinus bradycardia
   B. sinus arrest
   C. first-degree AV block
   D. junctional escape rhythm

5. Sinus bradycardia may be caused by:
   A. excessive inhibitory vagal tone on the SA node
   B. decrease in sympathetic tone on the SA node
   C. hypothermia
   D. all of the above

6. The heart rate in an asymptomatic bradycardia is _____ to _____ beats per minute.
   A. 30, 29
   B. 40, 49
   C. 50, 59
   D. 60, 69

7. A patient with marked sinus bradycardia who is symptomatic will likely have:
   A. hypothermia and chest pain
   B. hypotension and decreased cerebral perfusion
   C. hypoxia and increased central venous pressure (CVP)
   D. hypertension and decreased cerebral perfusion

8. Symptomatic sinus bradycardia must be promptly treated with:
   A. isoproterenol and epinephrine
   B. atropine and transcutaneous pacing
   C. lidocaine and oxygen
   D. dopamine and diltiazem (or verapamil)

9. An arrhythmia caused by episodes of failure in the automaticity of the SA node resulting in bradycardia or asystole is called:
   A. marked sinus arrhythmia
   B. Wenckebach phenomenon
   C. sinus arrest
   D. none of the above

10. Sinoatrial (SA) exit block may result from toxicity of the medication(s):
    A. quinidine
    B. digitalis
    C. propranolol
    D. all of the above

Atrial Arrhythmias

Wandering Atrial Pacemaker (WAP)

Premature Atrial Contractions (PACs)

Atrial Tachycardia (AT)

(Nonparoxysmal Atrial Tachycardia,

Paroxysmal Atrial Tachycardia [PAT])

Atrial Flutter (AF)

Atrial Fibrillation

OBJECTIVES

Upon completion of all or part of this chapter you should be able to complete the following objectives indicated by your instructor:

☐ **1.** Define and give the diagnostic characteristics, cause, and clinical significance of the following arrhythmias:

☐ Wandering atrial pacemaker (WAP)

☐ Premature atrial contractions (PAC)

☐ Atrial tachycardia (AT)

    ☐ Nonparoxysmal atrial tachycardia

    ☐ Paroxysmal atrial tachycardia (PAT)

☐ Paroxysmal supraventricular tachycardia (PSVT)

☐ Atrial flutter (AF)

☐ Atrial fibrillation

Wandering Atrial Pacemaker (WAP)

Definition

A **wandering atrial pacemaker (WAP)** (Figure 6-1) is an arrhythmia originating in pacemakers that shift back and forth between the SA node and an ectopic pacemaker in the atria or AV junction. It is characterized by P waves of varying size, shape, and direction in any given lead.

Diagnostic Characteristics

Heart rate: The heart rate is usually 60 to 100 beats per minute but may be slower. Usually, the heart rate gradually slows slightly when the pacemaker site shifts from the SA node to the atria or AV junction and increases as the pacemaker site shifts back to the SA node.

Rhythm: The rhythm is usually irregular, but, rarely, it may be regular.

Pacemaker site: The pacemaker site shifts back and forth between the SA node and an ectopic pacemaker in the atria or AV junction.

P waves: The P waves gradually change in size, shape, and direction over the duration of several beats. They vary in lead II from normal, positive (upright) P waves to abnormal, negative (inverted) P waves or even become buried in the QRS complexes as the pacemaker site shifts from the SA node to the atria or AV junction. These changes occur in reverse as the pacemaker site shifts back to the SA node. The P waves other than those arising in the SA node are **ectopic P waves (P′ waves).**

PR intervals: The duration of the PR intervals usually decreases gradually from about 0.20 second to about 0.12 second or less as the pacemaker site shifts from the SA node to the lower part of the atria or AV junction. The duration of the intervals then gradually increases as the pacemaker site shifts back to the SA node.

R-R intervals: The R-R intervals (and P-P intervals as well) are usually unequal, but they may be equal. They usually increase in duration as the pacemaker site shifts from the SA node to the atria or AV junction and decrease as the pacemaker shifts back to the SA node.

QRS complexes: The QRS complexes are normal unless a preexisting bundle branch block or anomalous AV conduction is present. A QRS complex normally follows each P wave.

Cause of Arrhythmia

A wandering atrial pacemaker may be a normal phenomenon seen in the very young or the aged and in athletes. It is caused in the majority of cases by the inhibitory vagal (parasympathetic) effect of respiration on the SA node and AV junction. It may also be caused by the administration of digitalis.

Clinical Significance

A wandering atrial pacemaker is usually not clinically significant, and treatment is not indicated. When the heart rate slows excessively, the signs and symptoms, clinical significance, and management are the same as those in symptomatic sinus bradycardia.

Notes

Wandering Atrial Pacemaker (WAP)

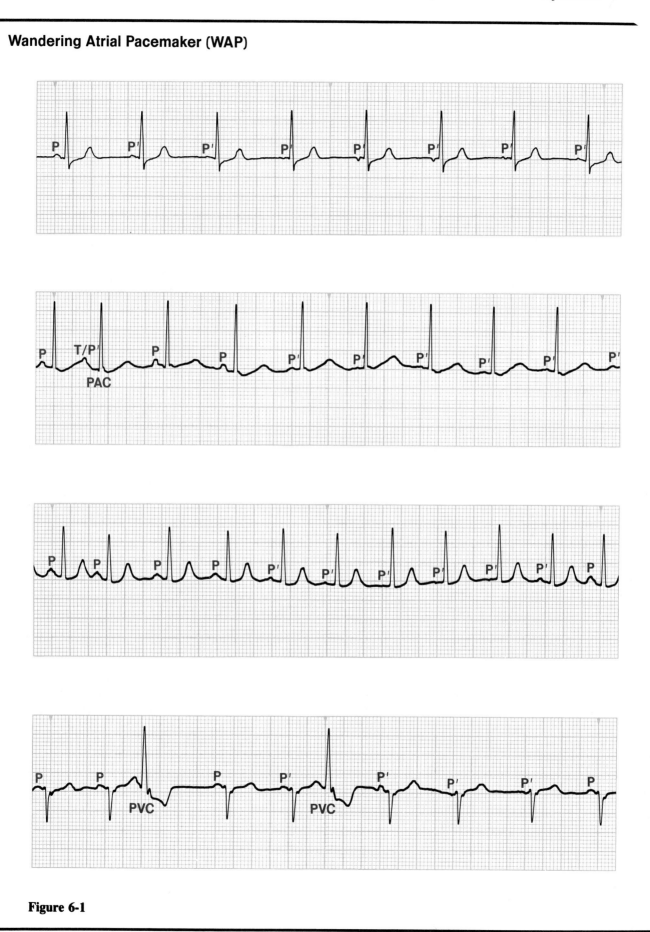

Figure 6-1

Premature Atrial Contractions (PACs)

Definition

A **premature atrial contraction (PAC)** (Figure 6-2) is an extra atrial contraction consisting of an abnormal (sometimes normal) P wave followed by a normal or abnormal QRS complex, occurring earlier than the next expected beat of the underlying rhythm. It is usually followed by a noncompensatory pause. Premature atrial contractions, which can originate in a single or multiple ectopic pacemakers in the atria, are also called **premature atrial beats (PABs)** or **complexes.**

Diagnostic Characteristics

Heart rate: The heart rate is that of the underlying rhythm.

Rhythm: The rhythm is irregular when **premature atrial contractions** are present.

Pacemaker site: The pacemaker site of the **PAC** is an ectopic pacemaker in any part of the atria outside the SA node. Premature atrial contractions may originate from a single ectopic pacemaker site or from multiple sites in the atria.

P waves: A premature atrial contraction is diagnosed when a P wave accompanied by a QRS complex occurs earlier than the next expected sinus P wave. The premature P wave is called an **ectopic P wave (P′).** Although the P′ waves of the PACs may resemble the normal sinus P waves, they are generally different. The size, shape, and direction of the P′ waves depend on the location of the pacemaker site. For example, they may appear positive (upright) and quite normal in lead II if the pacemaker site is near the SA node but negative (inverted) if the pacemaker site is near the AV junction, the result of retrograde atrial depolarization. P′ waves originating in the same atrial ectopic pacemaker are usually identical. The P′ waves precede the QRS complexes and are frequently buried in the preceding T waves, distorting them and often making these T waves more peaked and pointed than the other nonaffected ones. A P′ wave followed by a QRS complex is said to be a **conducted PAC.**

If the atrial ectopic pacemaker discharges too soon after the preceding QRS complex—early in diastole, for example—the AV junction or bundle branches may not be repolarized sufficiently to conduct the premature electrical impulse into the ventricles normally. Thus, being still **refractory** from conducting the previous electrical impulse, the AV junction or bundle branches may either slow the conduction of the premature electrical impulse, prolonging the PR interval (first-degree AV block), or block it completely (complete AV block). When complete AV block occurs, the P′ wave is not followed by a QRS complex. Such a PAC is called a **nonconducted** or **blocked PAC.** Nonconducted PACs are commonly the cause of unexpected pauses in the ECG, suggesting sinus arrest or sinoatrial (SA) exit block.

The interval between the P wave of the QRS complex preceding the PAC and the P′ wave of the PAC—the P-P′ interval—is typically shorter than the P-P interval of the underlying rhythm. Since the PAC usually depolarizes the SA node prematurely, the timing of the SA node is reset, causing the next cycle of the SA node to begin anew at this point. When this occurs, the next expected P wave of the underlying rhythm appears earlier than it would have if the SA node had not been disturbed. The resulting P′-P interval is called an **"incomplete compensatory pause"** or a **"noncompensatory pause."** This interval may be equal to the P-P interval of the underlying rhythm, or it may be slightly longer because of the depressing effect on the automaticity of the SA node brought on by its being depolarized prematurely. The interval between the P waves of the underlying rhythm preceding and following the PAC is less than twice the P-P interval of the underlying rhythm.

Less commonly, the SA node is not depolarized by the PAC so that its timing is not reset, allowing the next P wave of the underlying rhythm to appear at the time expected. Such a P′-P interval is said to be **"fully compensatory"** or a **"full compensatory pause."** In this case, the interval between the P waves of the underlying rhythm occurring before and after the PAC is twice the P-P interval of the underlying rhythm. A full compensatory pause may also occur, even if the SA node is prematurely depolarized, if the automaticity of the SA node is excessively depressed following its premature depolarization.

Premature Atrial Contractions (PACs)

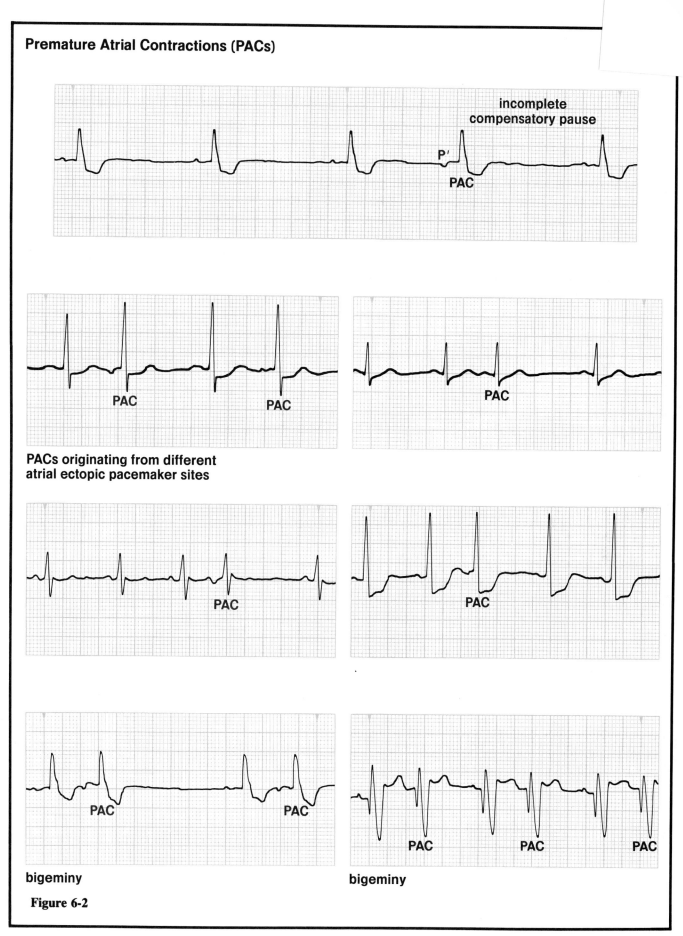

PACs originating from different
atrial ectopic pacemaker sites

bigeminy   bigeminy

Figure 6-2

PR intervals: The PR intervals of the PACs may be normal, but they usually differ from those of the underlying rhythm. The PR interval of a PAC varies from about 0.20 second when the pacemaker site is near the SA node to about 0.12 second when the pacemaker is near the AV junction. The PAC's PR interval may be greater than 0.20 second if there is a delay in AV conduction (first-degree AV block).

R-R and P-P intervals: The R-R intervals are unequal when premature atrial contractions are present. The interval between the P wave of the underlying rhythm preceding a PAC and the P′ wave of the PAC, the P-P′ interval **(coupling interval)**, varies depending on the ectopic pacemaker's rate of spontaneous depolarization and its location in the atria. Generally, the coupling intervals of PACs originating in the same ectopic pacemaker site are equal.

QRS complexes: The QRS complex of the PAC usually resembles that of the underlying rhythm because the conduction of the electrical impulse through the bundle branches is usually unchanged. If the atrial ectopic pacemaker discharges very soon after the preceding QRS complex, the bundle branches may not be repolarized sufficiently to conduct the electrical impulse of the PAC normally. If this occurs, the electrical impulse may only be conducted down one bundle branch, usually the left one, and blocked in the other, the right. The result is a wide and bizarre-appearing QRS complex that resembles a right bundle branch block. Such a PAC, called a **premature atrial contraction with aberrancy** (or **with aberrant ventricular conduction**), can mimic a premature ventricular contraction (see Premature Ventricular Contractions, page 168). Usually, a QRS complex follows each P′ wave **(conducted PACs)**, but a QRS complex may be absent because of a temporary complete AV block **(nonconducted PACs)**.

Frequency and pattern of occurrence of PACs: PACs may occur singly as **isolated beats** or consecutively as two or more beats **(group beats).** Two PACs in a row are called a **"couplet."** When three or more PACs occur consecutively, **atrial tachycardia** is considered to be present. PACs may alternate with the QRS complexes of the underlying rhythm **(atrial bigeminy)** or occur after every two

QRS complexes **(atrial trigeminy)** or after every three QRS complexes of the underlying rhythm **(atrial quadrigeminy).**

Cause of Arrhythmia

Common causes of PACs include an increase in catecholamines and sympathetic tone, infections, emotion, stimulants (e.g., alcohol, caffeine, and tobacco), sympathomimetic drugs (e.g., epinephrine, isoproterenol, and norepinephrine), electrolyte imbalance, hypoxia, or digitalis toxicity. PACs may also be associated with cardiovascular disease (such as myocardial ischemia, acute myocardial infarction, or early congestive heart failure) or with dilated or hypertrophied atria resulting from increased atrial pressure commonly caused by mitral stenosis or an atrial septal defect. Often, however, PACs may occur without apparent cause. The electrophysiologic mechanism responsible for PACs is either **enhanced automaticity** or **reentry.**

Clinical Significance

Isolated premature atrial contractions may occur in persons with apparently healthy hearts and are not significant. In persons with heart disease, however, frequent premature atrial contractions may indicate enhanced automaticity of the atria or a reentry mechanism resulting from a variety of causes, such as congestive heart failure or acute myocardial infarction. In addition, such PACs may warn of or initiate more serious supraventricular arrhythmias, such as atrial tachycardia, atrial flutter, atrial fibrillation, or paroxysmal supraventricular tachycardia.

If nonconducted premature atrial contractions are frequent and the heart rate is less than 50 beats per minute, the signs and symptoms, clinical significance, and management are the same as those of symptomatic sinus bradycardia.

Because premature atrial contractions with aberrancy often resemble premature ventricular contractions (see Premature Ventricular Contractions, page 168), care must be taken to identify such PACs correctly so as not to treat them inappropriately as PVCs.

Notes

Atrial Tachycardia (AT)
(Nonparoxysmal Atrial Tachycardia,
Paroxysmal Atrial Tachycardia [PAT])

Definition

Atrial tachycardia (AT) (Figure 6-3) is an arrhythmia originating in an ectopic pacemaker in the atria or the site of a rapid reentry circuit in the AV node with a rate between 160 to 240 beats per minute. It includes **nonparoxysmal atrial tachycardia** and **paroxysmal atrial tachycardia (PAT)**. PAT is often called **paroxysmal supraventricular tachycardia (PSVT)** when the site of origin (either atria or AV junction) cannot be determined with certainty.

Diagnostic Characteristics

Heart rate: The atrial rate is usually 160 to 240 beats per minute. The ventricular rate is usually the same as that of the atria, but it may be slower, often half the atrial rate because of a 2:1 AV block. **Atrial tachycardia** commonly starts and ends abruptly, occurring in paroxysms (**paroxysmal atrial tachycardia** or **PAT**), which may last from a few seconds to many hours and recur for many years. PAT is usually initiated by a premature atrial contraction. When atrial tachycardia does not start and end abruptly, it is called **nonparoxysmal atrial tachycardia.** By definition, three or more consecutive premature atrial contractions are considered to be atrial tachycardia. **Vagal maneuvers,** such as carotid sinus massage, by increasing the parasympathetic (vagal) tone, may either terminate paroxysmal atrial tachycardia abruptly, which it usually does, or slow it slightly. Vagal stimulation only slows the ventricular rate in nonparoxysmal atrial tachycardia.

Rhythm: The atrial rhythm is essentially regular. The ventricular rhythm is usually regular if the AV conduction ratio is constant, but it may be grossly irregular if a variable AV block is present.

Pacemaker site: The pacemaker site is an ectopic pacemaker in any part of the atria outside the SA node. Atrial tachycardia may occasionally originate in more than one atrial ectopic pacemaker site. One originating in three or more different ectopic pacemaker sites is called **multifocal atrial tachycardia (MAT).** The activity of the SA node is completely suppressed by atrial tachycardia.

P waves: The ectopic P waves in atrial tachycardia usually differ from normal sinus P waves. The size, shape, and direction of the P′ waves vary, depending on the location of the pacemaker site. They may appear positive (upright) and quite normal in lead II if the pacemaker site is near the SA node but negative (inverted) if they originate near the AV junction. The P′ waves are usually identical (except in multifocal atrial tachycardia) and precede each QRS complex. In multifocal atrial tachycardia, the P′ waves may vary in size, shape, and direction in each given lead. The P′ waves are often not easily identified because they are buried in the preceding T or U waves or QRS complexes. Normal sinus P waves are absent.

Note: Since it is often difficult to differentiate between paroxysmal atrial tachycardia and paroxysmal junctional tachycardia when the P′ waves are not clearly evident, the term **paroxysmal supraventricular tachycardia (PSVT)** is commonly used to indicate a paroxysmal tachycardia originating in the atria or AV junction without specifying the exact location of the ectopic pacemaker site.

P′ wave-QRS complex relationship: In most untreated atrial tachycardias not caused by digitalis intoxication whose atrial rate is less than 200 per minute, the AV conduction ratio is 1:1. When the atrial rate is greater than 200 per minute, a 2:1 AV conduction ratio is common. (A 2:1 AV conduction ratio indicates that for every two P′ waves, one is followed by a QRS complex.) When the AV block occurs only during the tachycardia, the arrhythmia is called **atrial tachycardia with block.** The cause of the AV block is the relatively long refractory period of the AV junction, which prevents the conduction of all the rapidly occurring atrial electrical impulses into the ventricles (**physiological AV block).**

If there is a preexisting AV block because of cardiac disease, if digitalis excess is the cause of the atrial tachycardia (e.g., nonparoxysmal atrial tachycardia), or if certain drugs (e.g., digitalis, propranolol, and diltiazem or verapamil) have been administered, 2:1 AV block may occur at atrial rates less than 200 per minute. Higher-degree AV block (e.g., 3:1, 4:1, and so forth) or variable AV block may also occur, particularly in nonparoxysmal atrial tachycardia caused by digitalis toxicity.

Atrial Tachycardia (AT)
(Nonparoxysmal Atrial Tachycardia, Paroxysmal Atrial Tachycardia [PAT])

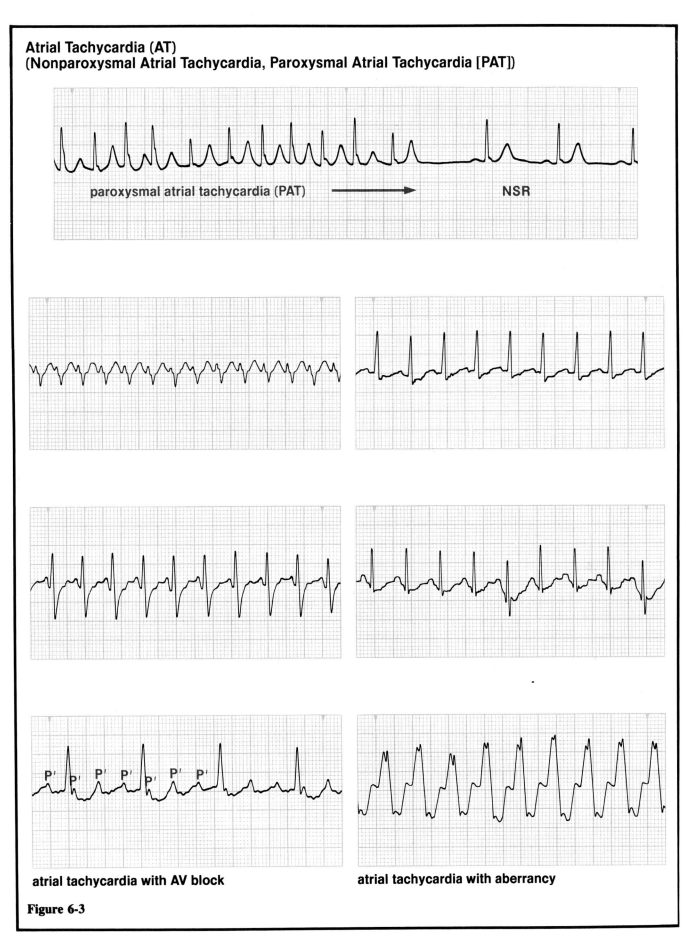

paroxysmal atrial tachycardia (PAT) ⟶ NSR

atrial tachycardia with AV block

atrial tachycardia with aberrancy

Figure 6-3

PR intervals: The PR intervals are usually normal and constant. Occasionally, however, the PR intervals are prolonged (greater than 0.20 second), particularly when the atrial rate is extremely rapid. This occurs when the atrial impulses reach the AV junction while it is in the relative refractory period, thereby increasing the AV conduction time. In addition, a preexisting first-degree AV block may be present. A shorter than normal PR interval may be present when atrial tachycardia is relatively slow or when it occurs in healthy young individuals. In multifocal atrial tachycardia, the PR intervals usually vary in each given lead.

R-R intervals: The R-R intervals are usually equal if the AV conduction ratio is constant (i.e., 2:1, 2:1, 2:1, and so forth). But if the AV conduction ratio varies (as in **atrial tachycardia with varying AV block,** i.e., 3:1, 2:1, 4:1, 3:1, and so forth), the R-R intervals will be unequal. The R-R intervals will also vary in each given lead if multifocal atrial tachycardia is present.

QRS complexes: The QRS complexes are normal unless a preexisting bundle branch block, aberrant ventricular conduction, or anomalous AV conduction is present. If the QRS complexes are abnormal only during the tachycardia, the arrhythmia is called **atrial tachycardia with aberrancy** (or **with aberrant ventricular conduction**). Atrial tachycardia with abnormal QRS complexes may resemble ventricular tachycardia (see Ventricular Tachycardia, page 172).

Cause of Arrhythmia

In general, the causes of atrial tachycardia are essentially the same as those of premature atrial contractions. Like PACs, atrial tachycardia may occur in persons with apparently healthy hearts as well as in those with diseased hearts. Most often atrial tachycardia occurs in patients with rheumatic heart disease, coronary artery disease (especially following an acute myocardial infarction), digitalis toxicity, or preexcitation syndrome.

Nonparoxysmal atrial tachycardia is most commonly caused by digitalis toxicity, in which case it is often associated with a 2:1 or higher-degree AV block or a varying AV block at relatively slow atrial rates for atrial tachycardia (less than 200 per minute). Atrial tachycardia with AV block may also occur in patients with significant heart disease such as coronary artery disease or cor pulmonale. Multifocal atrial tachycardia is most often associated with respiratory failure; it is rarely caused by digitalis excess. The electrophysiologic mechanism most likely responsible for nonparoxysmal atrial tachycardia is **enhanced automaticity,** whereas, for paroxysmal atrial tachycardia, it is a **reentry mechanism.**

Clinical Significance

The signs and symptoms in atrial tachycardia depend upon the presence or absence of heart disease, the nature of the heart disease, the ventricular rate, and the duration of the arrhythmia. Frequently, atrial tachycardia is accompanied by feelings of palpitations, nervousness, or anxiety. When the ventricular rate is very rapid, the ventricles are unable to fill completely during diastole, resulting in a significant reduction of the cardiac output and a decrease in perfusion of the brain and other vital organs. This may cause confusion, dizziness, lightheadedness, near-syncope or syncope, and, in patients with coronary artery disease, angina, congestive heart failure, or myocardial infarction.

In addition, since a rapid heart rate increases the workload of the heart, the oxygen requirements of the myocardium are usually increased in atrial tachycardia. Because of this, in addition to the consequences of decreased cardiac output, atrial tachycardia in acute myocardial infarction may increase myocardial ischemia and the frequency and severity of chest pain, bring about the extension of the infarct, cause congestive heart failure, hypotension, or cardiogenic shock, or predispose the patient to serious ventricular arrhythmias.

Symptomatic atrial tachycardia must be treated promptly to reverse the consequences of the reduced cardiac output and increased workload of the heart and to prevent the occurrence of serious ventricular arrhythmias.

Notes

Atrial Flutter (AF)

Definition

Atrial flutter (Figures 6-4 and 6-5) is an arrhythmia arising in an ectopic pacemaker or the site of a rapid reentry circuit in the atria, characterized by rapid abnormal atrial flutter (F) waves with a sawtooth appearance and, usually, a slower, regular ventricular response.

Diagnostic Characteristics

Heart rate: Usually, the atrial rate is between 240 and 360 (average, 300) **flutter (F) waves** per minute, but it may be slower or faster. The ventricular rate is commonly about 150 beats per minute (half the atrial rate because of a 2:1 AV block) in an **uncontrolled (untreated) atrial flutter** and about 60 to 75 in a **controlled (treated)** one or one with a preexisting AV block. Rarely, the ventricular rate may be over 240 beats per minute, the same as the atrial rate, if the atrial rate is relatively slow and a 1:1 AV conduction ratio is present. **Vagal maneuvers,** such as carotid sinus massage, often produce a slowing of the ventricular rate in stepwise increments.

Rhythm: The atrial rhythm is typically regular, but it may be irregular. The ventricular rhythm is usually regular if the AV conduction ratio is constant, but it may be grossly irregular if a variable AV block is present.

Pacemaker site: The pacemaker site is an ectopic pacemaker in part of the atria outside of the SA node. Commonly, it is located low in the atria near the AV node. The activity of the SA node is completely suppressed by atrial flutter.

Characteristics of atrial flutter waves (F waves):

1. Relationship to cardiac anatomy and physiology: An atrial flutter wave represents depolarization of the atria in an abnormal direction followed by atrial repolarization. Depolarization of the atria commonly begins near the AV node and progresses across the atria in a retrograde direction. Normal P waves are absent.

2. Onset and end: The onset and end of the flutter waves cannot be determined with certainty.

3. Components: The flutter wave consists of an abnormal atrial depolarization wave corresponding to an **ectopic P wave** followed by an **atrial T wave (Ta)** of atrial repolarization.

4. Direction: The first part of the flutter wave, corresponding to an ectopic P wave, is commonly negative (inverted) in lead II and followed by a positive (upright) atrial T wave.

5. Duration: The duration varies according to the rate of the flutter waves.

6. Amplitude: The amplitude, measured from peak to peak of the flutter wave, varies greatly: from less than 1 mm to over 5 mm.

7. Shape: The F waves have a **saw-toothed appearance.** The typical atrial flutter wave consists of a negative (inverted), V-shaped ectopic atrial wave immediately followed by an upright, peaked atrial T wave in lead II. An isoelectric line is seldom present between the waves. Typically, the first, downward part of the F wave is shorter and more abrupt than the second, upward part. Flutter waves are generally identical in shape and size in any given lead but may occasionally vary slightly. Atrial fibrillation may occur during atrial flutter and vice versa. Such a mixture of atrial flutter and fibrillation is called **"atrial flutter-fibrillation."**

8. F wave-QRS complex relationship: The F waves precede, are buried in, and follow the QRS complexes and may be superimposed on the T waves or ST segments. The AV conduction ratio in most untreated atrial flutters is commonly 2:1. This is because of the long refractory period of the AV junction, which prevents the conduction of all the rapidly occurring atrial electrical impulses into the ventricles **(physiological AV block).** (A 2:1 AV conduction ratio, for example, indicates that for every two F waves, one is followed by a QRS complex.) Rarely, the AV conduction ratio in untreated atrial flutter is 1:1. The AV block may be greater (i.e., 3:1, 4:1, and so forth) or even variable because of disease of the AV node, increased vagal (parasympathetic) tone, and certain drugs (e.g., digitalis, propranolol, and diltiazem or verapamil).

The AV conduction ratio is usually constant in any given lead, producing a regular ventricular

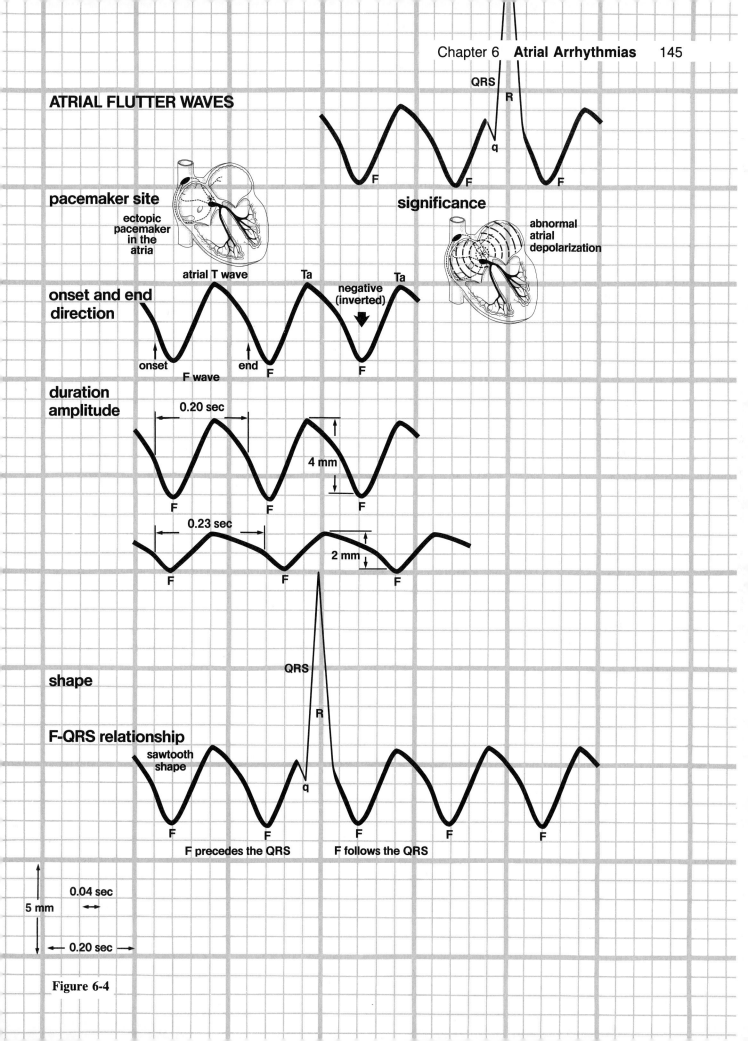

ATRIAL FLUTTER WAVES

QRS
R
q
F   F   F

pacemaker site

ectopic
pacemaker
in the
atria

significance

abnormal
atrial
depolarization

onset and end
direction

atrial T wave   Ta   Ta

negative
(inverted)

onset   end
F wave   F   F

duration
amplitude

0.20 sec

4 mm

F   F   F

0.23 sec

2 mm

F   F   F

shape

QRS

R

F-QRS relationship

sawtooth
shape

q

F   F   F   F   F

F precedes the QRS   F follows the QRS

0.04 sec

5 mm

0.20 sec

Figure 6-4

rhythm. If the AV conduction ratio varies, the ventricular rhythm will be irregular. When there is a 2:1 or 1:1 AV conduction ratio, the saw-toothed pattern of the F waves may be distorted by the QRS complexes and T waves, making the F waves difficult to recognize. On rare occasions when a complete AV block is present and the atria and ventricles beat independently, there is no set relation between the F waves and the QRS complexes. When this occurs, **atrioventricular (AV) dissociation** is present.

FR intervals: FR intervals are usually equal but may vary.

R-R intervals: The R-R intervals are equal if the AV conduction ratio is constant, but, if the AV conduction ratio varies, the R-R intervals are unequal.

QRS complexes: The QRS complexes are normal unless a preexisting bundle branch block, aberrant ventricular conduction, or anomalous AV conduction is present. Atrial flutter with a rapid ventricular response and abnormal QRS complexes may resemble ventricular tachycardia (see Ventricular Tachycardia, page 172).

Cause of Arrhythmia

Chronic (persistent) atrial flutter is most commonly seen in middle-aged and elderly persons with advanced rheumatic heart disease, particularly if mi-

tral or tricuspid valvular disease is present, and in those with coronary or hypertensive heart disease. **Transient (paroxysmal) atrial flutter** usually indicates the presence of cardiac disease; however, it may occasionally occur in apparently healthy persons. The arrhythmia may also be associated with the preexcitation syndrome, cardiomyopathy, thyrotoxicosis, digitalis toxicity (rarely), hypoxia, acute or chronic cor pulmonale, congestive heart failure, or damage to the SA node or atria because of pericarditis or myocarditis. Atrial flutter may be initiated by a premature atrial contraction. The electrophysiological mechanism responsible for atrial flutter is either **enhanced automaticity** or **reentry.**

Clinical Significance

The signs and symptoms and clinical significance of atrial flutter with a rapid ventricular response are the same as those of atrial tachycardia.

In addition, in 2:1 atrial flutter, in particular, the atria do not regularly contract and empty before each ventricular contraction, filling the ventricles during the last part of diastole, as they normally do. The loss of this **"atrial kick"** results in incomplete filling of the ventricles before they contract, causing a reduction of the cardiac output by as much as 25 percent.

Notes

Atrial Flutter (AF)

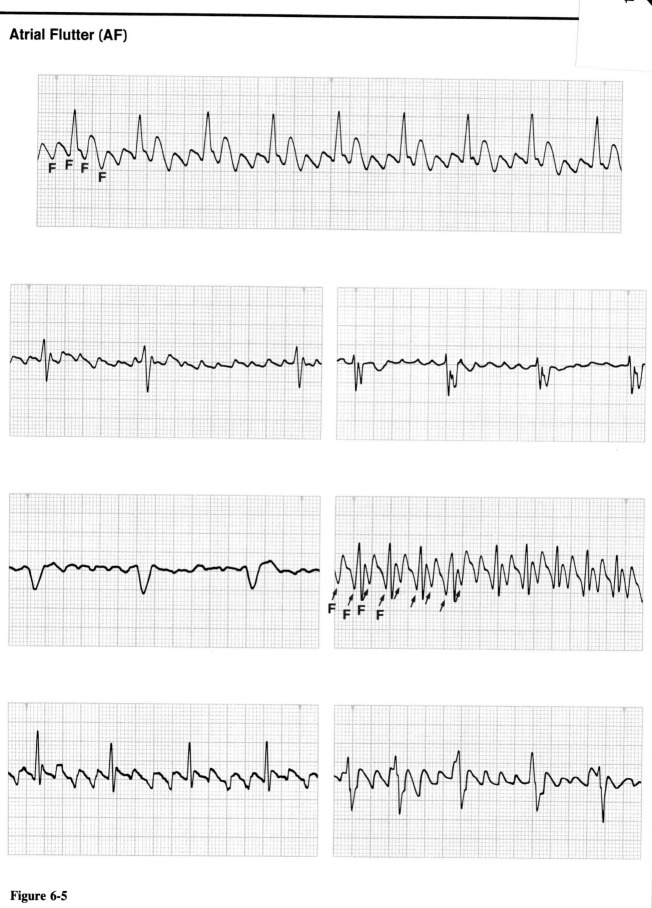

Figure 6-5

Atrial Fibrillation

Definition

Atrial fibrillation (Figures 6-6 and 6-7) is an arrhythmia arising in multiple ectopic pacemakers or sites of rapid reentry circuits in the atria, characterized by very rapid abnormal atrial fibrillation (f) waves and an irregular, often rapid ventricular response.

Diagnostic Characteristics

Heart rate: Typically, the atrial rate is 350 to 600 (average, 400) **fibrillation (f) waves** per minute, but it can be as high as 700. The ventricular rate is commonly about 160 to 180 (or as high as 200) beats per minute in an **uncontrolled (untreated) atrial fibrillation** and about 60 to 70 in a **controlled (treated)** one or one with a preexisting AV block. If the ventricular rate is greater than 100 per minute, atrial fibrillation is considered to be **"fast,"** and, if it is less than 60, it is considered **"slow."** Carotid sinus massage often slows the ventricular rate.

Rhythm: The atrial rhythm is irregularly (or grossly) irregular. The ventricular rhythm is almost always irregularly irregular in untreated atrial fibrillation.

Pacemaker site: The pacemaker sites, multiple ectopic pacemakers in the atria outside of the SA node, generate electrical impulses chaotically. The activity of the SA node is completely suppressed by atrial fibrillation.

Characteristics of atrial fibrillation waves (f waves):

1. Relationship to cardiac anatomy and physiology: Atrial fibrillation waves represent abnormal, chaotic, and incomplete depolarizations of small individual groups (or islets) of atrial muscle fibers. Since organized depolarizations of the atria are absent, P waves and organized atrial contractions are absent.

2. Onset and end: The onset and end of the f waves cannot be determined with certainty.

3. Direction: The direction of the f waves varies from positive (upright) to negative (inverted) at random.

4. Duration: The duration of the f waves varies greatly and cannot be determined with accuracy.

5. Amplitude: The amplitude varies from less than 1 millimeter to several millimeters. If the fibrillation waves are small (less than 1 mm), they are called **"fine" fibrillatory waves;** if they are large (1 mm or greater), they are called **"coarse" fibrillatory waves.** If the f waves are so small or "fine" that they are not recorded, the sections of the ECG between the QRS complexes may appear as a **wavy or flat (isoelectric) line.**

6. Shape: The f waves are irregularly shaped, rounded (or pointed), and dissimilar.

7. f Wave-QRS complex relationship: The f waves precede, are buried in, and follow the QRS complexes and are superimposed on the ST segments and T waves. Typically, in atrial fibrillation, fewer than one half or one third of the atrial electrical impulses are conducted through the AV junction into the ventricles, and these are at random. This results in a grossly irregular ventricular rhythm. The main reason for this is the long refractory period of the AV junction, which prevents the conduction of all the rapidly occurring atrial electrical impulses into the ventricles **(physiological AV block).**

R-R intervals: The R-R intervals are **typically unequal.** When atrial fibrillation is complicated by a second-degree, type I AV block, the R-R intervals progressively decrease in duration over a cycle of three or more R-R intervals, each cycle following an exceptionally wide R-R interval. When only two R-R intervals occur in a cycle, the ventricular rhythm assumes a roughly bigeminal appearance.

QRS complexes: The QRS complexes are normal unless a preexisting bundle branch block, aberrant ventricular conduction, or anomalous AV conduction is present. Atrial fibrillation with a rapid ventricular response and abnormal QRS complexes may resemble ventricular tachycardia, except for the irregular rhythm (see Ventricular Tachycardia, page 172).

Cause of Arrhythmia

Atrial fibrillation is commonly associated with advanced rheumatic heart disease (particularly with mitral stenosis), hypertensive or coronary heart dis-

ATRIAL FIBRILLATION WAVES

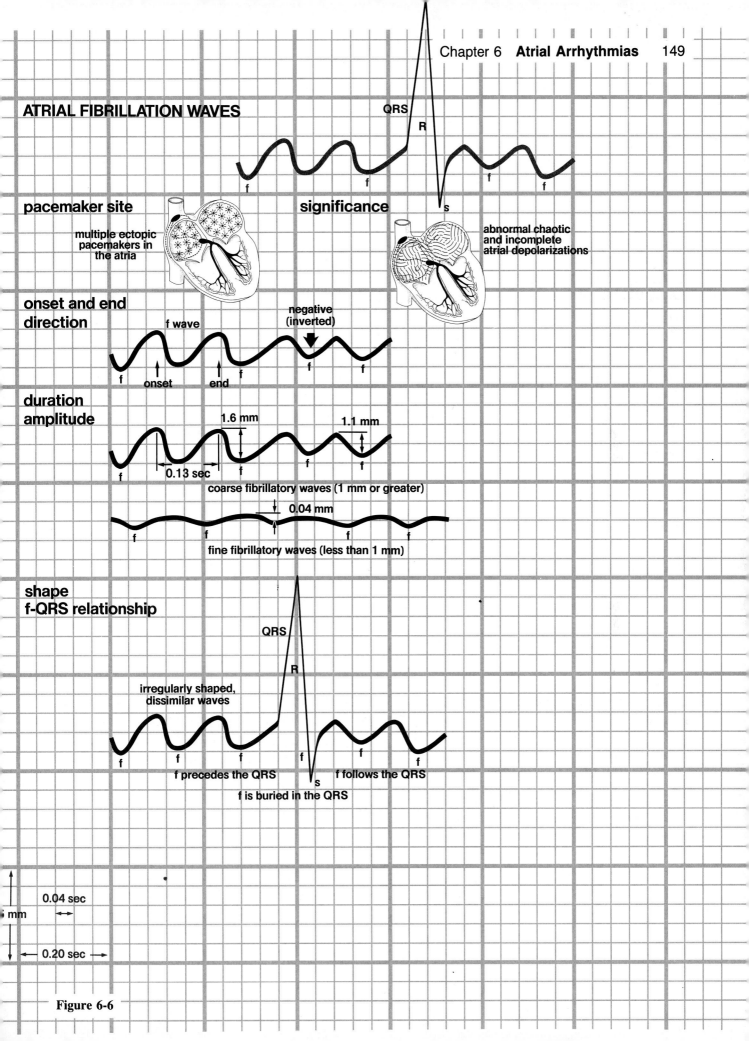

QRS

R

f   f   f

pacemaker site

multiple ectopic
pacemakers in
the atria

significance

s

abnormal chaotic
and incomplete
atrial depolarizations

**onset and end
direction**

f wave

negative
(inverted)

f   onset   end   f   f   f

**duration
amplitude**

1.6 mm   1.1 mm

0.13 sec

f   f   f   f

coarse fibrillatory waves (1 mm or greater)

0.04 mm

f   f   f   f   f

fine fibrillatory waves (less than 1 mm)

**shape
f-QRS relationship**

QRS

R

irregularly shaped,
dissimilar waves

f   f   f   f   f

s

f precedes the QRS   f follows the QRS

f is buried in the QRS

0.04 sec

mm

0.20 sec

Figure 6-6

ease (with or without acute myocardial infarction), and thyrotoxicosis. Less commonly, atrial fibrillation may occur in cardiomyopathy, acute myocarditis and pericarditis, chest trauma, and the preexcitation syndrome; it is rarely caused by digitalis toxicity. Whatever the underlying form of heart disease, atrial fibrillation is commonly associated with congestive heart failure. In a small percentage of cases, atrial fibrillation may occur in apparently normal individuals following excessive ingestion of alcohol and caffeine, during emotional stress, and sometimes without any apparent cause. Atrial fibrillation may be intermittent, even occurring in paroxysms as does paroxysmal atrial tachycardia, or it may be chronic (persistent). The electrophysiologic mechanism responsible for atrial fibrillation is either **enhanced automaticity** or **reentry.**

Clinical Significance

The signs and symptoms and clinical significance of atrial fibrillation with a rapid ventricular response are the same as those of atrial tachycardia.

In addition, in atrial fibrillation, the atria do not regularly contract and empty, filling the ventricles during the last part of diastole, as they normally do. The loss of this **"atrial kick"** results in incomplete filling of the ventricles before they contract, causing a reduction of the cardiac output by as much as 25 percent.

Atrial Fibrillation

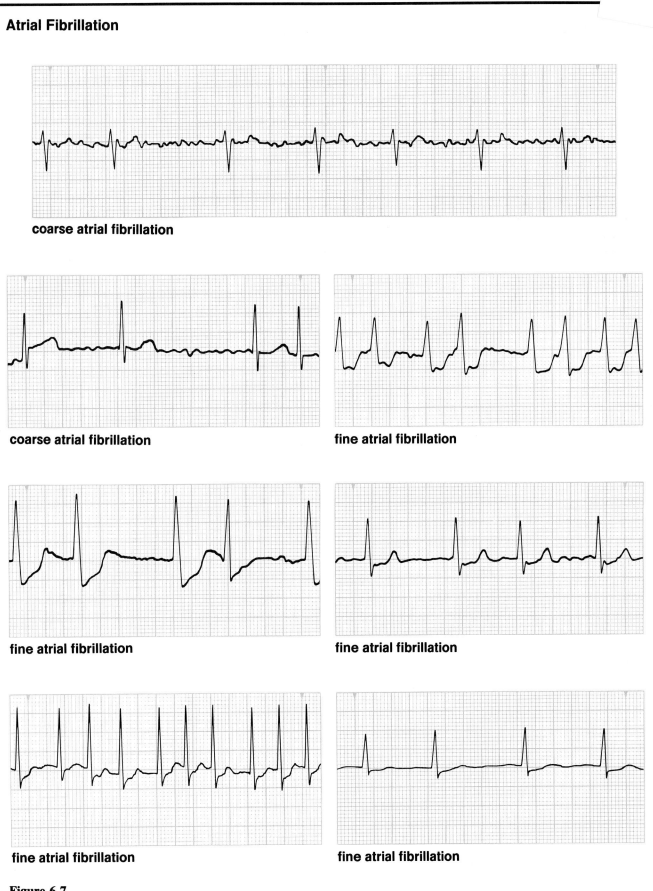

coarse atrial fibrillation

coarse atrial fibrillation

fine atrial fibrillation

fine atrial fibrillation

fine atrial fibrillation

fine atrial fibrillation

fine atrial fibrillation

Figure 6-7

1. An arrhythmia originating in pacemakers that shift back and forth between the SA node and an ectopic pacemaker in the atria or AV junction is called a(n):
   A. supraventricular tachycardia
   B. wandering atrial pacemaker
   C. alternating atrial flutter
   D. all of the above

2. The arrhythmia described in question number 1 may be a normal phenomenon seen in:
   A. the very young
   B. the elderly
   C. athletes
   D. all of the above

3. An extra atrial contraction consisting of an abnormal P wave followed by a normal or abnormal QRS complex, occurring earlier than the next beat of the underlying rhythm, is called:
   A. a premature junctional contraction
   B. a premature ventricular contraction
   C. a premature atrial contraction
   D. none of the above

4. A nonconducted or blocked PAC is:
   A. found in bradycardiac arrhythmias
   B. a P′ wave that is not followed by a QRS complex
   C. always symptomatic in patients
   D. none of the above

5. The QRS complex of the PAC usually resembles that of:
   A. the underlying rhythm
   B. a premature ventricular complex
   C. a right bundle branch block
   D. a left bundle branch block

6. Two PACs in a row are called:
   A. a reentry rhythm
   B. a couplet
   C. bigeminy
   D. atrial tachycardia

7. The electrophysiological mechanism responsible for PACs is:
   A. enhanced automaticity
   B. reentry
   C. all of the above
   D. none of the above

8. An arrhythmia originating in an ectopic pacemaker in the atria or the site of a rapid reentry circuit in the AV node with a rate between 160 and 240 beats per minute is called:
   A. atrial flutter
   B. junctional tachycardia
   C. sinus tachycardia
   D. atrial tachycardia

9. The reduction in cardiac output accompanying atrial tachycardia can cause:
   A. syncope
   B. lightheadedness
   C. dizziness
   D. all of the above

10. Atrial flutter is characterized by:
    A. an atrial rate slower than the ventricular rate
    B. flutter waves with a saw-toothed appearance
    C. an atrial rate between 160 and 240 beats per minute
    D. all of the above

CHAPTER 7

Junctional Arrhythmias

Premature Junctional Contractions (PJCs)

Junctional Escape Rhythm

Nonparoxysmal Junctional Tachycardia

(Accelerated Junctional Rhythm,

Junctional Tachycardia)

Paroxysmal Junctional Tachycardia (PJT)

OBJECTIVES

Upon completion of all or part of this chapter you should be able to complete the following objectives indicated by your instructor:

☐ **1.** Define and give the diagnostic characteristics, cause, and clinical significance of the following arrhythmias:
  ☐ Premature junctional contractions (PJCs)
  ☐ Junctional escape rhythm
  ☐ Paroxysmal junctional tachycardia (PJT)
  ☐ Nonparoxysmal junctional tachycardia
    ☐ Accelerated junctional rhythm
    ☐ Junctional tachycardia

Premature Junctional Contractions (PJCs)

Definition

A **premature junctional contraction (PJC)** (Figure 7-1) is an extra ventricular contraction that originates in an ectopic pacemaker in the AV junction, occurring before the next expected beat of the underlying rhythm. It consists of a normal or abnormal QRS complex with or without an abnormal P wave. If a P wave is present, it may precede or follow the QRS complex. Premature junctional contractions are also called premature junctional beats or complexes.

Diagnostic Characteristics

Heart rate: The heart rate is that of the underlying rhythm.

Rhythm: The rhythm is irregular when **premature junctional contractions** are present.

Pacemaker site: The pacemaker site of the **PJC** is an ectopic pacemaker in the AV junction.

P waves: P waves may or may not be associated with the PJCs. If they are present, they are abnormal P′ waves, varying in size, shape, and direction from normal P waves. The P′ waves may precede, be buried in, or, less commonly, follow the QRS complexes of the PJCs. A P′ wave that occurs before the QRS complex has most likely originated in the proximal part of the AV junction, whereas one occurring during or after the QRS complex, in the middle or distal part of the AV junction, respectively. If the P′ waves precede the QRS complexes, they may be buried in the preceding T waves, distorting them. If the P′ waves follow the QRS complexes, they are usually found in the ST segments. Since atrial depolarization occurs in a retrograde fashion, the P′ waves that precede or follow the QRS complexes are negative (inverted) in lead II. Absent P′ waves indicate that either (1) **retrograde atrial depolarizations** occurred during the QRS complexes or (2) atrial depolarizations have not occurred because of a **retrograde AV block** between the ectopic pacemaker site in the AV junction and the atria.

If the ectopic pacemaker in the AV junction discharges too soon after the preceding QRS complex, the premature P′ wave may not be followed by a QRS complex because the bundle of His or bundle branches may not be repolarized sufficiently to conduct an electrical wave into the ventricles (**nonconducted PJC).**

PR intervals: If the P′ waves of the PJCs precede the QRS complexes, the P′R intervals are usually abnormal (less than 0.12 second). Rarely, the P′R interval may be normal (0.12 to 0.20 second) or even prolonged (greater than 0.20 second) if there is a delay in the AV conduction (first-degree AV block) below the ectopic pacemaker site. If the P′ waves follow the QRS complexes, the RP′ intervals are usually less than 0.20 second.

R-R intervals: The R-R intervals are unequal when premature junctional contractions are present. The interval between the PJC and the preceding QRS complex (the pre-PJC interval) is shorter than the R-R interval of the underlying rhythm. A **full compensatory pause** commonly follows a PJC since the SA node is usually not depolarized by the PJC. Less commonly, the SA node is depolarized by the PJC, resulting in an **incomplete compensatory pause.** (See the discussion of full and incomplete compensatory pauses under Premature Atrial Contractions, page 136.)

QRS complexes: The QRS complex of the PJC usually resembles that of the underlying rhythm. If the ectopic pacemaker in the AV junction discharges too soon after the preceding QRS complex, the bundle branches may not be repolarized sufficiently to conduct the electrical impulse of the PJC normally. If this occurs, the electrical impulse may only be conducted down one bundle branch, usually the left one, and blocked in the other, the right, producing a wide and bizarre-appearing QRS complex that resembles a right bundle branch block. Such a premature junctional contraction, called a **premature junctional contraction with aberrancy** (or **with aberrant ventricular conduction**), can mimic a premature ventricular contraction (see Premature Ventricular Contractions, page 168). Usually, a QRS complex follows each premature P′ wave (**conducted PJC),** but a QRS complex may be absent because of a transient complete AV block below the ectopic pacemaker site in the AV junction (**nonconducted PJC).**

Premature Junctional Contractions (PJCs)

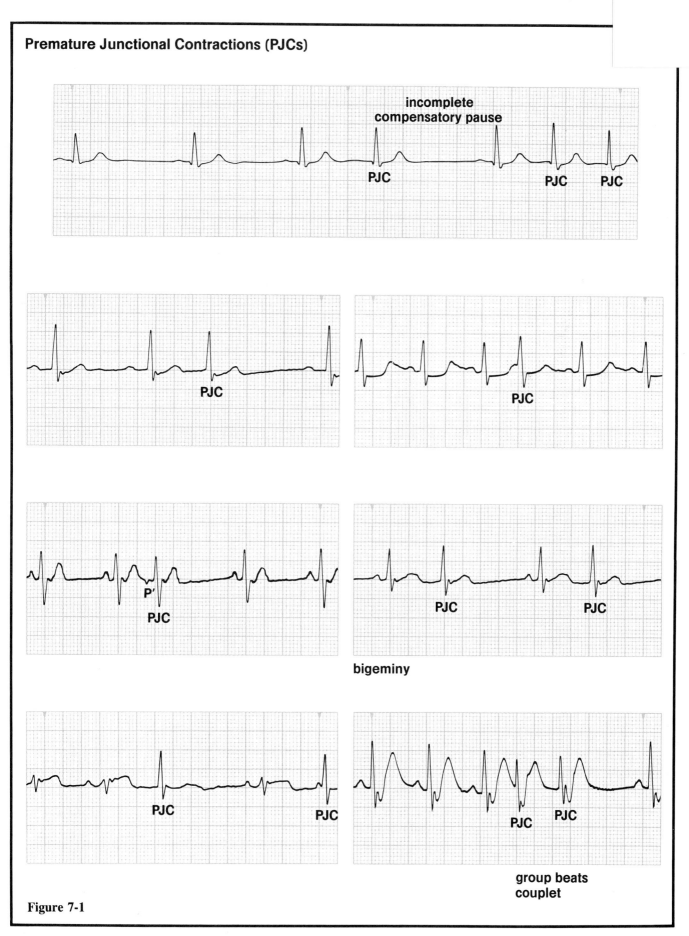

Figure 7-1

Frequency and pattern of occurrence of PJCs: PJCs may occur as **isolated beats** or consecutively as two or more beats **(group beats).** Two PJCs in a row are called a **"couplet."** When three or more PJCs occur consecutively, **junctional tachycardia** is considered to be present. PJCs may alternate with the QRS complexes of the underlying rhythm **(bigeminy)** or occur after every two QRS complexes **(trigeminy)** or after every three QRS complexes of the underlying rhythm **(quadrigeminy).**

Cause of Arrhythmia

Occasional PJCs may occur in a healthy person without apparent cause, but most commonly they are a result of digitalis toxicity and enhanced automaticity of the AV junction. Other causes are an increase in vagal (parasympathetic) tone on the SA node, an excessive dose of certain cardiac drugs (e.g., quinidine and procainamide) or sympathomimetic drugs (e.g., epinephrine, isoproterenol, and norepinephrine), hypoxia, congestive heart failure, or damage to the AV junction. The electrophysiological mechanism responsible for premature junctional contractions is either **enhanced automaticity** or **reentry.**

Clinical Significance

Isolated premature junctional contractions are not significant. However, if digitalis is being administered, PJCs may indicate digitalis toxicity and enhanced automaticity of the AV junction. Frequent PJCs, more than four to six per minute, may indicate an enhanced automaticity or a reentry mechanism in the AV junction and warn of the appearance of more serious junctional arrhythmias.

Because premature junctional contractions with aberrancy resemble premature ventricular contractions (see Premature Ventricular Contractions, page 168), such PJCs must be correctly identified so that the patient is not treated inappropriately.

Notes

Junctional Escape Rhythm

Definition

Junctional escape rhythm (Figure 7-2) is an arrhythmia originating in an escape pacemaker in the AV junction with a rate of 40 to 60 beats per minute. When less than three QRS complexes arising from the escape pacemaker are present, they are called **junctional escape beats** or **complexes.**

Diagnostic Characteristics

Heart rate: The heart rate is typically 40 to 60 beats per minute, but it may be less.

Rhythm: The ventricular rhythm is essentially regular.

Pacemaker site: The pacemaker site is an escape pacemaker in the AV junction.

P waves: P waves may be present or absent. If P waves are present but have no relation to the QRS complexes of the **junctional escape rhythm,** appearing independently at a rate different (typically slower) from that of the junctional rhythm, the pacemaker site is the SA node or an ectopic pacemaker in the atria. These P waves are usually positive (upright) in lead II. When the P waves occur independently of the QRS complexes, **atrioventricular (AV) dissociation** is present.

If the P waves regularly precede or follow the QRS complexes and are identical, the electrical impulses responsible for them have originated in the pacemaker site of the junctional escape rhythm. Such P' waves differ from normal P waves in size, shape, and direction. Since the atria depolarize retrogradely when the electrical impulses arise in the AV junction, the P' waves are negative (inverted) in lead II.

P' waves are absent in junctional escape rhythm if the P' waves occur during the QRS complexes, if a complete block in retrograde conduction is present, or if atrial flutter or fibrillation is the underlying atrial rhythm.

PR intervals: If the P' waves regularly precede the QRS complexes, the P'R intervals are abnormal (less than 0.12 second). If the P' waves regularly follow the QRS complexes, the RP' intervals are usually less than 0.20 second.

R-R intervals: The R-R intervals are usually equal.

QRS complexes: The QRS complexes are normal unless a preexisting bundle branch block is present. Junctional escape rhythm with abnormal QRS complexes may resemble ventricular escape rhythm.

Cause of Arrhythmia

Junctional escape rhythm is a normal response of the AV junction (1) when the rate of impulse formation of the dominant pacemaker (usually the SA node) becomes less than that of the escape pacemaker in the AV junction or (2) when the electrical impulses from the SA node or atria fail to reach the AV junction because of a sinus arrest, sinoatrial (SA) exit block, or third-degree (complete) AV block. Generally, when an electrical impulse fails to arrive at the AV junction within approximately 1.0 to 1.5 seconds, the escape pacemaker in the AV junction begins to generate electrical impulses at its inherent firing rate of 40 to 60 beats per minute. The result is one or more junctional escape beats or a junctional escape rhythm.

Clinical Significance

The signs and symptoms and clinical significance of junctional escape rhythm are the same as those in symptomatic sinus bradycardia. Symptomatic junctional escape rhythm must be treated promptly, preferably with a transcutaneous pacemaker, to reverse the consequences of the reduced cardiac output.

Notes

Junctional Escape Rhythm

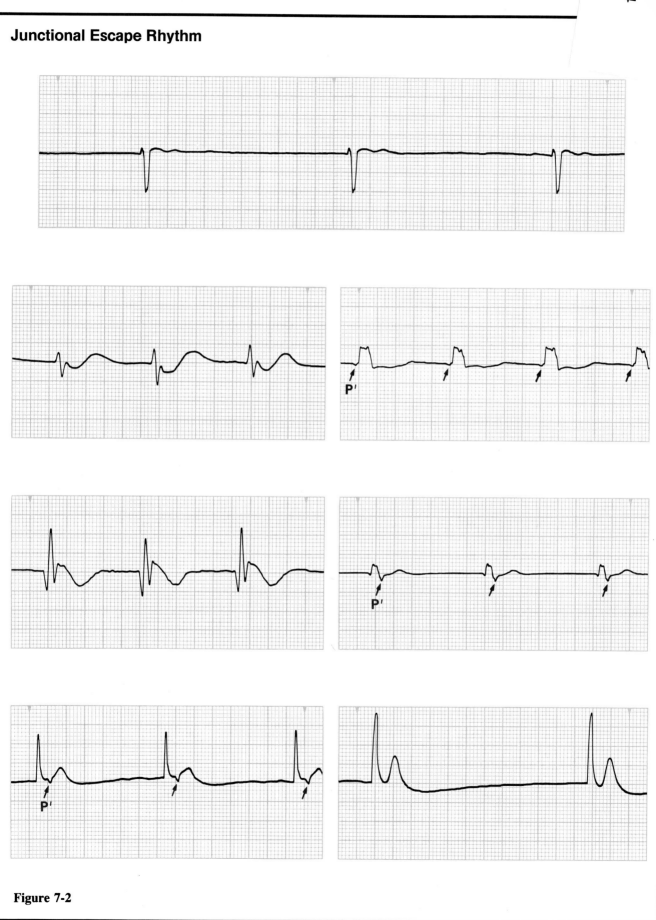

Figure 7-2

Nonparoxysmal Junctional Tachycardia
(Accelerated Junctional Rhythm, Junctional Tachycardia)

Definition

Nonparoxysmal junctional tachycardia (Figure 7-3) is an arrhythmia originating in an ectopic pacemaker in the AV junction with a regular rhythm and a rate of 60 to 150 beats per minute. It includes **accelerated junctional rhythm** and **junctional tachycardia.**

Diagnostic Characteristics

Heart rate: The heart rate is usually 60 to 130 beats per minute, but it may be greater than 130 beats per minute and as high as 150. **Nonparoxysmal junctional tachycardia** with a heart rate between 60 and 100 beats per minute is commonly called **accelerated junctional rhythm;** and one with a rate greater than 100 beats per minute, **junctional tachycardia.** The onset and termination of nonparoxysmal junctional tachycardia are usually gradual.

Rhythm: The rhythm is essentially regular.

Pacemaker site: The pacemaker site is an ectopic pacemaker in the AV junction.

P waves: P waves may be present or absent. If present, they may have no relation to the QRS complexes of the nonparoxysmal junctional tachycardia, appearing independently at a rate different from that of the junctional rhythm.

The pacemaker site of such P waves is the SA node or an ectopic pacemaker in the atria. These P waves are usually positive (upright) in lead II. When the P waves occur independently of the QRS complexes, **atrioventricular (AV) dissociation** is present.

If the P waves are identical and regularly precede or follow the QRS complexes, the electrical impulses responsible for them have originated in the pacemaker site of the nonparoxysmal junctional tachycardia. Such P′ waves differ from normal P waves in size, shape, and direction. Since the atria depolarize retrogradely when the electrical impulses arise in the AV junction, the P′ waves are negative (inverted) in lead II.

Nonparoxysmal Junctional Tachycardia
(Accelerated Junctional Rhythm, Junctional Tachycardia)

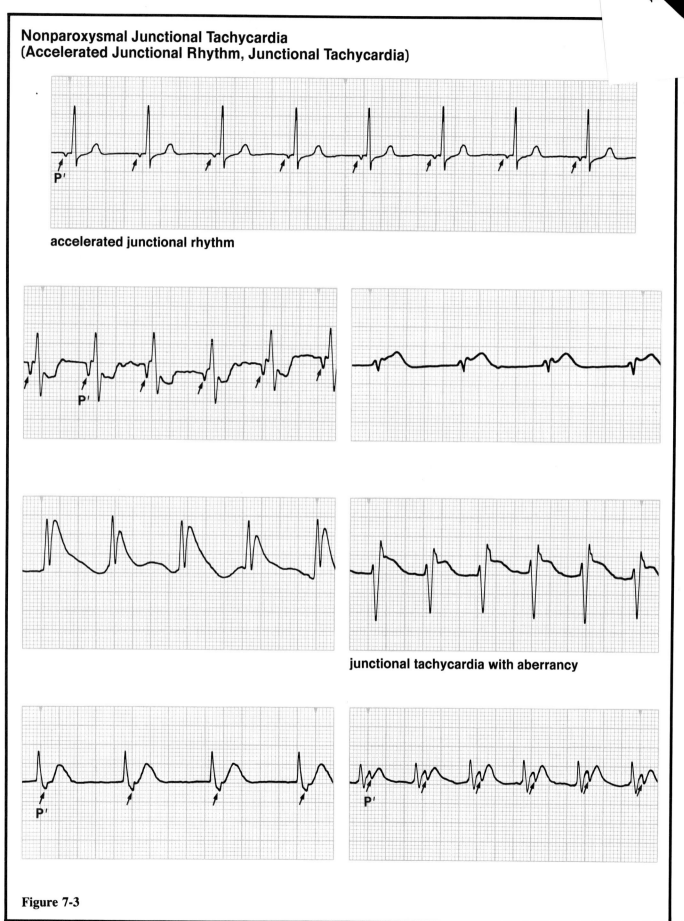

accelerated junctional rhythm

junctional tachycardia with aberrancy

Figure 7-3

P′ waves are absent in nonparoxysmal junctional tachycardia if the P′ waves occur during the QRS complexes, if a complete block in retrograde conduction is present, or if atrial flutter or fibrillation is the underlying atrial rhythm.

PR intervals: If the P′ waves regularly precede the QRS complexes, the P′R intervals are abnormal (less than 0.12 second). If the P′ waves regularly follow the QRS complexes, the RP′ intervals are usually less than 0.20 second.

R-R intervals: The R-R intervals are usually equal.

QRS complexes: The QRS complexes are normal unless a preexisting bundle branch block or aberrant ventricular conduction is present. If abnormal QRS complexes occur only when junctional tachycardia is present, the arrhythmia is called **junctional tachycardia with aberrancy** (or **aberrant ventricular conduction**).

Nonparoxysmal junctional tachycardia with abnormal QRS complexes may resemble accelerated idioventricular rhythm if the heart rate is 60 to 100 beats per minute (accelerated junctional rhythm), or it may resemble ventricular tachycardia if the heart rate is over 100 beats per minute (junctional tachycardia).

Cause of Arrhythmia

Nonparoxysmal junctional tachycardia is usually due to **enhanced automaticity** of the AV junction, unlike paroxysmal junctional tachycardia (PJT), which results from a **reentry mechanism.** Nonparoxysmal junctional tachycardia is most commonly a result of digitalis toxicity. Other common causes are excessive administration of catecholamines and damage to the AV junction from an inferior myocardial infarction or rheumatic fever. The arrhythmia may begin with one or more PJCs.

Clinical Significance

Nonparoxysmal junctional tachycardia is clinically significant because it commonly indicates dig-italis toxicity. The signs and symptoms and clinical significance of rapid nonparoxysmal junctional tachycardia are the same as those of atrial tachycardia.

In addition, in nonparoxysmal junctional tachycardia, the atria do not regularly contract and empty before each ventricular contraction, filling the ventricles during the last part of diastole, as they normally do. The loss of this **"atrial kick"** results in incomplete filling of the ventricles before they contract, causing a reduction of the cardiac output by as much as 25 percent.

Notes

Paroxysmal Junctional Tachycardia (PJT)

Definition

Paroxysmal junctional tachycardia (PJT) (Figure 7-4) is an arrhythmia originating in an ectopic pacemaker or the site of a rapid reentry circuit in the AV junction with a rate between 160 to 240 beats per minute. PJT is often called **paroxysmal supraventricular tachycardia (PSVT)** when the site of origin cannot be determined with certainty.

Heart rate: The heart rate is usually 160 to 240 beats per minute and constant. The heart rate, however, may be as low as 110 beats per minute or exceed 240 per minute. The onset and termination of **paroxysmal junctional tachycardia** are typically abrupt, the onset often being initiated by a premature atrial contraction. A brief period of asystole may follow the termination of the arrhythmia. The rate may be slower during the few beats after onset and before termination. Paroxysmal junctional tachycardia is characterized by repeated episodes (paroxysms) of tachycardia that last from a few minutes to many hours and recur for many years. **Carotid sinus massage** usually results in the abrupt termination of paroxysmal junctional tachycardia.

Rhythm: The rhythm is essentially regular.

Pacemaker site: The pacemaker site is an ectopic pacemaker in the AV junction.

P′ waves: P′ waves are often absent, being buried in the QRS complex. If present, they are identical and typically follow the QRS complexes. Rarely, the P′ waves precede the QRS complexes. The P′ waves are generally abnormal, differing from normal P waves in size, shape, and direction. Since atrial depolarization occurs in a retrograde fashion, the P′ waves are negative (inverted) in lead II.

PR intervals: If the P′ waves precede the QRS complexes, the P′R intervals are abnormal (less than 0.12 second). If the P′ waves follow the QRS complexes, the RP′ intervals are usually less than 0.20 second.

R-R intervals: The R-R intervals are usually equal.

QRS complexes: The QRS complexes are normal unless a preexisting bundle branch block or aberrant ventricular conduction is present. If abnormal QRS complexes occur only with the tachycardia, the arrhythmia is called **paroxysmal junctional tachycardia with aberrancy** (or **aberrant ventricular conduction**). Paroxysmal junctional tachycardia with abnormal QRS complexes may resemble ventricular tachycardia.

Cause of Arrhythmia

Paroxysmal junctional tachycardia may occur without apparent cause in healthy persons of any age with no apparent underlying heart disease. In susceptible persons, it may be precipitated by an increase in catecholamines and sympathetic tone, overexertion, stimulants (e.g., alcohol, coffee, and tobacco), electrolyte or acid-base abnormalities, hyperventilation, or emotional stress. The electrophysiological mechanism responsible for paroxysmal junctional tachycardia is a reentry mechanism.

Clinical Significance

The signs and symptoms and clinical significance of paroxysmal junctional tachycardia are the same as those of paroxysmal atrial tachycardia. In addition, syncope may occur after the termination of paroxysmal junctional tachycardia because of the asystole that may follow its termination.

Note: Since it is often difficult to differentiate between paroxysmal atrial tachycardia and paroxysmal junctional tachycardia when the P′ waves are not clearly evident, the term **paroxysmal supraventricular tachycardia (PSVT)** is commonly used to indicate a paroxysmal tachycardia originating in the atria or AV junction without specifying the exact location of the ectopic pacemaker site.

Notes

Paroxysmal Junctional Tachycardia (PJT)

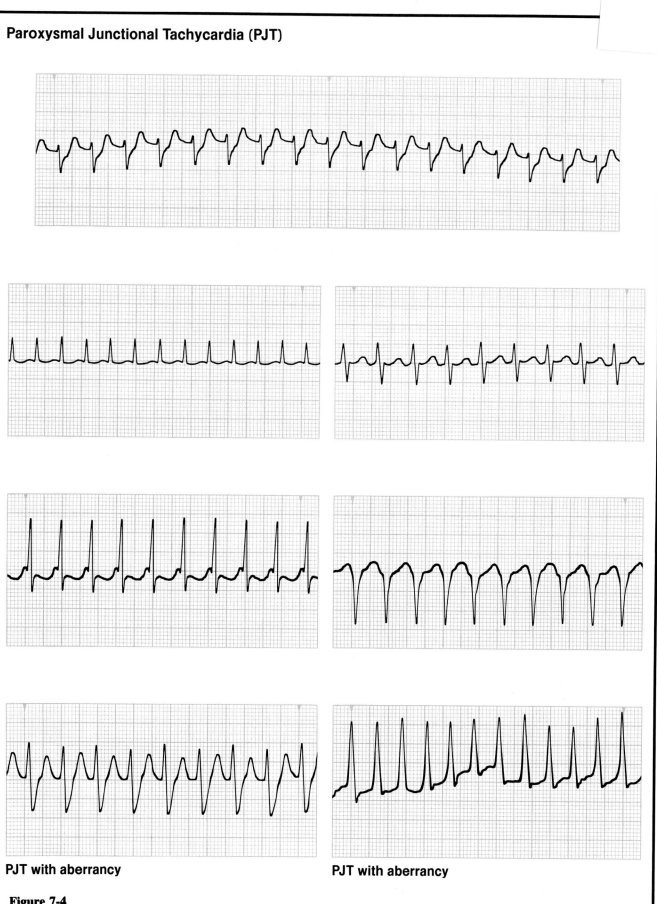

PJT with aberrancy   PJT with aberrancy

Figure 7-4

1. Absent P' waves in a junctional arrhythmia indicate:
   - A. retrograde atrial depolarizations occurred during the QRS complexes
   - B. atrial depolarizations have not occurred because of a retrograde AV block
   - C. either of the above
   - D. none of the above

2. If the ectopic pacemaker in the AV junction discharges too soon after the preceding QRS complex:
   - A. a premature ventricular contraction will occur
   - B. a premature atrial contraction with aberrancy occurs
   - C. the premature P' wave may not be followed by a QRS complex
   - D. none of the above

3. An extra contraction that originates in an ectopic pacemaker in the AV junction, occurring before the next expected beat of the underlying rhythm, is called:
   - A. a premature atrial contraction
   - B. a premature junctional contraction
   - C. a premature ventricular contraction
   - D. none of the above

4. The QRS complex of a PJC:
   - A. resembles a premature ventricular contraction if aberrant ventricular conduction is present
   - B. precedes or follows the P' wave associated with it
   - C. usually resembles that of the underlying rhythm
   - D. all of the above

5. Two PJCs in a row are called a:
   - A. trigeminy
   - B. couplet
   - C. reentry phenomenon
   - D. serious lethal rhythm

6. PJCs are caused by:
   - A. digitalis toxicity
   - B. increased parasympathetic tone on the SA node
   - C. sympathomimetic drugs
   - D. all of the above

7. More than four to six PJCs per minute may indicate:
   - A. enhanced automaticity in the AV junction
   - B. a reentry mechanism in the AV junction
   - C. that more serious junctional arrhythmias may occur
   - D. all of the above

8. An arrhythmia originating in an escape pacemaker in the AV junction with a rate of 40 to 60 beats per minute is called a(n):
   - A. agonal rhythm
   - B. junctional bradycardia
   - C. junctional escape rhythm
   - D. complete AV block

9. An arrhythmia consisting of narrow QRS complexes occurring at a rate of 55 beats per minute and P waves occurring independently at a slower rate is called:
   - A. a junctional escape rhythm
   - B. a supraventricular arrhythmia
   - C. atrioventricular (AV) dissociation
   - D. all of the above

10. The usual treatment for a symptomatic junctional escape rhythm is:
    - A. synchronized cardioversion
    - B. transcutaneous pacing
    - C. application of the anti-shock garment
    - D. none of the above

CHAPTER 8

Ventricular Arrhythmias

Premature Ventricular Contractions (PVCs)

Ventricular Tachycardia (VT)

Ventricular Fibrillation (VF)

Accelerated Idioventricular Rhythm (AIVR)

(Accelerated Ventricular Rhythm,

Idioventricular Tachycardia,

Slow Ventricular Tachycardia)

Ventricular Escape Rhythm

(Idioventricular Rhythm)

Ventricular Asystole

(Cardiac Standstill)

OBJECTIVES

Upon completion of all or part of this chapter you should be able to complete the following objectives indicated by your instructor:

☐ **1.** Define and give the diagnostic characteristics, cause, and clinical significance of the following arrhythmias:

☐ Premature ventricular contractions (PVCs)

☐ Ventricular tachycardia (VT)

☐ Ventricular fibrillation (VF)

☐ Accelerated idioventricular rhythm (AIVR)

☐ Ventricular escape rhythm

☐ Ventricular asystole

Premature Ventricular Contractions (PVCs)

Definition

A **premature ventricular contraction (PVC)** (Figure 8-1) is an extra ventricular contraction consisting of an abnormally wide and bizarre QRS complex that originates in an ectopic pacemaker in the ventricles. It occurs earlier than the expected beat of the underlying rhythm and is usually followed by a compensatory pause.

Diagnostic Characteristics

Heart rate: The heart rate is that of the underlying rhythm.

Rhythm: The rhythm is typically irregular when **premature ventricular contractions** are present.

Pacemaker site: The pacemaker site of the **PVC** is an ectopic pacemaker in the ventricles, specifically in the bundle branches, Purkinje network, or ventricular myocardium. Premature ventricular contractions may originate from a single ectopic pacemaker site **(unifocal PVCs)** or from multiple sites in the ventricles **(multifocal PVCs).**

P waves: P waves may be present or absent. If present, they are usually of the underlying rhythm and have no relation to the PVCs. Typically, the PVCs do not disturb the P-P cycle of the underlying rhythm so that the P waves continue without disruption during and after the PVCs, occurring at their expected time. Uncommonly, the electrical impulse responsible for the PVC enters the atria, depolarizing them retrogradely. This results in a P′ wave that follows the QRS complex of the PVC at an RP′ interval of about 0.20 second, but often the P′ wave is buried in the QRS complex. Since atrial depolarization occurs in a retrograde fashion, these P′ waves are negative (inverted) in lead II. The electrical impulse of the PVC may also depolarize the SA node, momentarily suppressing it, so that the next P wave of the underlying rhythm appears later than expected.

Often the P waves of the underlying rhythm are obscured by the PVCs, but sometimes they appear as notches on the ST segment or T wave of the PVCs. This provides a clue that the premature ectopic complex is a PVC and not a premature atrial contraction with aberrant ventricular conduction. In a premature atrial contraction, a P wave typically precedes the QRS complex (see Premature Atrial Contractions, page 136).

PR intervals: No PR intervals are associated with the PVCs.

R-R intervals: The R-R intervals are unequal when PVCs are present. The R-R interval between the PVC and the preceding QRS complex of the underlying rhythm is usually shorter than that of the underlying rhythm. This R-R interval is called the **coupling interval.** PVCs with the same coupling interval in a given ECG lead usually originate from the same ectopic pacemaker site.

A **full compensatory pause** commonly follows a PVC since the SA node is often not depolarized by the PVC (i.e., the P wave of the underlying rhythm that follows the PVC appears at the expected time). Consequently, the interval between the P waves of the underlying rhythm occurring before and after the PVC is twice the P-P interval of the underlying rhythm.

Rarely, when the SA node is depolarized by the PVC, an **incomplete compensatory pause** occurs. (See the discussion of full and incomplete compensatory pause under Premature Atrial Contractions, page 136.)

A combination of a full compensatory pause and a P wave of the underlying rhythm superimposed on a premature ectopic beat with a wide and bizarre QRS complex helps to make a positive diagnosis of a PVC.

QRS complexes: The QRS complex of the PVC typically appears prematurely (and without a preceding ectopic P wave) before the next expected QRS complex of the underlying rhythm. The QRS complex is nearly always 0.12 second or greater in duration, and, because of the abnormal direction and sequence of ventricular depolarization, it is distorted and bizarre, often with notching, appearing different from the QRS complex of the underlying rhythm. It is usually followed by an abnormal ST segment and a large T wave, opposite in direction to the major deflection of the QRS complex.

The shape of a PVC often resembles that of a right or left bundle branch block. (See Chapter 10, Bundle Branch and Fascicular Blocks.) For example, the QRS complex of a PVC originating from

Premature Ventricular Contractions (PVCs)

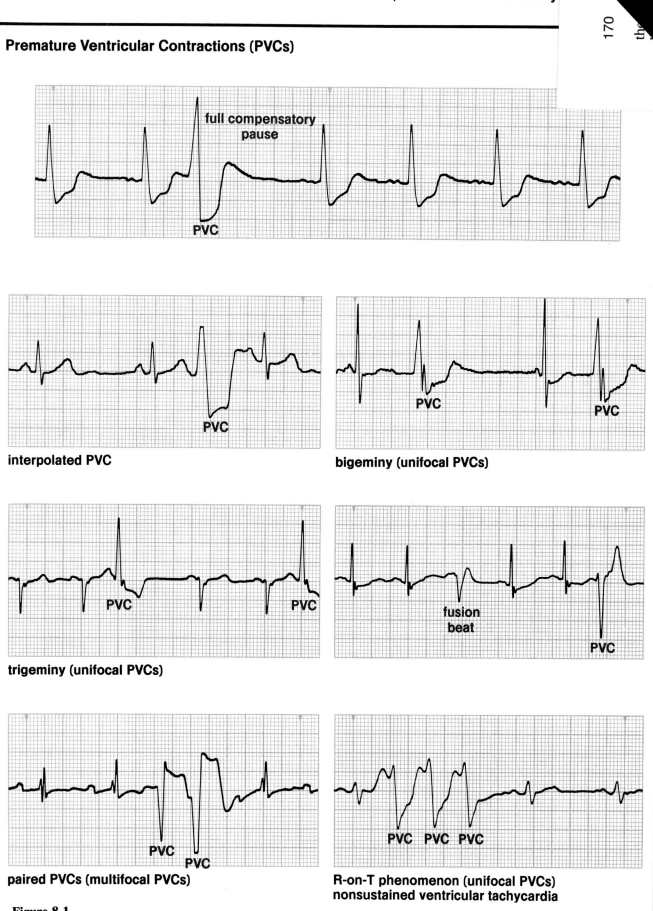

Figure 8-1

the left ventricle resembles that of a right bundle branch block. Likewise, a PVC originating in the right ventricle has a QRS complex resembling that of a left bundle branch block. However, the QRS complex of a PVC arising from a bundle branch appears only slightly bizarre (**fascicular PVC**). A PVC arising from the ventricles near the bifurcation of the bundle of His may appear relatively normal.

The QRS complexes of PVCs that originate from the same ectopic pacemaker site are usually identical in any given lead (**unifocal or uniform PVCs**). Such PVCs usually have equal (**constant**) coupling intervals. Occasionally, unifocal PVCs may differ from each other because of changing depolarization pathways within the ventricles—a common abnormality present in severe myocardial disease. Such PVCs arising from the same pacemaker site with constant coupling intervals but differing QRS complexes are called **multiform PVCs.** PVCs originating in two or more ectopic pacemaker sites characteristically have different QRS complexes and varying coupling intervals in the same lead. Such PVCs are called **multifocal PVCs.**

When a PVC occurs at about the same time that an electrical impulse of the underlying rhythm is activating the ventricles, depolarization of the ventricles occurs simultaneously in two directions. This results in a QRS complex that has the characteristics of both the PVC and the QRS complex of the underlying rhythm. Such a QRS complex is called a **ventricular fusion beat.** The presence of ventricular fusion beats provides evidence in favor of a premature ectopic contraction being ventricular in origin and not supraventricular with aberrant ventricular conduction.

Frequency and pattern of occurrence of PVCs: The PVCs may be **infrequent** (less than five beats per minute) or **frequent** (five or more beats per minute). They may occur singly (**isolated**) or in groups of two or more in succession. Groups of two or more PVCs are called **"ventricular group beats"** or **"bursts"** or **"salvos"** of PVCs. Two PVCs in a row are called **"paired PVCs"** or a **"couplet."** A group of three or more consecutive PVCs is considered to be **ventricular tachycardia.**

If PVCs alternate with the QRS complexes of the underlying rhythm, **ventricular bigeminy** is present. If, in ventricular bigeminy, the PVCs follow the QRS complexes of the underlying rhythm at precisely the same intervals, **coupling** is said to be present. **Ventricular trigeminy** occurs when there

is one PVC for every two QRS complexes of the underlying rhythm or one QRS complex of the underlying rhythm for every two PVCs.

The term *R-on-T phenomenon* is used to indicate that a PVC has occurred during the **vulnerable period of ventricular repolarization** (i.e., the relative refractory period of the ventricles coincident with the **peak of the T wave).** During this period, the myocardium is at its greatest **electrical nonuniformity,** a condition where some of the ventricular muscle fibers may be completely repolarized, others may be only partially repolarized, while still others may be completely refractory. Stimulation of the ventricles at this point by an intrinsic electrical impulse such as that generated by a PVC or by an extrinsic impulse from a cardiac pacemaker or an electrical countershock may result in nonuniform conduction of the electrical impulse through the muscle fibers. Some of the fibers will be able to conduct the electrical impulse normally while others will only be able to conduct them slowly or not at all. Thus, a **reentry mechanism** will be established that may precipitate repetitive ventricular contractions and result in ventricular tachycardia or fibrillation. (See Chapter 1 for a discussion of the reentry mechanism, page 15.)

A PVC that occurs at about the same time that a ventricular depolarization of the underlying rhythm is expected to occur is called an **end-diastolic PVC.** This usually results in a **ventricular fusion beat.** End-diastolic PVCs tend to occur when the underlying rhythm is relatively rapid.

A PVC occurring between two normally conducted QRS complexes without greatly disturbing the underlying rhythm is called an **interpolated PVC.** This tends to occur when the underlying rhythm is relatively slow. The R-R interval that includes the PVC is often slightly greater than that of the underlying rhythm, but a full compensatory pause usually does not occur.

Some PVCs, based on their frequency and pattern of occurrence, are more prone than others to initiate life-threatening arrhythmias, particularly following an acute myocardial infarction or ischemic episode. These PVCs, the **warning arrhythmias,** include:

- **PVCs falling on the T wave** (the **R-on-T phenomenon**)
- **Multiform** and **multifocal PVCs**
- **Frequent PVCs** of more than five or six per minute
- **Ventricular group beats** with bursts or salvos of two, three, or more

Cause of Arrhythmia

PVCs may occur in healthy persons with apparently healthy hearts and without apparent cause. PVCs, especially if they are frequent, may be caused by an increase in catecholamines and sympathetic tone (as in emotional stress), an increase in vagal (parasympathetic) tone, stimulants (e.g., alcohol, caffeine, and tobacco), excessive administration of digitalis or sympathomimetic drugs (e.g., epinephrine, isoproterenol, and norepinephrine), hypoxia, acidosis, hypokalemia, or congestive heart failure. PVCs frequently occur in acute myocardial infarction. The electrophysiologic mechanism responsible for PVCs in the above conditions is either **enhanced automaticity** or **reentry.**

Clinical Significance

Isolated premature ventricular contractions in patients with no underlying heart disease usually have no significance and require no treatment. In the presence of heart disease, such as an acute myocardial infarction or ischemic episode, and drug (e.g., digitalis) intoxication, however, PVCs may indicate the presence of enhanced ventricular automaticity, a reentry mechanism, or both, and may herald the appearance of such life-threatening arrhythmias as ventricular tachycardia or fibrillation.

Although warning arrhythmias have been recognized as high-risk factors in triggering ventricular tachycardia or fibrillation, any PVC can trigger these lethal arrhythmias in patients with an acute myocardial infarction or ischemic episode. For this reason, **all** PVCs should be treated immediately when they occur under these conditions.

At times, premature atrial and junctional contractions with aberrant ventricular conduction may mimic PVCs.

Notes

Ventricular Tachycardia (VT)

Definition

Ventricular tachycardia (VT, V TACH) (Figure 8-2) is an arrhythmia originating in an ectopic pacemaker in the ventricles with a rate between 110 and 250 beats per minute. The QRS complexes are abnormally wide and bizarre.

Diagnostic Characteristics

Heart rate: The heart rate is over 100 beats per minute, usually between 110 and 250 beats per minute. **Ventricular tachycardia** exists if three or more consecutive premature ventricular contractions are present, occurring at a rate greater than 100 beats per minute. The onset and termination of ventricular tachycardia may or may not be abrupt. Ventricular tachycardia may occur in paroxysms of three or more PVCs separated by the underlying rhythm (**nonsustained ventricular tachycardia** or **paroxysmal ventricular tachycardia**) or persist for a long period of time (**sustained ventricular tachycardia**).

Rhythm: The rhythm is usually regular, but it may be slightly irregular.

Pacemaker site: The pacemaker site of ventricular tachycardia is an ectopic pacemaker in the bundle branches, Purkinje network, or ventricular myocardium.

P waves: P waves may be present or absent. If present, they usually have no set relation to the QRS complexes of the ventricular tachycardia, appearing between the QRS complexes at a rate different from that of the ventricular tachycardia. The pacemaker site of such P waves is the SA node or an ectopic or escape pacemaker in the atria or AV junction. These P waves may be positive (upright) or negative (inverted) in lead II. P waves are often difficult to detect in ventricular tachycardia, especially if it is rapid. When the P waves occur independently of the QRS complexes, **atrioventricular (AV) dissociation** is present. Rarely, identical P waves regularly follow the QRS complexes. The electrical impulses responsible for them have most likely originated in the ectopic pacemaker site of the ventricular tachycardia. Such P' waves differ from normal P waves in size, shape, and direction. Since the atria are depolarized in a retrograde manner by the electrical impulse entering the atria from the

ventricles through the AV junction (**retrograde AV conduction**), the P' waves are negative (inverted) in lead II.

PR intervals: If P waves are present and occur independently of the QRS complexes, no PR intervals are present. If P' waves regularly follow the QRS complexes, the RP' intervals are usually less than 0.20 second.

R-R intervals: The R-R intervals may be equal or vary slightly.

QRS complexes: The QRS complexes exceed 0.12 second and are usually distorted and bizarre, often with notching. They are followed by large T waves, opposite in direction to the major deflection of the QRS complexes. Usually, the QRS complexes are identical, but, occasionally, one or more QRS complexes differ in size, shape, and direction, especially at the onset or end of ventricular tachycardia. These are most likely **fusion beats.** (See the discussion of fusion beats under Premature Ventricular Contractions, page 170.)

Occasionally, an electrical impulse of the underlying rhythm is conducted from the atria to the ventricles through the AV junction producing a normal-appearing QRS complex (0.10 second or less) among the abnormal QRS complexes of the ventricular tachycardia. Such a QRS complex is called a **capture beat.** The R-R interval between the QRS complex of the ventricular tachycardia preceding the capture beat and the QRS complex of the capture beat is usually less than that of the ventricular tachycardia. The presence of capture or ventricular fusion beats provides evidence that the tachycardia is most likely ventricular in origin and not a supraventricular tachycardia with aberrant ventricular conduction.

When there are two distinctly different forms of QRS complexes alternating with each other (indicating that there are two ventricular ectopic pacemakers), the arrhythmia is called **bidirectional ventricular tachycardia.** When the QRS complexes in a ventricular tachycardia differ markedly from beat to beat, the arrhythmia is called **multiform ventricular tachycardia.** Another form of ventricular tachycardia characterized by QRS complexes that gradually change back and forth from one shape and direction to another over a series of beats is called **torsade de pointes.** This term, literally translated from French, means **"twisting around a point."**

Ventricular Tachycardia (VT)

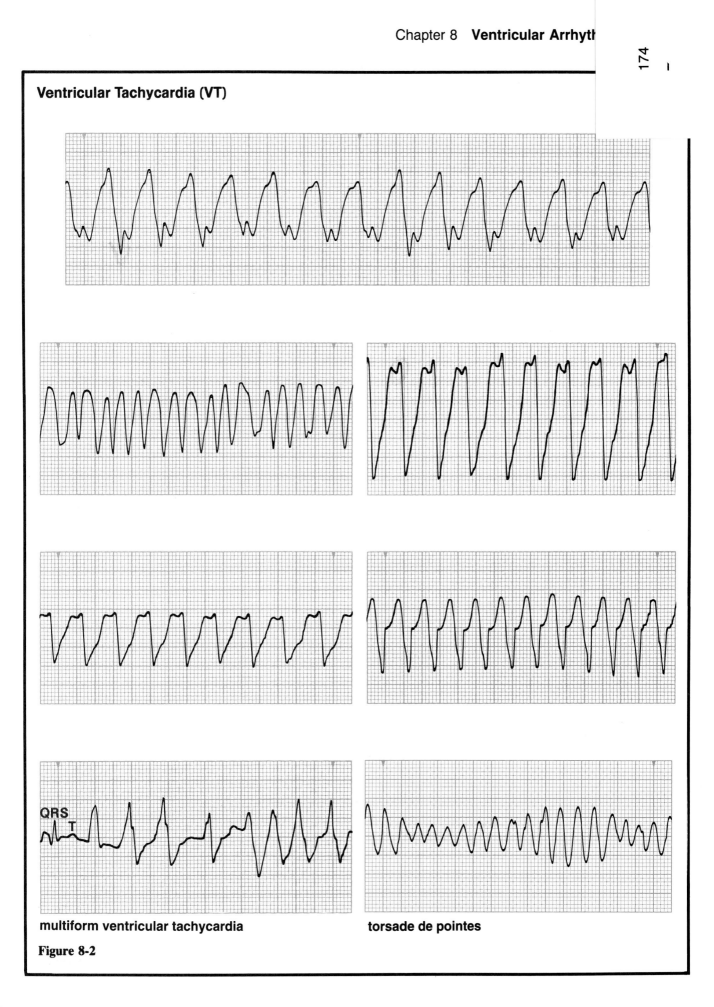

multiform ventricular tachycardia   torsade de pointes

Figure 8-2

Cause of Arrhythmia

Ventricular tachycardia usually occurs in the presence of significant cardiac disease. Most commonly, it occurs in coronary artery disease, particularly in the setting of acute myocardial infarction and especially if hypoxia or acidosis is present. Digitalis toxicity is also a common cause of ventricular tachycardia. The arrhythmia also occurs in such cardiac conditions as cardiomyopathy, mitral valve prolapse, and congestive heart failure. The ventricles are particularly vulnerable to ventricular tachycardia when the **QT interval** is prolonged from various causes, including excess of certain drugs (e.g., quinidine, procainamide, disopyramide, phenothiazines, and tricyclic antidepressants), bradyarrhythmias (e.g., marked sinus bradycardia and third-degree AV block with slow ventricular escape rhythm), electrolyte disturbances (e.g., hypokalemia), liquid protein diets, and central nervous system disorders (e.g., subarachnoid hemorrhage and intracranial trauma). The **torsade de pointes** form of ventricular tachycardia is particularly prone to occur following administration of such antiarrhythmic agents as disopyramide, quinidine, and procainamide or other agents that prolong the QT interval. The electrophysiologic mechanism responsible for ventricular tachycardia is either **enhanced automaticity** or **reentry.**

A premature ventricular contraction can initiate ventricular tachycardia when the PVC occurs during the **vulnerable period of ventricular repolarization** coincident with the **peak of the T wave,** i.e., the **R-on-T phenomenon.** (See the discussion of vulnerable period under Premature Ventricular Contractions, page 170.) Often ventricular tachycardia may occur without preexisting or precipitating premature ventricular contractions.

Clinical Significance

The signs and symptoms in ventricular tachycardia vary, depending on the nature and severity of the underlying cardiac disease, such as acute myocardial infarction or congestive heart failure. Ventricular tachycardia may cause or aggravate existing angina pectoris, acute myocardial infarction, or congestive heart failure; produce hypotension or shock; or terminate in ventricular fibrillation or asystole. The patient with ventricular tachycardia may often experience feelings of impending death.

In ventricular tachycardia, the atria do not regularly contract and empty before each ventricular contraction, filling the ventricles during the last part of diastole, as they normally do. The loss of this **"atrial kick"** results in incomplete filling of the ventricles before they contract, causing a reduction of the cardiac output by as much as 25 percent. This reduction in cardiac output often compounds the already low cardiac output frequently seen in the diseased hearts in which ventricular tachycardia tends to occur.

Because ventricular tachycardia is considered a life-threatening arrhythmia, often initiating or degenerating into ventricular fibrillation or asystole, **ventricular tachycardia must be treated immediately!**

At times, a supraventricular tachycardia (e.g., sinus, atrial, and junctional tachycardias, atrial flutter, and paroxysmal supraventricular tachycardia) with wide QRS complexes caused by a preexisting bundle branch block, aberrant ventricular conduction, or anomalous AV conduction may mimic ventricular tachycardia. Atrial fibrillation with wide QRS complexes and a rapid ventricular rate may also mimic ventricular tachycardia, but usually the grossly irregular rhythm of atrial fibrillation provides a clue to its true identity.

The presence of certain features common to ventricular tachycardia, namely, atrioventricular (AV) dissociation, a QRS-complex duration greater than 0.12 second (and especially if it is greater than 0.14 second), and capture or ventricular fusion beats, helps to differentiate ventricular tachycardia from a supraventricular tachycardia with wide QRS complexes. A **12-lead ECG** or **lead MCL**$_1$ is also helpful in making a differentiation in this situation.

Notes

Ventricular Fibrillation (VF)

Definition

Ventricular fibrillation (VF, V-FIB) (Figures 8-3 and 8-4) is an arrhythmia arising in numerous ectopic pacemakers in the ventricles, characterized by very rapid abnormal ventricular fibrillation (f) waves and no QRS complexes.

Diagnostic Characteristics

Heart rate: No coordinated ventricular beats are present. The ventricles contract from about 300 to 500 times a minute in an unsynchronized, uncoordinated, and haphazard manner. The fibrillating ventricles are often described as resembling a **"bag of worms."**

Rhythm: The rhythm is grossly (totally) irregular.

Pacemaker site: The pacemaker sites of **ventricular fibrillation** are multiple ectopic pacemakers in the Purkinje network and ventricular myocardium.

Characteristics of ventricular fibrillation waves (VF waves):

1. Relationship to cardiac anatomy and physiology: Ventricular fibrillation waves represent abnormal, chaotic, and incomplete ventricular depolarizations caused by haphazard depolarization of small individual groups (or islets) of muscle fibers. Since organized depolarizations of the atria and ventricles are absent, distinct P waves, QRS complexes, ST segments, and T waves and organized atrial and ventricular contractions are absent.

2. Onset and end: The onset and end of the ventricular fibrillation waves often cannot be determined with certainty.

3. Direction: The direction of the ventricular fibrillation waves varies at random from positive (upright) to negative (inverted).

4. Duration: The duration of ventricular fibrillation waves cannot be measured with certainty.

5. Amplitude: The amplitude varies from less than 1 mm to about 10 mm. Generally, if the ventricular fibrillation waves are small (less than 3 mm), the arrhythmia is called **"fine" ventricular fibrillation.** If the ventricular fibrillation waves are large (greater than 3 mm), it is called **"coarse" ventricular fibrillation.** If the ventricular fibrillation waves are so small or "fine" that they are not recorded, the ECG appears as a **wavy or flat (isoelectric) line** resembling **ventricular asystole.**

6. Shape: The ventricular fibrillation waves are of varying shape: bizarre, rounded or pointed, and markedly dissimilar.

VENTRICULAR FIBRILLATION WAVES

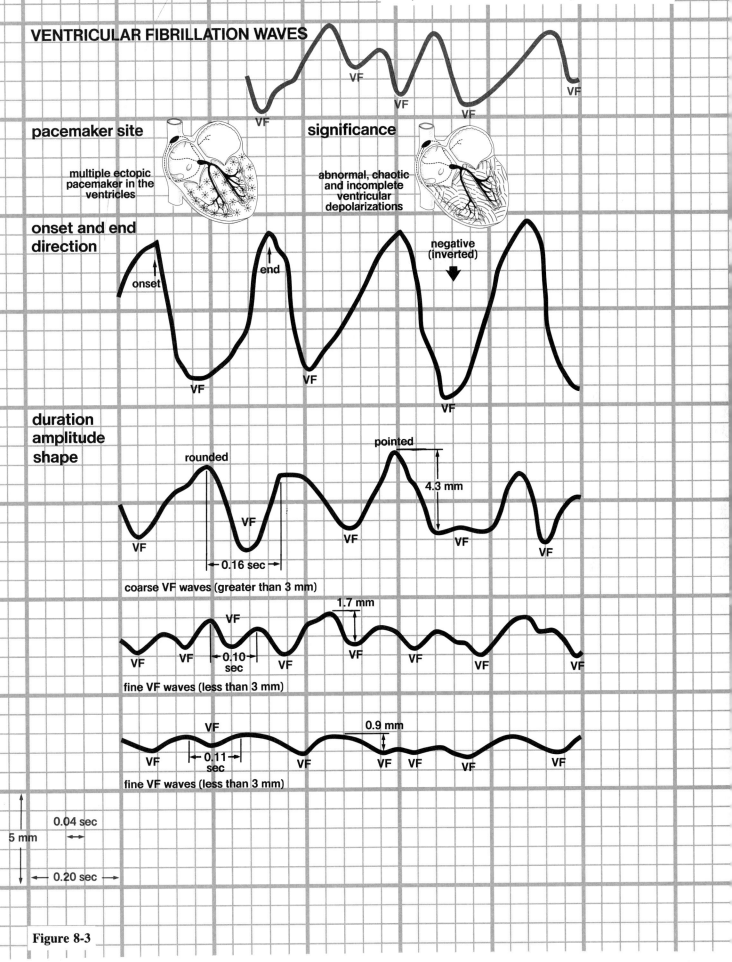

VF

VF

VF

VF

pacemaker site

multiple ectopic pacemaker in the ventricles

significance

abnormal, chaotic and incomplete ventricular depolarizations

onset and end direction

onset

end

negative (inverted)

VF

VF

VF

duration amplitude shape

rounded

pointed

4.3 mm

VF

VF

VF

VF

VF

←— 0.16 sec —→

coarse VF waves (greater than 3 mm)

VF

1.7 mm

VF   VF   ←0.10→   VF   VF   VF   VF   VF
                sec

fine VF waves (less than 3 mm)

VF   0.9 mm

VF   ├ 0.11 ┤   VF   VF   VF   VF   VF
        sec

fine VF waves (less than 3 mm)

5 mm   0.04 sec

←— 0.20 sec —→

Figure 8-3

PR intervals: PR intervals are absent.

R-R intervals: R-R intervals are absent.

QRS complexes: QRS complexes are absent.

Cause of Arrhythmia

Ventricular fibrillation, one of the most common causes of cardiac arrest, usually occurs in the presence of significant cardiac disease, most commonly in coronary artery disease, myocardial ischemia, and acute myocardial infarction and in third-degree AV block with a slow ventricular escape rhythm. The arrhythmia also occurs frequently as a terminal event in many cardiac, medical, and traumatic conditions. It may occur in cardiomyopathy, mitral valve prolapse, and cardiac trauma (penetrating or blunt). The arrhythmia may also be caused by an excessive dose of digitalis, quinidine, or procainamide; hypoxia; acidosis; or electrolyte imbalance (e.g., hypokalemia and hyperkalemia). Ventricular fibrillation may also occur during anesthesia, cardiac and noncardiac operations, cardiac catheterization, and cardiac pacing and following cardioversion or accidental electrocution. The electrophysiological mechanism responsible for ventricular fibrillation is either **enhanced automaticity** or **reentry.**

A premature ventricular contraction can initiate ventricular fibrillation when the PVC occurs during the **vulnerable period of ventricular repolarization** coincident with the **peak of the T wave** (i.e., the **R-on-T phenomenon**), particularly when electrical stability of the heart has been altered by ischemia or acute myocardial infarction. (See the discussion of vulnerable period under Premature Ventricular Contractions, page 170.) Sustained ventricular tachycardia may also precipitate ventricular

fibrillation. Often ventricular fibrillation may begin without preexisting or precipitating premature ventricular contractions or ventricular tachycardia.

Clinical Significance

Organized ventricular depolarization and contraction and, consequently, cardiac output cease at the moment ventricular fibrillation occurs. Ventricular fibrillation results in faintness, followed within seconds by loss of consciousness, seizures, apnea, and, if the arrhythmia remains untreated, death. **Ventricular fibrillation must be treated immediately!**

The significance of coarse versus fine ventricular fibrillation is that coarse ventricular fibrillation, indicating a recent onset of the arrhythmia, is more apt to be reversed by defibrillation shock than is fine ventricular fibrillation, which indicates that the arrhythmia has been present for some time. Sometimes the distinction between coarse and fine ventricular fibrillation cannot be made because of the limitations of the monitoring equipment.

Since fine ventricular fibrillation may resemble ventricular asystole, ventricular fibrillation must be correctly identified using at least two ECG leads (i.e., lead II and lead I or III) so that the patient is not inappropriately treated for ventricular asystole.

In addition, ECG artifacts produced by loose or dry electrodes, broken ECG leads, or patient movement or muscle tremor may also resemble ventricular fibrillation. A rapid assessment of the patient, including a check of the patient's pulse, must be performed immediately upon the electrocardiographic onset of ventricular fibrillation to confirm the arrhythmia before treating the patient for cardiac arrest.

Notes

Ventricular Fibrillation (VF)

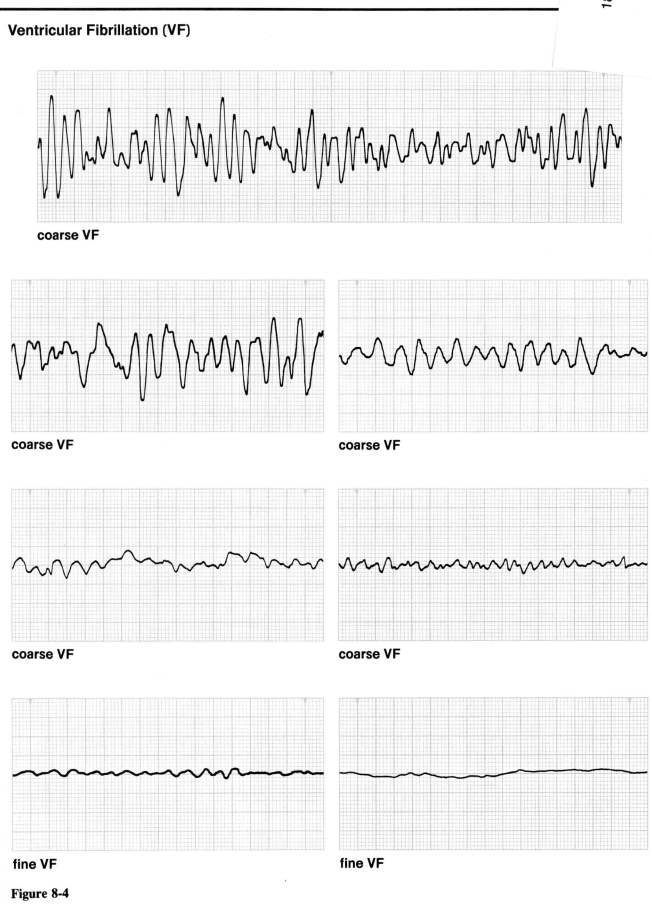

coarse VF

coarse VF

coarse VF

coarse VF

coarse VF

fine VF

fine VF

Figure 8-4

Accelerated Idioventricular Rhythm (AIVR)
(Accelerated Ventricular Rhythm, Idioventricular Tachycardia, Slow Ventricular Tachycardia)

Definition

Accelerated idioventricular rhythm (AIVR) (Figure 8-5) is an arrhythmia originating in an ectopic pacemaker in the ventricles with a rate between 40 to 100 beats per minute.

Diagnostic Characteristics

Heart rate: The heart rate is between 40 and 100 beats per minute. The onset and termination of **accelerated idioventricular rhythm** are usually gradual, but the arrhythmia may begin abruptly following a premature ventricular contraction.

Rhythm: The rhythm is essentially regular, but it may be irregular.

Pacemaker site: The pacemaker site is an ectopic pacemaker in the bundle branches, Purkinje network, or ventricular myocardium.

P waves: P waves may be present or absent. If present, they have no relation to the QRS complexes of the accelerated idioventricular rhythm, appearing independently at a rate different from that of the QRS complexes **(atrioventricular [AV] dissociation).**

The pacemaker site of such P waves is the SA node or an ectopic or escape pacemaker in the atria or AV junction. These P waves may be positive (upright) or negative (inverted) in lead II.

PR intervals: If P waves are present and occur independently of the QRS complexes, no PR intervals are present.

R-R intervals: The R-R intervals may be equal or may vary.

QRS complexes: The QRS complexes typically exceed 0.12 second and are bizarre, but they may be only slightly wider than normal (greater than 0.10 second but less than 0.12 second) if the pacemaker site is in the bundle branches below the bundle of His. **Fusion beats** may be present if a supraventricular rhythm is present and particularly if its rate is about the same as that of the accelerated idioventricular rhythm. When this occurs, the cardiac rhythm alternates between the supraventricular rhythm and the accelerated idioventricular rhythm. Fusion beats most commonly occur at the onset and end of the arrhythmia. (See the discussion of fusion beats under Premature Ventricular Contractions, page 170.)

Cause of Arrhythmia

Accelerated idioventricular rhythm is relatively common in acute myocardial infarction. It occurs (1) when the firing rate of the dominant pacemaker (usually the SA node) or escape pacemaker in the AV junction becomes less than that of the ventricular ectopic pacemaker or (2) when a sinus arrest, sinoatrial (SA) exit block, or third-degree (complete) AV block develops. Accelerated idioventricular rhythm may also result from digitalis toxicity. The electrophysiological mechanism responsible for accelerated idioventricular rhythm is probably **enhanced automaticity.**

Clinical Significance

Accelerated idioventricular rhythm occurring in acute myocardial infarction usually requires no treatment since it is self-limited in most cases. Because it does not affect the course or prognosis of the myocardial infarction, it is considered relatively benign.

Notes

Accelerated Idioventricular Rhythm (AIVR)
(Accelerated Ventricular Rhythm, Idioventricular
Tachycardia, Slow Ventricular Tachycardia)

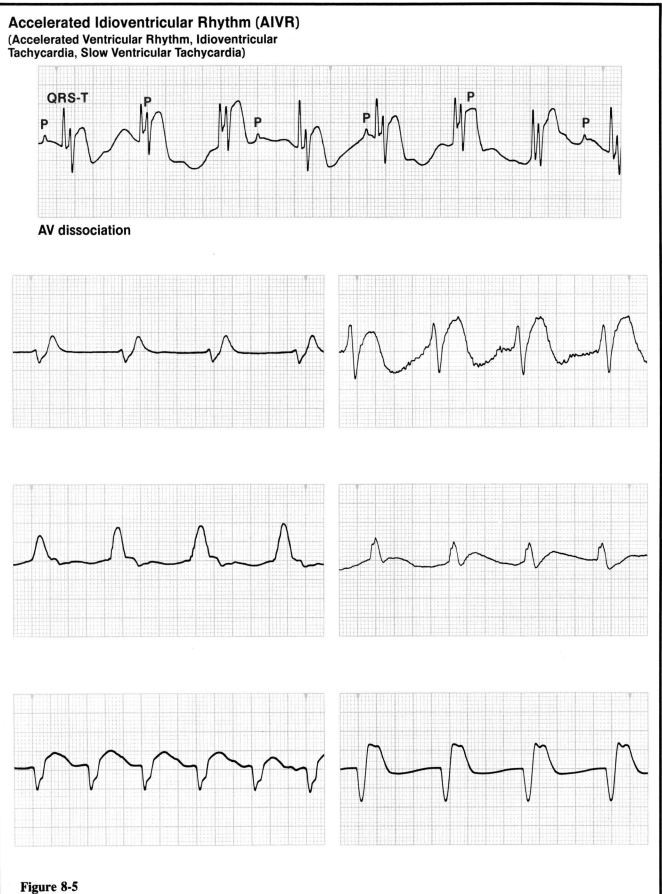

AV dissociation

Figure 8-5

Ventricular Escape Rhythm
(Idioventricular Rhythm)

Definition

Ventricular escape rhythm (Figure 8-6) is an arrhythmia originating in an escape pacemaker in the ventricles with a rate of less than 40 beats per minute. When less than three QRS complexes arising from the escape pacemaker are present, they are called **ventricular escape beats** or **complexes.**

Diagnostic Characteristics

Heart rate: The heart rate is less than 40 beats per minute, usually between 30 and 40 beats per minute, but it may be less.

Rhythm: The rhythm is usually regular, but it may be irregular.

Pacemaker site: The pacemaker site of **ventricular escape rhythm** is an escape pacemaker in the bundle branches, Purkinje network, or ventricular myocardium.

P waves: P waves may be present or absent. If present, they have no set relation to the QRS complexes of the ventricular escape rhythm, appearing independently at a rate different from that of the QRS complexes. The pacemaker site of such P waves is the SA node or an ectopic or escape pacemaker in the atria or AV junction. These P waves may be positive (upright) or negative (inverted) in lead II.

They precede, are buried in, or follow the QRS complexes haphazardly. When the atria and ventricles thus beat independently, **atrioventricular (AV) dissociation** is present.

PR intervals: PR intervals are absent.

R-R intervals: The R-R intervals may be equal or may vary.

QRS complexes: The QRS complexes exceed 0.12 second and are bizarre. Sometimes the shape of the QRS complexes varies in any given lead.

Cause of Arrhythmia

Ventricular escape rhythm usually occurs (1) when the rate of impulse formation of the dominant pacemaker (usually the SA node) and escape pacemaker in the AV junction becomes less than that of the escape pacemaker in the ventricles or (2) when the electrical impulses from the SA node, atria, and AV junction fail to reach the ventricles because of a sinus arrest, sinoatrial (SA) exit block, or third-degree (complete) AV block. Generally, when an electrical impulse fails to arrive in the ventricles within approximately 1.5 to 2.0 seconds, an escape pacemaker in the ventricles takes over at its inherent firing rate of 30 to 40 beats per minute. The result is one or more ventricular escape beats or a ventricular escape rhythm.

Ventricular escape rhythm also occurs in advanced heart disease and is often the cardiac arrhythmia that is present in a dying heart, the so-called **agonal rhythm,** just before the appearance of the final arrhythmia, ventricular asystole.

Clinical Significance

Ventricular escape rhythm is generally symptomatic. Hypotension with marked reduction in cardiac output and decreased perfusion of the brain and other vital organs may occur, resulting in syncope, shock, or congestive heart failure. Ventricular escape rhythm must be treated promptly, preferably with a transcutaneous pacemaker to reverse the consequences of the reduced cardiac output.

Notes

Ventricular Escape Rhythm
(Idioventricular Rhythm)

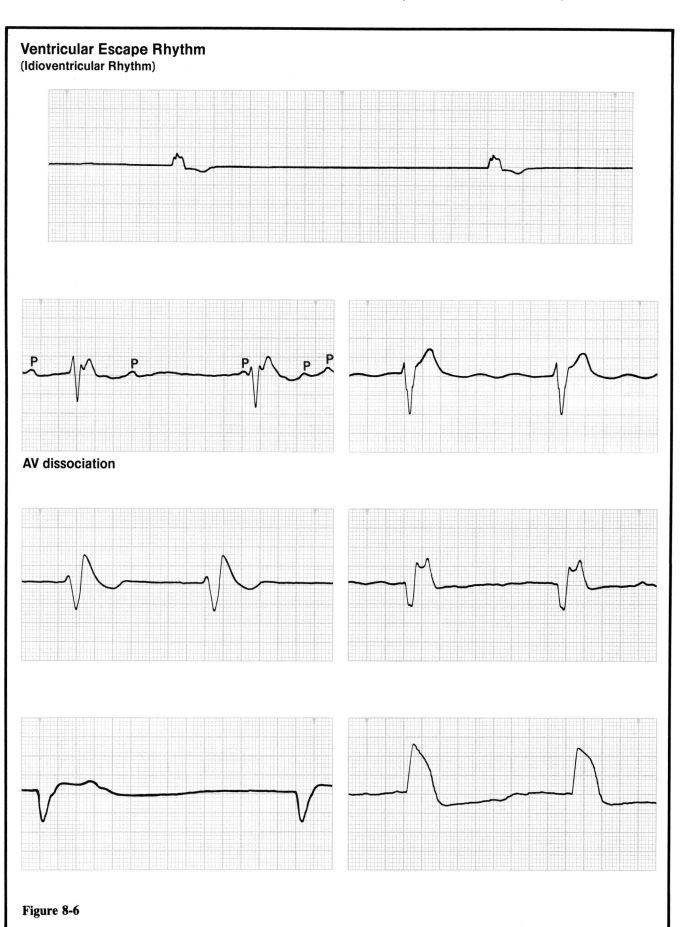

AV dissociation

Figure 8-6

Ventricular Asystole
(Cardiac Standstill)

Definition

Ventricular asystole (Figure 8-7) is the absence of all electrical activity within the ventricles.

Diagnostic Characteristics

Heart rate: Heart rate is absent.

Rhythm: Rhythm is absent.

Pacemaker site: A pacemaker site in the ventricles is absent. If P waves are present, their pacemaker site is the SA node or an ectopic or escape pacemaker in the atria or AV junction.

P waves: P waves may be present or absent.

PR intervals: PR intervals are absent.

R-R intervals: R-R intervals are absent.

QRS complexes: QRS complexes are absent.

Cause of Arrhythmia

Ventricular asystole, one of the common causes of cardiac arrest, may occur in advanced cardiac disease as a primary event when the dominant pacemaker (usually the SA node) and/or the escape pacemaker in the AV junction fail to generate electrical impulses or when the electrical impulses are blocked from entering the ventricles because of a third-degree (complete) AV block and an escape pacemaker in the ventricles fails to take over. In the dying heart, ventricular asystole is usually the final arrhythmia following ventricular tachycardia, ventricular fibrillation, electromechanical dissociation, or ventricular escape rhythm. Ventricular asystole may also follow the termination of tachyarrhythmias by whatever means—drugs or **defibrillation shock** or **synchronized countershock.**

Clinical Significance

Organized ventricular depolarization and contraction and, consequently, cardiac output are absent in ventricular asystole. The occurrence of sudden ventricular asystole in a conscious person results in faintness, followed within seconds by loss of consciousness, seizures, and apnea **(Adams-Stokes syndrome),** and, if the arrhythmia remains untreated, death. Ventricular asystole must be treated immediately.

Electromechanical dissociation (EMD) is the absence of effective ventricular contraction, cardiac output, and pulse in the presence of an ECG—a life-threatening condition. See discussion of EMD under Pulseless Electrical Activity (PEA) in Chapter 13.

Notes

Ventricular Asystole
(Cardiac Standstill)

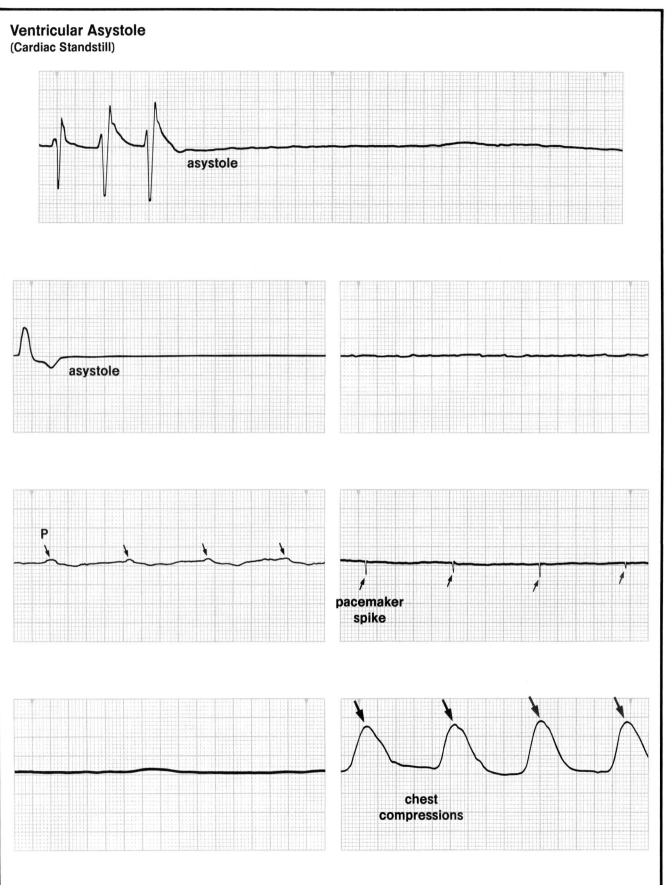

Figure 8-7

1. An extra contraction consisting of an abnormally wide and bizarre QRS complex originating in an ectopic pacemaker in the ventricles is called a:
   A. PAC
   B. PJC
   C. PVC
   D. none of the above

2. Identical premature ventricular contractions that originate from a single ectopic pacemaker site are called:
   A. multifocal
   B. unifocal
   C. multiform
   D. isolated

3. A PVC may:
   A. trigger ventricular fibrillation if it occurs on the T wave
   B. depolarize the SA node, momentarily suppressing it, so that the next P wave of the underlying rhythm appears later than expected
   C. all of the above
   D. none of the above

4. A PVC that appears relatively normal usually originates:
   A. near the bifurcation of the bundle of His
   B. in the Purkinje network
   C. in the AV junction
   D. in the SA node

5. A QRS that has characteristics of both the PVC and a QRS complex of the underlying rhythm is called a(n):
   A. fascicular PVC
   B. multifocal PVC
   C. ventricular fusion beat
   D. isolated PVC

6. Groups of two or more PVCs are called:
   A. ventricular group beats
   B. bursts
   C. salvos
   D. all of the above

7. A reentry mechanism may precipitate:
   A. repetitive ventricular contractions
   B. ventricular tachycardia
   C. ventricular fibrillation
   D. all of the above

8. PVCs may be caused by:
   A. stimulants
   B. hyperkalemia
   C. a decrease in sympathetic tone
   D. alkalosis

9. A form of ventricular tachycardia characterized by QRS complexes that gradually change back and forth from one shape and direction to another over a series of beats is called:
   A. multiform ventricular tachycardia
   B. torsade de pointes
   C. bigeminy
   D. none of the above

10. When the ventricles contract between 300 and 500 times a minute in an unsynchronized, uncoordinated manner, the immediate treatment is:
    A. pacing
    B. bretylium
    C. defibrillation
    D. lidocaine

CHAPTER
9

AV Blocks

First-degree AV Block

Second-degree AV Block

Type I AV Block (Wenckebach)

Second-degree AV Block

Type II AV Block

Second-degree AV Block

2:1 and High-degree (Advanced) AV Block

Third-degree AV Block (Complete AV Block)

Pacemaker Rhythm

OBJECTIVES

Upon completion of all or part of this chapter you should be able to complete the following objectives indicated by your instructor:

☐ **1.** Define and give the diagnostic characteristics, cause, and clinical significance of the following arrhythmias:

☐ First-degree AV block

☐ Second-degree, Type I AV block (Wenckebach)

☐ Second-degree, Type II AV block

☐ Second-degree, 2:1 and high-degree (advanced) AV block

☐ Third-degree (complete AV block)

☐ Pacemaker rhythm

First-degree AV Block

Definition

First-degree AV block (Figure 9-1) is an arrhythmia in which there is a constant delay in the conduction of electrical impulses, usually through the AV node. It is characterized by abnormally prolonged PR intervals that are greater than 0.20 second and constant.

Diagnostic Characteristics

Heart rate: The heart rate is that of the underlying sinus or atrial rhythm. The **atrial** and **ventricular rates** are typically the same.

Rhythm: The rhythm is that of the underlying rhythm.

Pacemaker site: The pacemaker site is that of the underlying rhythm.

P waves: The P waves are identical and precede each QRS complex.

PR intervals: The PR intervals are abnormal (greater than 0.20 second) and usually do not vary from beat to beat.

R-R intervals: The R-R intervals are those of the underlying rhythm.

QRS complexes: The QRS complexes are usually normal, but they may be abnormal (rarely) because of a preexisting bundle branch block. Typically, the AV conduction ratio is 1:1, that is, a QRS complex follows each P wave.

Cause of Arrhythmia

First-degree AV block usually represents a delay in the conduction of the electrical impulses through the AV node, and, thus, the QRS complexes are typically normal—unless a preexisting bundle branch block is present. Infrequently, the AV block may occur below the AV node (**infranodal**) in the His-Purkinje system of the ventricles (i.e., bundle of His or bundle branches). Although first-degree AV block may appear without any apparent cause, it occurs commonly in acute inferior myocardial infarction because of the effect of an increase in vagal (parasympathetic) tone and ischemia on the AV node. It can also occur as the result of an increase in vagal tone from whatever cause or from digitalis toxicity.

Clinical Significance

First-degree AV block produces no signs or symptoms per se and requires no treatment. Because it can progress to a higher-degree AV block, the patient requires observation and ECG monitoring.

Notes

First-degree AV Block

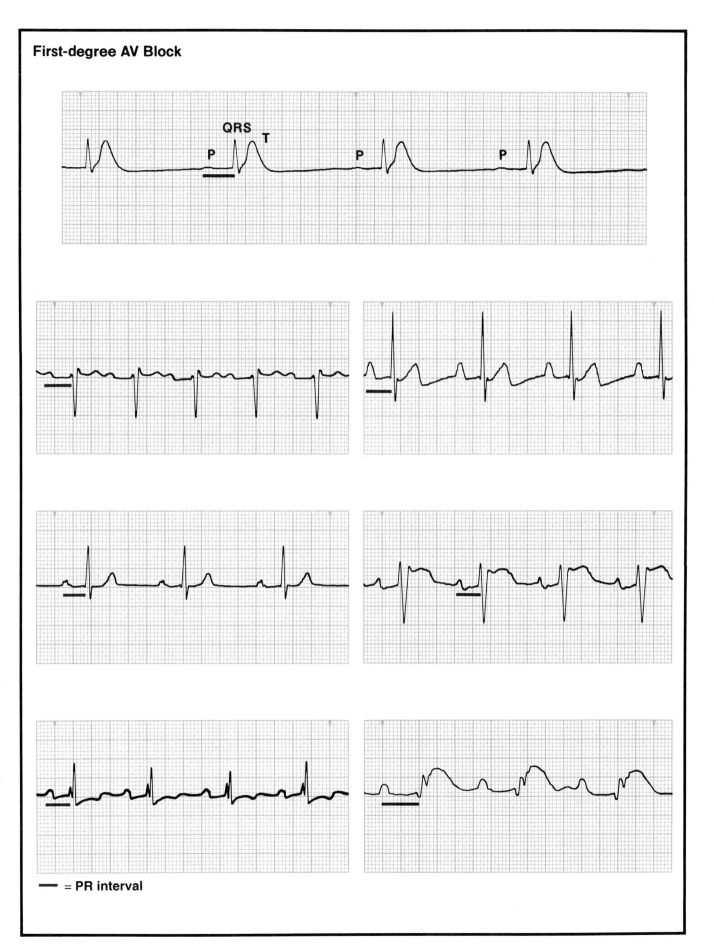

= PR interval

Figure 9-1

Second-degree AV Block
Type I AV Block (Wenckebach)

Definition

Second-degree, type I AV block (Wenckebach) (Figure 9-2) is an arrhythmia in which there is a progressive delay, following each P wave, in the conduction of electrical impulses through the AV node until conduction is completely blocked. This arrhythmia is characterized by progressive lengthening of the PR intervals until a QRS complex fails to appear after a P wave. The sequence of increasing PR intervals and absent QRS complex is repetitive.

Diagnostic Characteristics

Heart rate: The **atrial rate** is that of the underlying sinus or atrial rhythm. The **ventricular rate** is typically less than the atrial rate.

Rhythm: The **atrial rhythm** is essentially regular. The **ventricular rhythm** is usually irregular.

Pacemaker site: The pacemaker site is that of the underlying rhythm.

P waves: The P waves are identical and precede the QRS complexes when they occur.

PR intervals: The PR intervals gradually lengthen until a QRS complex fails to appear after a P wave (**nonconducted P wave** or **dropped beat**). Following the pause produced by the nonconducted P wave, the sequence begins anew.

R-R intervals: The R-R intervals are unequal. As the PR intervals gradually lengthen, the R-R intervals typically decrease gradually until the P wave is not conducted. The cycle then repeats itself. The reason for the progressive decrease in the R-R intervals is that the PR intervals do not increase in such increments as to maintain the R-R intervals at the same duration as that of the first one immediately following the nonconducted P wave. This characteristic cyclic decrease in the R-R intervals may also be seen in atrial fibrillation complicated by a Wenckebach block.

Rarely, the R-R interval may remain constant until the nonconduction of the P wave. The R-R interval that includes the nonconducted P wave is usually less than the sum of two of the R-R intervals of the underlying rhythm.

QRS complexes: The QRS complexes are typically normal, but they may be abnormal (rarely) because of a preexisting bundle branch block. Commonly, the AV conduction ratio is 5:4, 4:3, or 3:2 but may be 6:5, 7:6, and so forth. An AV conduction ratio of 5:4, for example, indicates that for every five P waves, four are followed by QRS complexes. The repetitive sequence of two or more beats in a row followed by a dropped beat is called **group beating.** The AV conduction ratio may be fixed or may vary in any given lead.

Cause of Arrhythmia

Type I second-degree AV block most commonly represents defective conduction of the electrical impulses through the AV node, and, thus, the QRS complexes are typically normal unless a preexisting bundle branch block is present. The AV block may infrequently occur below the AV node (**infranodal**) in the His-Purkinje system of the ventricles (i.e., bundle of His or bundle branches). Type I second-degree AV block often occurs as does first-degree AV block in acute inferior myocardial infarction because of the effect of an increase in vagal (parasympathetic) tone and ischemia on the AV node. It also may be caused by acute infections, such as rheumatic fever and acute myocarditis; increased vagal tone from whatever cause; drug toxicity (e.g., digitalis, propranolol, and diltiazem or verapamil); or electrolyte imbalance.

Clinical Significance

Type I second-degree AV block is usually transient and reversible. Although it produces few if any symptoms per se, it can progress to a higher-degree AV block. For this reason, the patient requires observation and ECG monitoring. Type I AV block does respond to atropine if it is necessary to increase the heart rate.

Notes

Second-degree AV Block
Type I AV Block (Wenckebach)

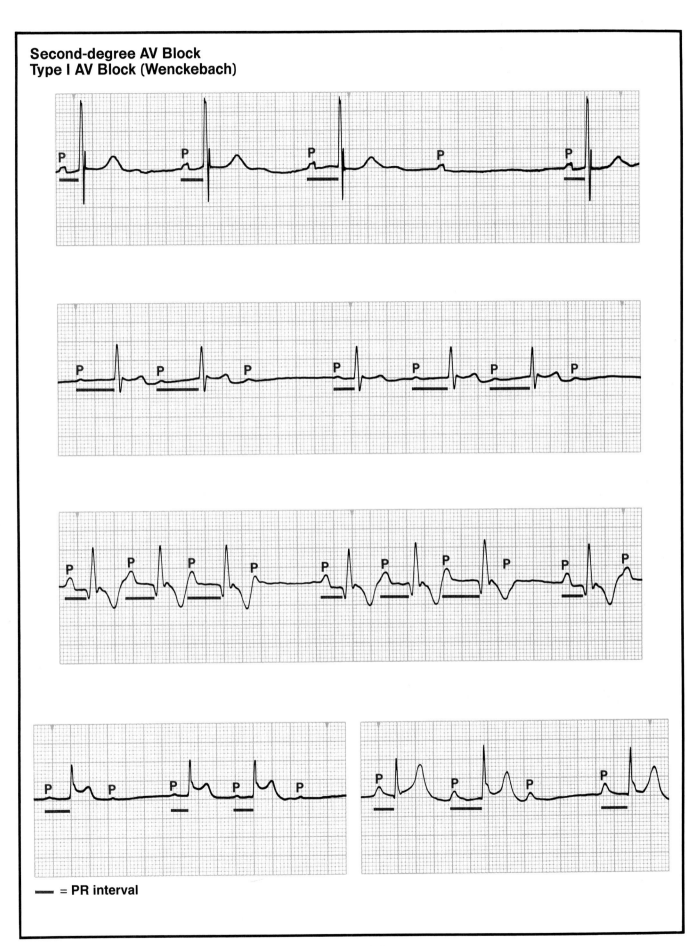

■ = PR interval

Figure 9-2

Second-degree AV Block
Type II AV Block

Definition

Second-degree, type II AV block (Figure 9-3) is an arrhythmia in which a complete block of conduction of the electrical impulses occurs in one bundle branch and an intermittent block in the other. This produces an AV block characterized by regularly or irregularly absent QRS complexes, commonly producing an AV conduction ratio of 4:3 or 3:2, and a bundle branch block.

Diagnostic Characteristics

Heart rate: The **atrial rate** is that of the underlying sinus, atrial, or junctional rhythm. The **ventricular rate** is typically less than the atrial rate.

Rhythm: The **atrial rhythm** is essentially regular. The **ventricular rhythm** is usually irregular.

Pacemaker site: The pacemaker site is that of the underlying rhythm.

P waves: The P waves are identical and precede the QRS complexes when they occur.

PR intervals: The PR intervals may be normal or abnormal (greater than 0.20 second). They are usually constant.

R-R intervals: The R-R intervals are equal except for those that include the **nonconducted P waves (dropped beats);** these are equal to or slightly less than twice the R-R interval of the underlying rhythm.

QRS complexes: The QRS complexes are typically abnormal (greater than 0.12 second) because of a bundle branch block. Rarely, the QRS complex may be normal (0.10 second or less) if the AV block is at the level of the bundle of His and a preexisting bundle branch block is not present. Commonly, the AV conduction ratio is 4:3 or 3:2 but may be 5:4,

6:5, 7:6, and so forth. An AV conduction ratio of 4:3, for example, indicates that for every four P waves, three are followed by QRS complexes. The repetitive sequence of two or more beats in a row followed by a dropped beat is called **group beating.** The AV conduction ratio may be fixed, or it may vary within any given lead.

Cause of Arrhythmia

Type II second-degree AV block usually occurs below the bundle of His and represents an intermittent block of conduction of the electrical impulses through one bundle branch and a complete block in the other. This produces an intermittent AV block with abnormally wide and bizarre QRS complexes. Commonly, type II second-degree AV block is the result of extensive damage to the bundle branches following an acute anteroseptal myocardial infarction, and, unlike type I second-degree AV block, not the result of an acute inferior myocardial infarction or increased vagal (parasympathetic) tone or drug toxicity on the AV node. Rarely, the AV block occurs at the level of the bundle of His. When this occurs, the QRS complexes are normal (0.10 second or less) unless a preexisting bundle branch block is present.

Clinical Significance

The signs and symptoms of type II second-degree AV block with excessively slow heart rates are the same as those in symptomatic sinus bradycardia. Because type II second-degree AV block is more serious than type I AV block, often progressing to a third-degree AV block and even ventricular asystole, a transcutaneous pacemaker is indicated immediately, whether or not symptoms are present, especially in the setting of an acute anteroseptal myocardial infarction. Atropine is usually ineffective in reversing a type II AV block.

Notes

Second-degree AV Block
Type II AV Block

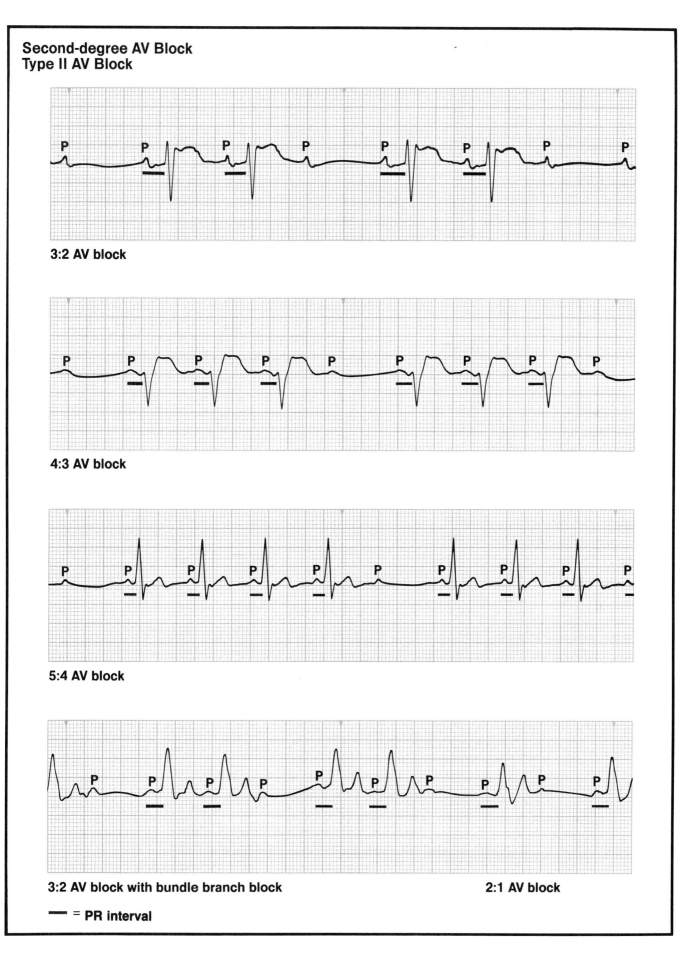

3:2 AV block

4:3 AV block

5:4 AV block

3:2 AV block with bundle branch block   **2:1 AV block**

━━ = PR interval

Figure 9-3

Second-degree AV Block
2:1 and High-degree (Advanced) AV Block

Definition

Second-degree, 2:1 and high-degree (advanced) AV block (Figure 9-4) is an arrhythmia caused by the defective conduction of electrical impulses through the AV node or the bundle branches, or both. This produces an AV block characterized by regularly or irregularly absent QRS complexes, commonly producing an AV conduction ratio of 2:1 or greater, with or without a bundle branch block.

Diagnostic Characteristics

Heart rate: The **atrial rate** is that of the underlying sinus, atrial, or junctional rhythm. The **ventricular rate** is typically less than the atrial rate.

Rhythm: The **atrial rhythm** is essentially regular. The **ventricular rhythm** may be regular or irregular. The ventricular rhythm is irregular when the AV block is intermittent or when the AV conduction ratio is variable.

Pacemaker site: The pacemaker site is that of the underlying rhythm.

P waves: The P waves are identical and precede the QRS complexes when they occur.

PR intervals: The PR intervals may be normal or abnormal (greater than 0.20 second); they are constant.

R-R intervals: The R-R intervals may be equal or may vary.

QRS complexes: The QRS complexes may be normal or abnormal because of a bundle branch block. Commonly, the AV conduction ratios are even numbers, such as 2:1, 4:1, 6:1, 8:1, and so forth, but may be uneven numbers, such as 3:1 or 5:1. The AV block is identified by the AV conduction ratio present (e.g., 2:1, 3:1, 4:1, or 6:1 AV block). A

3:1 or higher AV block is called a **high-degree (or advanced) AV block.** An AV conduction ratio of 3:1, for example, indicates that for every three P waves, one is followed by a QRS complex. The AV conduction ratio may be fixed, or it may vary in any given lead.

Cause of Arrhythmia

2:1 and high-degree AV block with normal QRS complexes usually represents defective conduction of the electrical impulses through the AV node and is often associated with a **second-degree, type I AV block.** It is commonly caused by an acute inferior myocardial infarction, myocarditis, digitalis toxicity, or electrolyte imbalance.

2:1 and high-degree AV block with wide QRS complexes usually represents defective conduction of the electrical impulses through the bundle branches and is often associated with a **second-degree, type II AV block.** This type of AV block is commonly caused by an acute anteroseptal myocardial infarction.

Clinical Significance

When the heart rate is excessively slow in 2:1 and high-degree AV block, the signs and symptoms are the same as those in symptomatic sinus bradycardia. 2:1 and high-degree AV block with normal QRS complexes may often be transient; however, 2:1 and high-degree AV block with wide QRS complexes frequently progresses to a third-degree AV block.

A transcutaneous pacemaker is indicated in all symptomatic patients with 2:1 and high-degree AV block and in asymptomatic patients with wide QRS complexes, especially in the setting of an acute anteroseptal myocardial infarction. 2:1 and high-degree AV block with normal QRS complexes usually responds to atropine.

Notes

Second-degree AV Block
2:1 and High-degree (Advanced) AV Block

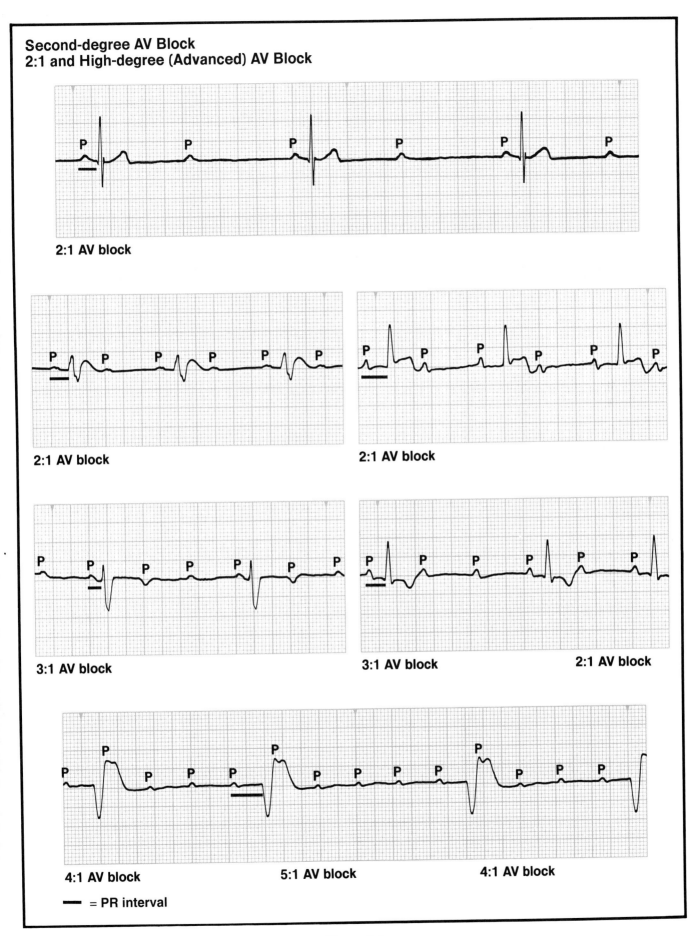

2:1 AV block

2:1 AV block

2:1 AV block

3:1 AV block

3:1 AV block

2:1 AV block

4:1 AV block

5:1 AV block

4:1 AV block

▬ = PR interval

Figure 9-4

Third-degree AV Block
(Complete AV Block)

Definition

Third-degree AV block (Figure 9-5) is the complete absence of conduction of the electrical impulses through the AV node, bundle of His, or bundle branches, characterized by independent beating of the atria and ventricles.

Diagnostic Characteristics

Heart rate: The **atrial rate** is that of the underlying sinus, atrial, or junctional rhythm. The **ventricular rate** is typically 40 to 60 beats per minute, but it may be as slow as 30 to 40 or less. The ventricular rate is usually less than the atrial rate.

Rhythm: The **atrial rhythm** may be regular or irregular, depending on the underlying sinus, atrial, or junctional rhythm. The **ventricular rhythm** is essentially regular. The atrial and ventricular rhythms are independent of each other (**atrioventricular [AV] dissociation**).

Pacemaker site: If P waves are present, they may have originated in the SA node or an ectopic pacemaker in the atria or AV junction. The pacemaker site of the QRS complexes is an escape pacemaker in the AV junction, bundle branches, or Purkinje network, below the AV block. Generally, if the third-degree AV block is at the level of the AV node, the escape pacemaker is usually infranodal, in the bundle of His. If the third-degree AV block is at the level of the bundle of His or bundle branches, the escape pacemaker is in the ventricles distal to the site of the AV block. If the escape pacemaker is in the AV junction (i.e., **junctional escape rhythm**), the heart rate is 40 to 60 beats per minute. If the escape pacemaker is in the ventricles, i.e., bundle branches or Purkinje network (**ventricular escape rhythm**), the heart rate is 30 to 40 beats per minute or less.

P waves: P waves or atrial flutter or fibrillation waves may be present. When present, they have no relation to the QRS complexes, appearing independently at a rate different from that of the QRS complexes (**AV dissociation**).

PR intervals: The PR intervals vary widely since the P waves and QRS complexes occur independently.

R-R and P-P intervals: The R-R intervals are usually equal and independent of the P-P intervals.

QRS complexes: The QRS complexes typically exceed 0.12 second and are bizarre if the escape pacemaker site is in the ventricles or if the escape pacemaker site is in the AV junction and a preexisting bundle branch block is present. But the QRS complexes may be normal (0.10 second or less) if the pacemaker site is above the bundle branches in the AV junction and no bundle branch block is present.

Cause of Arrhythmia

Third-degree AV block represents a complete block of the conduction of the electrical impulses from the atria to the ventricles at the level of the AV node, bundle of His, or bundle branches. It may be **transient and reversible** or **permanent.**

Transient and reversible third-degree AV block is usually associated with normal QRS complexes and a heart rate of 45 to 60 beats per minute (i.e., **junctional escape rhythm**). It is commonly due to a complete block of conduction of the electrical impulses through the AV node. This can result from ischemia of the AV node associated with an acute inferior myocardial infarction, increased vagal (parasympathetic) tone, acute myocarditis, digitalis or propranolol toxicity, or electrolyte imbalance.

Permanent or chronic third-degree AV block is usually associated with wide QRS complexes and a heart rate of 30 to 40 beats per minute or less (i.e., **ventricular escape rhythm**). It is commonly due to a complete block of conduction of electrical impulses through both bundle branches. The most likely causes are acute anteroseptal myocardial infarction and chronic degenerative changes in the bundle branches present in the elderly. Permanent third-degree AV block usually does not result from increased vagal (parasympathetic) tone or drug toxicity.

Third-degree AV Block
(Complete AV Block)

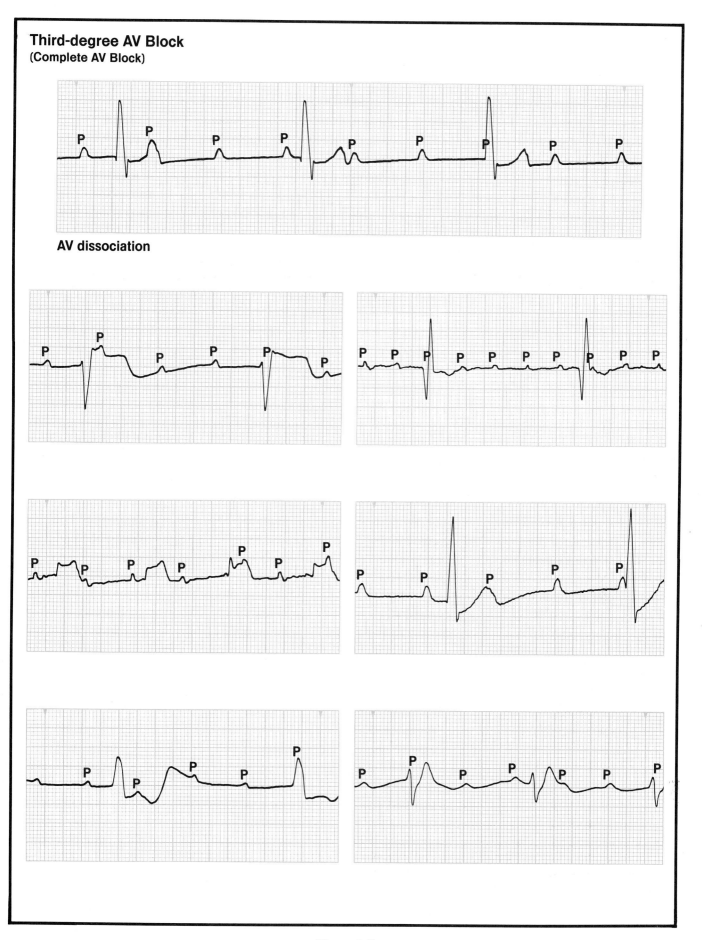

AV dissociation

Figure 9-5

Clinical Significance

The signs and symptoms of third-degree AV block are the same as those in symptomatic sinus bradycardia, except that third-degree AV block can be more ominous, especially when it is associated with wide and bizarre QRS complexes. If an AV junctional or ventricular escape pacemaker does not take over after a sudden onset of third-degree AV block, ventricular asystole will occur. This results in faintness, followed within seconds by loss of consciousness, seizures, and apnea **(Adams-Stokes syndrome),** and death if an escape pacemaker does not respond or ventricular asystole is not treated immediately.

A transcutaneous pacemaker is required immediately for the treatment of symptomatic third-degree AV block with wide QRS complexes (regardless of cause) and for asymptomatic third-degree AV block with wide QRS complexes in a setting of an acute anteroseptal myocardial infarction. Third-degree AV block with narrow QRS complexes does respond to atropine occasionally if it is caused by an acute inferior myocardial infarction.

Notes

Pacemaker Rhythm

Definition

A **pacemaker rhythm** (Figure 9-6) consists of the beats and rhythm produced by a cardiac pacemaker.

Types of Pacemakers

There are two basic kinds of pacemakers: **fixed rate** and **demand.**

- **Fixed rate pacemakers** are designed to fire constantly at a preset rate without regard to the patient's own electrical activity of the heart.
- **Demand pacemakers** have a sensing device that senses the heart's electrical activity and fires at a preset rate only when the heart's electrical activity drops below a predetermined rate level.

Pacemakers can be either **single-chamber pacemakers** that pace either the ventricles or atria or **dual-chambered pacemakers** that pace both the atria and ventricles. Examples of commonly used pacemakers from each category are described below and their **Intersociety Commission for Heart Disease Resources (ICHD) code** is noted.

- The **first of the three letters** of the code indicates which chamber is paced: **A** = atria, **V** = ventricles, **D** = both atria and ventricles.
- The **second letter** indicates which chamber is sensed: **A** = atria, **V** = ventricles, **D** = both atria and ventricles.
- The **third letter** indicates the response of the pacemaker to a P wave or QRS complex: **I** = pacemaker output is inhibited by the P wave or QRS complex, **D** = pacemaker output is inhibited by a QRS complex and triggered by a P wave.

Single Chamber Pacemakers:

Atrial demand pacemaker (AAI). A pacemaker that senses spontaneously occurring P waves and **paces the atria** when they do not appear.

Ventricular demand pacemaker (VVI). A pacemaker that senses spontaneously occurring QRS complexes and **paces the ventricles** when they do not appear.

Dual Chamber Pacemakers:

Atrial synchronous ventricular pacemaker (VDD). A pacemaker that senses spontaneously occurring P waves and QRS complexes and **paces the ventricles** when QRS complexes fail to appear after spontaneously occurring P waves, as in complete AV block. In this type of pacemaker, the pacing of the ventricles is synchronized with the P waves, so that the ventricular contractions follow the atrial contractions in a normal sequence.

AV sequential pacemaker (DVI). A pacemaker that senses spontaneously occurring QRS complexes and **paces both the atria and ventricles** (the atria first, followed by the ventricles after a short delay) when QRS complexes do not appear.

Optimal sequential pacemaker (DDD). A pacemaker that senses spontaneously occurring P waves and QRS complexes and (1) **paces the atria** when P waves fail to appear, as in sick sinus syndrome, and (2) **paces the ventricles** when QRS complexes fail to appear after spontaneously occurring or paced P waves. In this type of pacemaker, like the VDD pacemaker, the pacing of the ventricles is synchronized with the atrial activity so that the ventricular contractions follow the atrial contractions in a normal sequence.

Diagnostic Features

Heart rate: The heart rate produced by a permanently implanted **cardiac pacemaker** is usually between 60 and 70 beats per minute, depending on its preset rate of firing. If the pacemaker rate is greater than 90 beats per minute, it is probably malfunctioning.

Rhythm: The ventricular rhythm produced by a pacemaker that is pacing constantly is regular. The ventricular rate may be irregular when the pacemaker is pacing on demand.

Pacemaker site: The pacing site of a cardiac pacemaker is an electrode usually located in the tip of the pacemaker lead, commonly positioned in the apex of the right ventricular cavity (**ventricular pacemaker),** in the right atrium (**atrial pacemaker),** or in both (**dual chamber pacemaker).**

Pacemaker spikes: The electrical discharge from a cardiac pacemaker produces a narrow, often biphasic spike. A pacemaker lead positioned in the atria produces a pacemaker spike followed by a small, often flattened P wave; a pacemaker lead positioned in the ventricles produces a wide (0.12 second or greater) and bizarre QRS complex. A P wave or QRS complex following a pacemaker spike indicates **"capturing"** by the cardiac pacemaker. A pacemaker spike not followed by a P wave or QRS complex indicates that the pacemaker is discharging but not capturing. In a fixed rate pacemaker, the pacemaker spikes occur at regular intervals. In a demand pacemaker, the pacemaker spikes in the atria and/or ventricles occur at regular intervals or occur intermittently interspersed with the patient's own electrical activity of the heart.

P waves: P waves may be present or absent. If present, they may be spontaneously occurring or induced by a pacemaker lead positioned in the atria. When not followed by inherent QRS complexes, spontaneously occurring P waves are usually followed by pacemaker-induced QRS complexes. This indicates that a dual chamber VDD or DDD pacemaker is present. A narrow, often biphasic spike— the pacemaker spike—precedes pacemaker-induced P waves. These P waves may be followed by the inherent QRS complexes or pacemaker-induced QRS complexes as seen in dual chamber DVI or DDD pacemakers. A ventricular pacemaker usually does not produce a retrograde, inverted P wave.

PR intervals: The PR intervals of the underlying rhythm may be normal (0.12 to 0.20 second) or abnormal depending on the arrhythmia. The PR intervals in atrial synchronous and dual-paced, AV sequential pacemakers are within normal limits.

R-R intervals: The R-R intervals of the pacemaker rhythm are equal. When the pacemaker-induced QRS complexes are interspersed among the patient's normally occurring QRS complexes, the R-R intervals are unequal.

QRS complexes: The QRS complexes of the underlying rhythm may be normal (0.10 second or less in width) or abnormal. Pacemaker-induced QRS complexes are typically greater than 0.12 second in width and bizarre. Preceding each pacemaker-induced QRS complex is a narrow deflection, often biphasic, the pacemaker spike, representing the electrical discharge of the pacemaker. If only the atria are being paced, the QRS complexes are those of the underlying rhythm. These are normal unless a preexisting bundle branch block is present.

Clinical Significance

A pacemaker rhythm indicates that the patient's heart is being electronically paced. Cardiac pacemakers are usually permanently implanted in patients to correct an underlying third-degree AV block or episodes of symptomatic bradycardia. Usually a 2 ½- to 3-inch diameter bulge is present in the upper, anterior chest wall, indicating an implanted cardiac pacemaker.

The presence of pacemaker spikes followed by a QRS complex indicates that the patient's heart rate is being regulated by a cardiac pacemaker. When a normal or wide and bizarre QRS complex follows every pacemaker spike or every paced P wave (as seen in single-chamber pacing) or every pair of pacemaker spikes (as seen in dual-chamber pacing), the pacemaker is apparently functioning normally even if the patient's own P waves and QRS complexes are interspersed between the pacemaker spikes and associated QRS complexes.

Some of the problems that can occur with cardiac pacemakers include:
- Presence of pacemaker spikes that are not followed by P waves or QRS complexes indicates a malfunctioning pacemaker, one whose electric impulses are unable to stimulate the heart to depolarize. The failure to capture most likely results from the current output of the pacemaker being adjusted too low.
- Complete absence of pacemaker spikes in the presence of bradycardia or ventricular asystole indicates battery failure.
- A pacemaker spike rate of over 300 per minute causing a ventricular tachyarrhythmia can occur in older models of pacemakers. This indicates a malfunction in the electrical impulse generating circuit, usually the result of low battery power. Such a malfunctioning pacemaker is known as a runaway pacemaker.
- Failure of a demand pacemaker to shut off when the patient has adequate electrical activity of the heart indicates a failure in the pacemaker's sensing circuit. The danger here is that the pacemaker spikes may fall on the vulnerable period of the cardiac cycle, triggering a life-threatening arrhythmia.

No treatment is necessary if the cardiac pacemaker is functioning properly. Appropriate treatment may be necessary if the pacemaker is malfunctioning and an underlying bradyarrhythmia, ventricular asystole, or ventricular fibrillation is

Pacemaker Rhythm

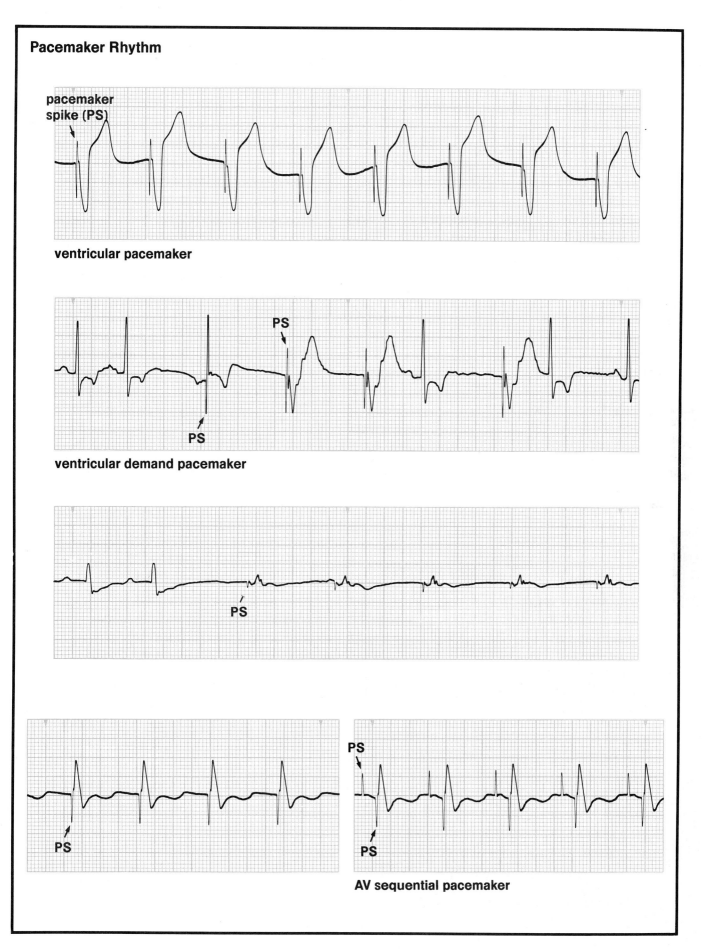

pacemaker
spike (PS)

ventricular pacemaker

PS

PS

ventricular demand pacemaker

PS

PS

PS

PS

PS

AV sequential pacemaker

Figure 9-6

present. Lidocaine may be administered without inhibiting the heart's response to the pacemaker. When delivering a defibrillatory shock or countershock, the defibrillator paddles should be placed about 2 inches away from the cardiac pacemaker and not directly over it.

Notes

CHAPTER REVIEW QUESTIONS

1. An arrhythmia that occurs commonly in acute inferior myocardial infarction because of the effect of an increase in vagal (parasympathetic) tone and ischemia on the AV node is called:
   A. chronic third-degree AV block
   B. second-degree, type II AV block
   C. first-degree AV block
   D. ventricular tachycardia

2. An arrhythmia in which there is a progressive delay following each P wave in the conduction of electrical impulses through the AV node until the conduction of electrical impulses is completely blocked is called a:
   A. first-degree AV block
   B. second-degree, type I AV block
   C. second-degree, type II AV block
   D. third-degree AV block

3. Second-degree, type I AV block is usually transient and reversible yet the patient should be monitored and observed because:
   A. it can progress to a higher degree AV block
   B. it can progress to ventricular tachycardia
   C. it is symptomatic
   D. none of the above

4. An arrhythmia in which a complete block of conduction of electrical impulses occurs in one bundle branch and an intermittent block in the other is called:
   A. first-degree AV block
   B. second-degree, type I AV block
   C. second-degree, type II AV block
   D. third-degree AV block

5. If a second-degree, type II AV block presents in the setting of an acute anteroseptal MI, the immediate treatment is:
   A. a transcutaneous pacemaker
   B. atropine
   C. an isoproterenol drip
   D. none of the above

6. A high-degree or advanced AV block has an AV conduction ratio of:
   A. 8:1 or greater
   B. 4:1 or 6:1
   C. 3:1 or 4:1
   D. all of the above

7. The absence of conduction of electrical impulses through the AV node, bundle of His, or bundle branches, characterized by independent beating of the atria and ventricles, is called a:
   A. second-degree, type I AV block
   B. second-degree, type II AV block
   C. third-degree AV block
   D. first-degree AV block

8. An escape pacemaker in the AV junction has a firing rate of _____ beats per minute.
   A. 100 to 120
   B. 80 to 100
   C. 60 to 80
   D. 40 to 60

9. If an AV junctional or ventricular escape pacemaker does not take over a sudden onset of third-degree AV block, ventricular asystole will occur, resulting in:
   A. ventricular escape rhythm
   B. Adams-Stokes syndrome
   C. bundle branch block
   D. atrial arrest

10. A pacemaker that senses spontaneous occurring P waves and QRS complexes and paces the atria when P waves fail to appear and paces the ventricles when QRS complexes fail to appear after spontaneously occurring or paced P waves is called a(n):
    A. optimal sequential pacemaker (DDD)
    B. AV sequential pacemaker (DVI)
    C. atrial synchronous ventricular pacemaker (VDD)
    D. ventricular demand pacemaker (VVI)

CHAPTER 10

Bundle Branch and Fascicular Blocks

Upon completion of all or part of this chapter you should be able to complete the following objectives indicated by your instructor:

☐ **1.** Name and identify the AV node and the parts of the electrical conduction system within the ventricles on an anatomical drawing.

☐ **2.** Define ventricular activation time (VAT) and intrinsicoid deflection.

☐ **3.** Name the artery or arteries that supply the following structures of the electrical conduction system:
- ☐ Interventricular septum
  - ☐ Posterior portion
  - ☐ Anterior portion
  - ☐ Middle portion
- ☐ AV node
- ☐ Bundle of His
  - ☐ Proximal part
  - ☐ Distal part
- ☐ Right bundle branch
  - ☐ Proximal part
  - ☐ Distal part
- ☐ Left bundle branch
  - ☐ Main stem
  - ☐ Left anterior fascicle
  - ☐ Left posterior fascicle

☐ **4.** Describe the anatomical features and the blood supply that make the following structures vulnerable or not vulnerable to disruption:
- ☐ Right bundle branch
- ☐ Left bundle branch
- ☐ Left anterior fascicle
- ☐ Left posterior fascicle

☐ **5.** List five major causes of bundle branch and fascicular blocks.

☐ **6.** Identify the location of the myocardial infarctions that may result in the following:
- ☐ Right bundle branch block
- ☐ Left bundle branch block
- ☐ Left anterior fascicular block
- ☐ Left posterior fascicular block

☐ **7.** Indicate the significance of the following:
- ☐ Bundle branch or fascicular block by itself
- ☐ Bundle branch or fascicular block complicating an acute myocardial infarction
- ☐ Bundle branch block complicated by a first- or second-degree AV block
- ☐ Right bundle branch block and left posterior fascicular block occurring together

☐ **8.** Give the treatment and the reason for it for the following:
- ☐ A bundle branch or fascicular block occurring alone
- ☐ A bundle branch block complicated by (1) a fascicular block or (2) a first-degree or second-degree AV block, occurring alone or in the setting of an acute myocardial infarction
- ☐ A bundle branch block progressing to a third-degree AV block in the setting of an acute myocardial infarction

☐ **9.** Discuss the pathophysiology, causes, and ECG characteristics in the following bundle branch and fascicular blocks:
- ☐ Right bundle branch block
- ☐ Left bundle branch block
- ☐ Left anterior fascicular block
- ☐ Left posterior fascicular block

Anatomy and Physiology of the Electrical Conduction System

The electrical conduction system located below the **AV node** and within the ventricles, the **His-Purkinje system of the ventricles,** consists of the **bundle of His,** the **right** and **left bundle branches,** and the **Purkinje network,** the terminal portion of the electrical conduction system composed of extremely fine **Purkinje fibers** (Figure 10-1).

The long, thin, round **right bundle branch (RBB)** runs down the right side of the interventricular septum to conduct the electrical impulses to the right ventricle. The **left bundle branch (LBB),** which consists of a short, thick, flat **left common bundle branch** (or **main stem**) and two main divisions—the **left anterior** and **posterior fascicles,** conducts the electrical impulses to the left ventricle, including the interventricular septum. The relatively long, thin **left anterior fascicle (LAF)** occupies the left side of the anterior wall of the interventricular septum. It conducts the electrical impulses from the main stem of the left bundle branch to the anterior and lateral walls of the left ventricle. The short, broad **left posterior fascicle (LPF),** which runs down the posterior wall of the interventricular septum, conducts the electrical impulses to the posterior wall of the left ventricle.

Normally, the electrical impulses progress through the right bundle branch and left bundle branch and its fascicles simultaneously, causing first the depolarization of the interventricular septum and then the synchronous depolarization of the right and left ventricles. The electrical activity generated by the depolarization of the smaller right ventricle is buried in that generated by the left ventricle.

The time that it takes for depolarization of the interventricular septum, the right ventricle, and most of the left ventricle, up to and including the endocardial to epicardial depolarization of the left ventricular wall under the facing lead, is commonly called the **ventricular activation time (VAT)** (Figure 10-2), or the **preintrinsicoid deflection** or **intrinsicoid deflection time (IDT).** The **VAT** is measured from the onset of the QRS complex to the peak of the last R wave in the QRS complex. Normally, it is **less than 0.05 second** in the left precordial leads V_5 and V_6. The rest of the QRS com-

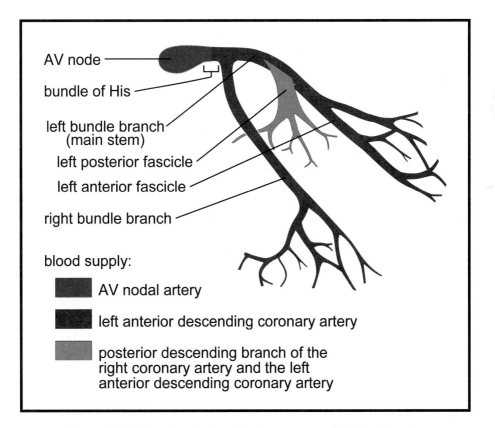

AV node

bundle of His

left bundle branch
  (main stem)

left posterior fascicle

left anterior fascicle

right bundle branch

blood supply:

AV nodal artery

left anterior descending coronary artery

posterior descending branch of the
right coronary artery and the left
anterior descending coronary artery

Figure 10-1. The electrical conduction system and its blood supply.

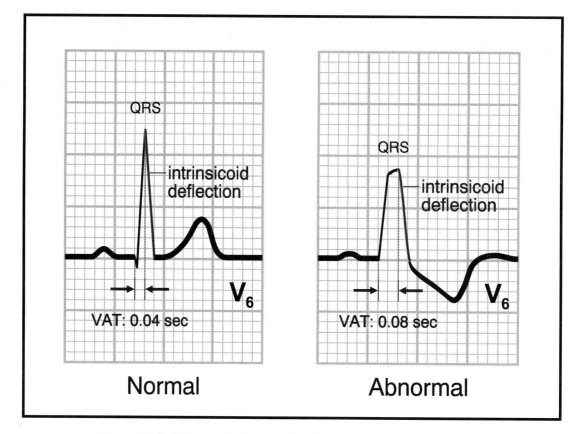

Figure 10-2. The ventricular activation time and intrinsicoid deflection.

plex, from the peak of the R wave to the onset of the ST segment, or the J point, represents the final depolarization of the left ventricle progressing away from the facing lead. The downstroke of the R wave, which begins at the peak of the R wave and ends at the J point or tip of the following S wave, is called the **intrinsicoid deflection.** The ventricular activation time is prolonged in left bundle branch block and left ventricular hypertrophy.

Blood Supply to the Electrical Conduction System

The **anterior portion of the interventricular septum** is supplied by the *left anterior descending coronary artery (LAD)* of the *left coronary artery (LCA);* the **posterior portion of the septum,** by the *posterior descending coronary artery;* and the **middle portion,** by both of these arteries. The *posterior descending coronary artery* arises from the *right coronary artery (RCA)* in 85 to 90 percent of the hearts and from the *left circumflex coronary artery* the other 10 to 15 percent of the time.

The main blood supply of the **AV node** and **proximal part of the bundle of His** is the *AV node artery* which, like the *posterior descending coronary artery,* arises from the *right coronary artery* in 85 to 90 percent of the hearts and, in the other 10 to 15 percent, from the *left circumflex coronary artery.* Occasionally, the *AV node artery* also supplies the **distal part of the bundle of His,** the **proximal part of the right bundle branch,** and the **main stem of the left bundle branch.**

The *left anterior descending coronary artery* by way of its branches, particularly the *septal perforator arteries,* is the main blood supply, in most hearts, to the **distal part of the bundle of His,** the entire **right bundle branch** (including the proximal and distal parts), the **main stem of the left bundle branch,** and the **left anterior fascicle.** The **left posterior fascicle** is supplied by both the *posterior descending coronary artery* and the *left anterior descending coronary artery.*

Table 10-1 summarizes the blood supply to the various parts of the electrical conduction system.

Table 10-1. The electrical conduction system and its primary and alternate blood supply

Electrical conduction system	Primary blood supply	Alternate blood supply
AV Node	AV node artery	None
Bundle of His		
Proximal	AV node artery	None
Distal	LAD	AV node artery
Right Bundle Branch		
Proximal	LAD	AV node artery
Distal	LAD	None
Left Bundle Branch		
Main Stem	LAD	AV node artery
Left Anterior Fascicle	LAD	None
Left Posterior Fascicle	LAD and PDA	None

LAD: Left anterior descending coronary artery by way of the septal perforator arteries.
PDA: Posterior descending coronary artery.

Pathophysiology of Bundle Branch and Fascicular Blocks

The relatively thin **right bundle branch** is more vulnerable to disruption than the **left bundle branch** with its short, thick, wide main stem and widely spread fascicles. A relatively small lesion can disrupt the right bundle branch and cause a block whereas a much more widespread lesion is necessary to block the less vulnerable main stem of the left bundle branch.

The **left anterior fascicle** of the left bundle branch, like the right bundle branch, is also thin and vulnerable to disruption. The **left posterior fascicle,** on the other hand, because it is short and thick and supplied by both the right coronary artery and left anterior descending coronary artery, is rarely disrupted.

Right and left bundle branch block may be present in a heart with a normal intact and viable septum and in one whose septum has been damaged, for example, by an anteroseptal myocardial infarction.

Causes of Bundle Branch and Fascicular Blocks

Although bundle branch and fascicular blocks may be present on rare occasions in normal hearts, they are usually the result of heart disease. Common causes of bundle branch and fascicular blocks are:

- **Ischemic heart disease** affecting the interventricular septum within which the bundle branch or fascicle lies.
- **Idiopathic degenerative disease of the electrical conduction system** with fibrosis and/or sclerosis and disruption of the conduction fibers (Lenegre's disease and Lev's disease).
- **Cardiomyopathy,** a primary disease of the myocardium affecting the bundle branches, often of unknown etiology.
- **Severe left ventricular hypertrophy (LVH)** from whatever cause, such as hypertensive heart disease, may result in left bundle branch block.
- **Acute myocardial infarction.** The relationships between the area of acute myocardial infarction and the associated bundle branch and fascicular blocks are as follows:
  - **Right bundle branch block** primarily occurs secondary to an **anteroseptal myocardial infarction** and, rarely, to an **inferior myocardial infarction.**
  - **Left bundle branch block** may occur secondary to either an **anteroseptal** or **inferior myocardial infarction.**
  - **Left anterior fascicular block** occurs secondary to an **anteroseptal myocardial infarction.**
  - **Left posterior fascicular block** is relatively rare in acute myocardial infarction since both the left anterior descending coronary artery and the right coronary artery have to be occluded for left posterior fascicular block to occur.

- **Miscellaneous causes,** some of which are **acute** and some, **chronic,** include:
  - Acute congestive heart failure, acute pulmonary embolism or infarction, acute pericarditis or myocarditis.
  - Aortic valve disease, cardiac tumors, and syphilitic, rheumatic, and congenital heart disease.
  - Trauma, including cardiac catheterization, coronary angiography, and cardiac surgery.
  - Potassium overdose.

Significance of Bundle Branch and Fascicular Blocks

A **bundle branch** or **fascicular block** by itself is not significant and requires no treatment. The underlying heart disease that produced the bundle branch or fascicular block usually determines the prognosis.

In general, a bundle branch or fascicular block complicating an **acute anteroseptal myocardial infarction** indicates a more serious condition than an acute myocardial infarction without one, often requiring a temporary transcutaneous pacemaker. The incidence of **pump failure** and **life-threatening arrhythmias,** such as **sustained ventricular tachycardia** and **ventricular fibrillation,** is much higher in patients with an acute myocardial infarction complicated by a bundle branch block than in those who do not have such a complication. For this reason, the mortality rate in such patients is several times higher than in those with uncomplicated acute myocardial infarction.

A **bundle branch block** may occasionally progress to a **third-degree (complete) (AV) block** in the setting of an acute myocardial infarction, requiring a temporary transcutaneous pacemaker. This is most likely to happen when a **first- or second-degree AV block** complicates a right or left bundle branch block occurring during the early stages of the infarction. The progression of right bundle branch block to complete AV block occurs twice as often as that of left bundle branch block, especially when right bundle branch block is associated with a fascicular block. The occurrence of a complete AV block in the setting of an acute myocardial infarction is an ominous sign, indicating the involvement of both the left anterior descending coronary artery of the left coronary artery and the posterior descending artery of the right coronary artery. Complete AV block, in this instance, is usually transient, however, lasting about 1 to 2 weeks.

Left anterior and **posterior fascicular blocks** are usually benign and rarely progress to complete left bundle branch block unless they are secondary to an acute myocardial infarction. A left posterior fascicular block occurring with a right bundle branch block, although rare, signifies a poor prognosis since occlusion of both the right coronary artery and the left anterior descending coronary artery must occur for this to happen.

Treatment of Bundle Branch and Fascicular Blocks

Specific treatment is usually not indicated for a bundle branch or fascicular block if it is present alone and not the result of an acute myocardial infarction.

A transcutaneous pacemaker is indicated for the treatment of a right or left bundle branch block under the following conditions:

- If a new right or left bundle branch block or an alternating bundle branch block (one in which a right bundle branch block alternates with a left bundle branch block) results from an acute myocardial infarction.
- If a bundle branch block is complicated by a fascicular block, a first- or second-degree AV block, or both, especially in the setting of an acute myocardial infarction.
- If a bundle branch block progresses to a complete AV block, especially in the setting of an acute myocardial infarction.

Right Bundle Branch Block

Pathophysiology

In **right bundle branch block** (Figure 10-3), the electrical impulses are prevented from entering the right ventricle directly because of the disruption of conduction of the electrical impulses through the right bundle branch. Right bundle branch block may be present in a heart with a normally intact and viable interventricular septum or in one without an intact septum, as would result following an anteroseptal myocardial infarction. The ECG characteristics of the two right bundle branch blocks differ significantly.

In **right bundle branch block with a normally intact and viable interventricular septum,** the electrical impulses travel rapidly down the left bundle branch (1), into the interventricular septum and left ventricle, as they normally do, while progressing slowly across the interventricular septum from left to right to enter the right ventricle after a short delay. Consequently, the interventricular septum and left ventricle depolarize first in a normal way: the septum from left to right (2); the left ventricle from right to left (3). Following left ventricular depolarization, the right ventricle depolarizes in a normal direction: from left to right (4).

The electrical forces generated by the depolarization of the right ventricle in right bundle branch block occur after those of the interventricular septum and left ventricle and travel in a normal direction, i.e., anteriorly and to the right, toward lead V_1. Because of the delay in the depolarization of the right ventricle, the QRS complex is typically greater than 0.10 second in duration and bizarre in shape

and appearance. When it is 0.12 second or greater in duration, it is said to be **complete;** when between 0.10 and 0.11 second, **incomplete.** The term *right bundle branch block* used alone signifies a "complete" right bundle branch block.

In **right bundle branch block without an intact interventricular septum,** depolarization of the nonviable interventricular septum does not occur. The depolarization of the left and right ventricles, however, occurs as it does above in a right bundle branch block with an intact septum.

Causes of Right Bundle Branch Block

Right bundle branch block may be present in healthy individuals with apparently normal hearts without any apparent cause. Common causes of *chronic* right bundle branch block are:
- Coronary and hypertensive heart disease
- Cardiac tumors
- Cardiomyopathy and myocarditis
- Syphilitic, rheumatic, and congenital heart disease (atrial septal defect)
- Cardiac surgery
- Congenital right bundle branch block
- Idiopathic degenerative disease of the electrical conduction system (i.e., Lenegre's disease and Lev's disease)

Common causes of *acute* right bundle branch block are:
- Acute anteroseptal myocardial infarction
- Acute pulmonary embolism or infarction
- Acute congestive heart failure
- Acute pericarditis or myocarditis

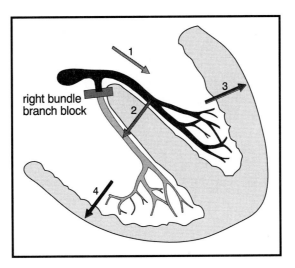

ECG Characteristics

QRS Complexes:

Duration: The duration of the QRS complex in **complete right bundle branch block** is 0.12 second or greater; in **incomplete right bundle branch block,** the duration of the QRS complex is 0.10 to 0.11 second.

QRS axis: The QRS axis may be normal or deviated to the right, i.e., right axis deviation: $> +90$ degrees. If left axis deviation is present $(> -30$ degrees), both right bundle branch block and left anterior fascicular block are present.

QRS pattern in right bundle branch block with an intact interventricular septum: In right bundle branch block, the electrical forces of depolarization of the right ventricle occur abnormally late, following those of the interventricular septum and left ventricle. These right ventricular electrical forces are directed anteriorly and to the right and last more than 40 msec (≥ 0.04 sec), producing the typical late broad, or **"terminal,"** **R** and **S waves** in various leads. The combined electrical forces of the left ventricle and delayed right ventricle produce the typical **wide biphasic QRS complexes of right bundle branch block.**

Q waves: Normal small **septal q waves** are present in leads I, aVL, and V_5-V_6, reflecting the normal depolarization of the interventricular septum.

R waves: Small **r waves** are present in the right precordial leads V_1-V_2, reflecting the normal depolarization of the interventricular septum. Wide and slurred, tall **"terminal" R waves** are present in lead aVR and the right precordial leads V_1-V_2. This produces the classical **triphasic rSR′ pattern of RBBB** (or the **"M"** or **"rabbit ears" pattern**) in leads V_1-V_2.

S waves: Deep and slurred **"terminal" S waves** are present in leads I and aVL and the left precordial leads V_5-V_6. This produces the typical **qRS pattern of RBBB** in leads V_5-V_6.

QRS pattern in right bundle branch block without an intact interventricular septum: In right bundle branch block without an intact and viable interventricular septum, the initial normal depolarization of the interventricular septum does not occur. The result is the absence of **initial small r waves** in the precordial leads V_1-V_2 and **septal q waves** in leads I, aVL, and V_5-V_6. Consequently, the classical triphasic **rSR′ pattern of RBBB** is replaced by a **QSR pattern** in V_1-V_2.

ST Segments: **ST segment depression** may be present in leads V_1-V_3.

T Waves: **T wave inversion** may be present in leads V_1-V_3.

Note: "Terminal" means the last 0.04 second of the QRS complex.

Notes

Right Bundle Branch Block

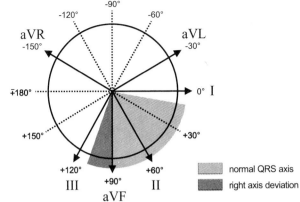

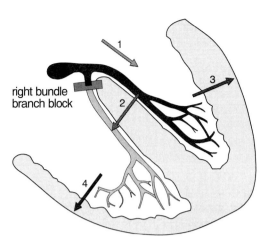

right bundle branch block

With an intact interventricular septum

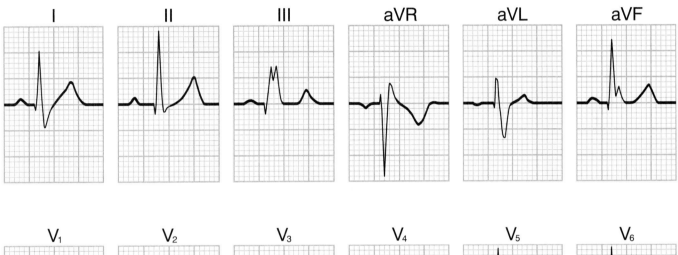

Without an intact interventricular septum

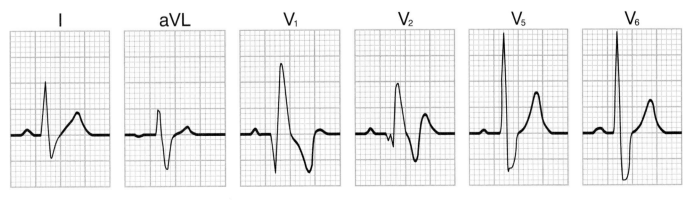

Figure 10-3. Right bundle branch block.

Summary of the ECG Characteristics in Right Bundle Branch Block:

With an Intact Interventricular Septum

Lead V₁

Wide QRS complex with a classic **triphasic rSR′** pattern:

- Initial **small r wave** (Normal interventricular septal depolarization)
- **Deep, slurred S wave** (Normal left ventricular depolarization)
- Late **(terminal) tall R′ wave** (Delayed right ventricular depolarization)

Leads I, aVL, V₅-V₆

Wide QRS complex with a **qRS** pattern:

- Initial **small q wave** (Normal interventricular septal depolarization)
- **Tall R wave** (Normal left ventricular depolarization)
- Late **(terminal) deep, slurred S wave** (Delayed right ventricular depolarization)

QRS axis

Normal QRS axis or right axis deviation (**+90°** to **+110°**).

Without an Intact Interventricular Septum

Lead V₁

Wide QRS complex with a **QSR** pattern:

- **Absent initial small r wave** (Absent interventricular septal depolarization)
- **Deep QS wave** (Normal left ventricular depolarization)
- Late **(terminal) tall R wave** (Delayed right ventricular depolarization)

Leads I, aVL, V₅-V₆

Wide QRS complex with an **RS** pattern:

- **Tall R wave** (Normal left ventricular depolarization)
- Late **(terminal) deep, slurred S wave** (Delayed right ventricular depolarization)

QRS axis

Normal QRS axis or right axis deviation (**+90°** to **+110°**).

With an intact interventricular septum

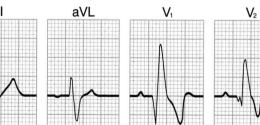

Without an intact interventricular septum

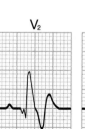
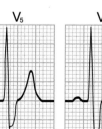

Left Bundle Branch Block

Pathophysiology

In **left bundle branch block** (Figure 10-4), the electrical impulses are prevented from entering the left ventricle directly because of the disruption of conduction of the electrical impulses through the left bundle branch. Although left bundle branch block may be present in a heart with a normally intact and viable interventricular septum, it usually occurs in hearts without an intact septum, as would result following an anteroseptal myocardial infarction. The ECG characteristics of the two left bundle branch blocks differ somewhat.

In **left bundle branch block with a normally intact and viable interventricular septum,** the electrical impulses travel rapidly down the right bundle branch (1), into the right ventricle, as they normally do, while progressing slowly across the interventricular septum from right to left into the left ventricle. Consequently, the interventricular septum depolarizes first in an abnormal way, from right to left (2), and either anteriorly or posteriorly. This is followed by the depolarization of the right ventricle in a normal way, left to right (3), and then, depolarization of the left ventricle in a normal direction: from right to left (4).

The electrical forces generated by the depolarization of the left ventricle in left bundle branch block occur after those of the interventricular septum and right ventricle and travel in a normal leftward direction, away from lead V_1. Since the electrical impulses enter the left ventricle from the right via the interventricular septum instead of the left bundle branch, as they normally do, the depolarization of the left ventricle occurs slightly behind schedule, but in an essentially normal sequence.

Because of the delay in the depolarization of the left ventricle, the **ventricular activation time** is greater than 0.05 second and the QRS complex is typically greater than 0.10 second in duration and abnormal in shape and appearance. When the QRS complex is 0.12 second or greater in duration, the left bundle branch block is said to be **complete;** when between 0.10 and 0.11 second, **incomplete.** The term *left bundle branch block* used alone signifies a "complete" left bundle branch block.

In **left bundle branch block without an intact interventricular septum,** depolarization of the non-viable interventricular septum does not occur. The depolarization of the left and right ventricles, however, occurs as it does above in a left bundle branch block with an intact septum.

Causes of Left Bundle Branch Block

Left bundle branch block, unlike right bundle branch block, always indicates a diseased heart, being extremely unusual in healthy hearts. In general, left bundle branch block is more common than is right bundle branch block in elderly individuals with diseased hearts. Common causes of *chronic* left bundle branch block are:

- Hypertensive heart disease (the most common cause) and coronary artery disease
- Cardiomyopathy and myocarditis
- Syphilitic, rheumatic, and congenital heart disease and aortic stenosis from whatever cause
- Cardiac tumors
- Idiopathic degenerative disease of the electrical conduction system (i.e., Lenegre's disease and Lev's disease)

Common causes of *acute* left bundle branch block are:

- Acute anteroseptal myocardial infarction
- Acute congestive heart failure
- Acute pericarditis or myocarditis

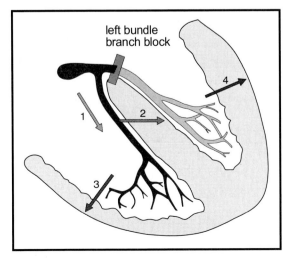

ECG Characteristics

QRS Complexes:

Duration: The duration of the QRS complex in **complete left bundle branch block** is 0.12 second or greater; in **incomplete left bundle branch block,** the duration of the QRS complex is 0.10 to 0.11 second.

QRS axis: The QRS axis may be normal, but it is commonly deviated to the left (i.e., left axis deviation: > -30 degrees).

QRS pattern in left bundle branch block with an intact interventricular septum: In left bundle branch block, the electrical forces of depolarization of the left ventricle occur abnormally late, following those of the right ventricle. The electrical forces produced by the depolarization of the left ventricle are directed leftward and last more than 40 msec (≥ 0.04 sec), producing the typical broad R and S waves in the various leads. The combined electrical forces of the right ventricle and delayed left ventricle produce the typical **wide monophasic QRS complexes of left bundle branch block.**

Q waves: **Septal q waves** are *absent* in leads I and aVL and the left precordial leads V_5-V_6 where they normally occur. Their absence results from the depolarization of the interventricular septum in an abnormal direction, from right to left.

R waves: **Small to relatively tall, narrow R waves** are present in leads V_1-V_3 when the interventricular septum depolarizes from *right to left and anteriorly.* This occurs in about two thirds of the left bundle branch blocks. These R waves in leads V_1-V_3 give the typical appearance of a **"poor R-wave progression"** across the precordial leads. In the other third

of the left bundle branch blocks, where the interventricular septum depolarizes from *right to left and posteriorly,* R waves are absent in leads V_1-V_3.

Tall, wide slurred R waves are present in leads I and aVL and the left precordial leads V_5-V_6. The R waves may be **notched** or have an **rsR′ pattern.** The **ventricular activation time** is prolonged up to 0.07 second or more, particularly in lead aVL and the left precordial leads V_5-V_6.

S waves: **Deep, wide S waves** are present in leads V_1-V_3, producing the typical **rS** or **QS complexes.** Because of these waves, an anteroseptal myocardial infarction may be mistakenly diagnosed. S waves are absent in leads I and aVL and the left precordial leads V_5-V_6.

QRS pattern in left bundle branch block without an intact interventricular septum: In left bundle branch block without an intact interventricular septum, the initial depolarization of the septum from right to left does not occur. This leaves the initial electrical forces of right ventricular depolarization (from left to right) unopposed so that significant **narrow r waves** may be present in leads V_1 and V_2, and **small q waves,** in leads I and aVL and the left precordial leads V_5-V_6.

ST Segments: **ST segment depression** is present in leads I and aVL and the left precordial leads V_5-V_6. **ST segment elevation** is present in leads V_1-V_3.

T Waves: **T wave inversion** is present in leads I and aVL and the left precordial leads V_5-V_6. **T wave elevation** is present in leads V_1-V_3.

Notes

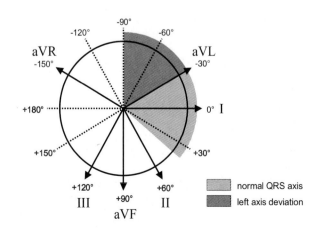

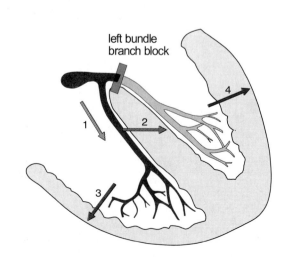

Left Bundle Branch Block

With an intact interventricular septum

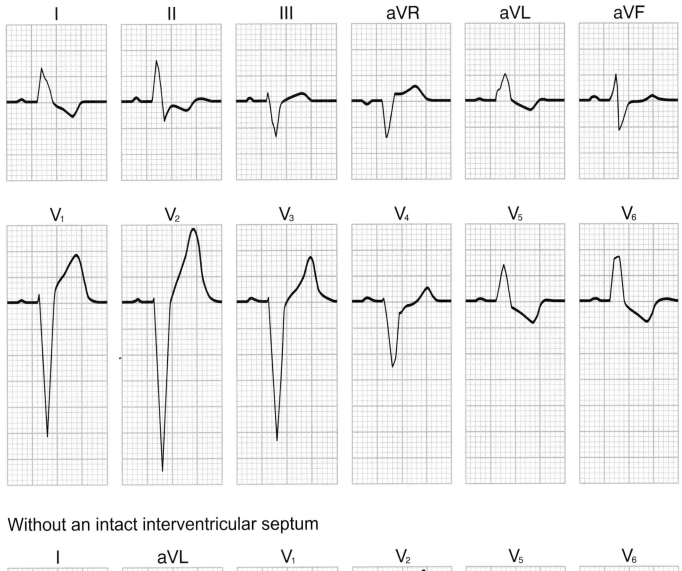

Without an intact interventricular septum

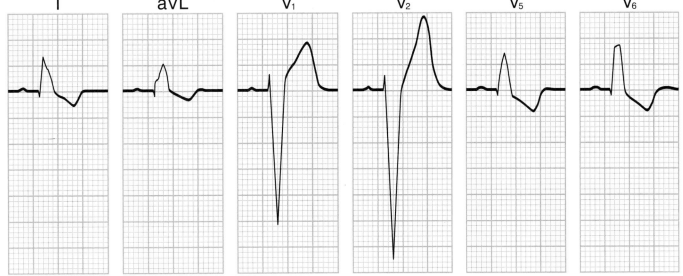

Figure 10-4. Left bundle branch block.

Summary of the ECG Characteristics in Left Bundle Branch Block:

With an Intact Interventricular Septum

Lead V₁

Wide QRS complex with an **rS** or **QS** pattern:

- Initial **small r wave** (Abnormal interventricular septal depolarization from right to left and anteriorly)
- **Deep, wide S wave** (Delayed, essentially normal left ventricular depolarization)

OR

- **Absent R wave** (Abnormal interventricular septal depolarization from right to left and posteriorly)
- **Deep, wide QS wave** (Delayed, essentially normal left ventricular depolarization)

Leads I, aVL, V₅-V₆

Wide QRS complex with an **R** or **rsR′** pattern:

- **Tall, wide, slurred R wave with or without notching and/or an rsR′ pattern** with a **prolonged ventricular activation time.** (Delayed, essentially normal left ventricular depolarization)

QRS axis

Normal QRS axis or left axis deviation (**−30°** to **−90°**).

Without an Intact Interventricular Septum

Leads V₁ and V₂

Wide QRS complex with an **rS** pattern:

- **Small narrow r wave** (Unopposed normal right ventricular depolarization)
- **Deep, wide S wave** (Delayed, essentially normal left ventricular depolarization)

Leads I, aVL, V₅-V₆

Wide QRS complex with a **qR** pattern:

- **Small q wave** (Unopposed normal right ventricular depolarization)
- **Tall, wide, slurred R wave with or without notching and/or an rsR′ pattern** with a **prolonged ventricular activation time.** (Delayed, essentially normal left ventricular depolarization)

QRS axis

Normal QRS axis or left axis deviation (**−30°** to **−90°**).

Left Bundle Branch Block

With an intact interventricular septum

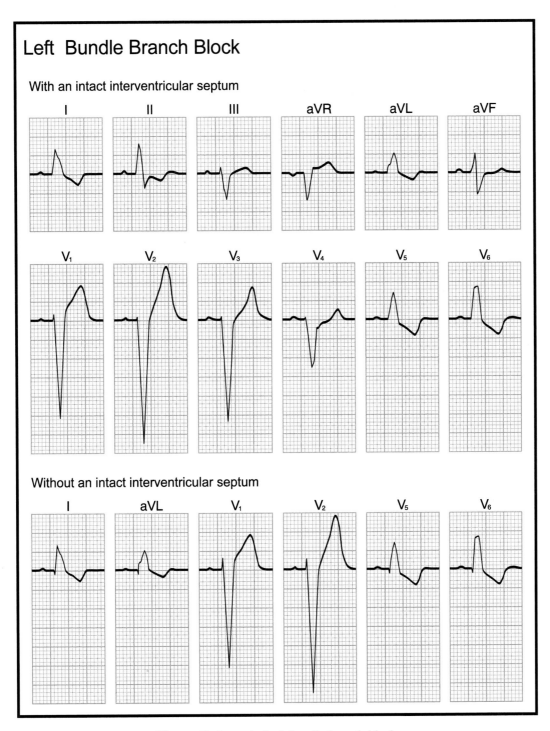

Without an intact interventricular septum

Figure 10-4, cont. Left bundle branch block.

Left Anterior Fascicular Block
(Left Anterior Hemiblock)

Pathophysiology

In **left anterior fascicular block** (Figure 10-5), the electrical impulses are prevented from entering the anterior and lateral walls of the left ventricle directly. The electrical impulses travel rapidly down the left posterior fascicle (1) into the interventricular septum and posterior wall of the left ventricle and then, after a very slight delay, into the anterior and lateral walls of the left ventricle. At the same time, the electrical impulses travel down the right bundle branch (1) into the right ventricle in a normal way.

The interventricular septum depolarizes first in a normal direction, from left to right (2). This is followed by the depolarization of the right ventricle (3) and the posterior wall of the left ventricle (3a), followed almost instantly by depolarization of the anterior and lateral walls of the left ventricle (3b).

Since there is no appreciable delay between the depolarization of the posterior and anterolateral walls of the left ventricle, the QRS complex is of normal duration. The electrical forces generated by the depolarization of the anterior and lateral walls of the left ventricle travel in an **upward** and **leftward direction,** producing a **marked left axis deviation.**

Causes of Left Anterior Fascicular Block

The most common cause of left anterior fascicular block is acute anteroseptal myocardial infarction, alone or in combination with a right bundle branch block.

ECG Characteristics
QRS Complexes:

Duration: Normal, less than 0.10 second in duration.

QRS axis: The QRS axis is typically deviated to the left, i.e., left axis deviation ($-30°$ to $-90°$).

QRS pattern: The QRS complexes appear **normal without unusual notching or any delay in the ventricular activation time.** The electrical forces of depolarization of the anterolateral area of the left ventricle, somewhat delayed by 40 msec (≥ 0.04 sec), are directed upward and leftward. The presence of an initial **small q wave** in lead I and an initial **small r wave** in lead III (q_1r_3 **pattern**) is an indication of a left anterior fascicular block.

Q waves: Initial **small q waves** are present in leads I and aVL and absent in leads II, III, and aVF.

R waves: Initial **small r waves are present** in leads II, III, and aVF.

S waves: The **S waves** are typically deep and larger than the **R waves** in leads II, III, and aVF.

Note: These findings relative to the QRS complexes are significant only in the absence of other causes of left axis deviation:
- **Left ventricular hypertrophy**
- **Inferior (diaphragmatic) myocardial infarction** with Q waves in leads II, III, and aVF
- **Chronic obstructive pulmonary disease (COPD)**

ST Segments: Normal.

T Waves: Normal.

Notes

Left Anterior Fascicular Block

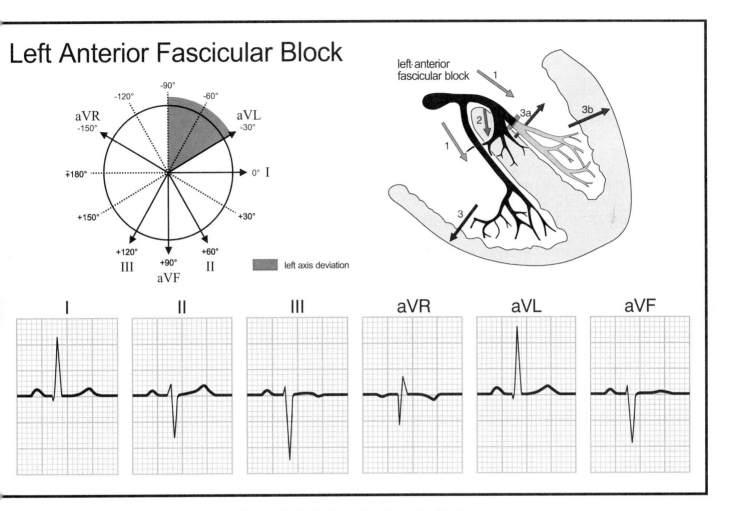

Figure 10-5. Left anterior fascicular block.

Left Posterior Fascicular Block
(Left Posterior Hemiblock)

Pathophysiology

In **left posterior fascicular block** (Figure 10-6), the electrical impulses are prevented from entering the interventricular septum and posterior wall of the left ventricle directly. The electrical impulses travel rapidly down the left anterior fascicle (1) into the anterior and lateral walls of the left ventricle and then, after a very slight delay, into the posterior wall of the left ventricle. At the same time, the electrical impulses travel down the right bundle branch (1) into the right ventricle in a normal way and into the interventricular septum.

The interventricular septum depolarizes first in an abnormal direction, from right to left (2). This is followed by the depolarization of the right ventricle (3) and the anterior and lateral walls of the left ventricle (3a), followed almost instantly by depolarization of the posterior wall of the left ventricle (3b).

Since there is no appreciable delay between the depolarization of the anterolateral and posterior walls of the left ventricle, the QRS complex is of normal duration. The electrical forces generated by the depolarization of the posterior wall of the left ventricle travel in a **downward** and **rightward direction,** producing a **marked right axis deviation.**

Causes of Left Posterior Fascicular Block

Left posterior fascicular block is rare, but it can occur in an extensive acute myocardial infarction involving the left anterior descending artery and the posterior descending branch of the right coronary artery. Left posterior fascicular block can occur alone or in combination with a right bundle branch block.

ECG Characteristics
QRS Complexes:

Duration: Normal, less than 0.10 second in duration.

QRS axis: The QRS axis is typically deviated to the right, i.e., right axis deviation (**+110°** to **+180°**).

QRS pattern: The QRS complexes appear **normal without unusual notching or any delay in the ventricular activation time.** The electrical forces of depolarization of the posterior part of the left ventricle, somewhat delayed by 40 msec ($\geq$ 0.04 sec), are directed downward and rightward. The presence of an initial **small q wave** in lead III and an initial **small r wave** in lead I (**q_3r_1 pattern**) is an indication of a left posterior fascicular block.

> *Q waves:* Initial **small q waves** are present in leads II, III, and aVF and absent in leads I, aVL, and V_5-V_6.

> *R waves:* Initial **small r waves** are present in leads I and aVL; and **tall R waves,** in leads II, III, and aVF.

> *S waves:* **Deep S waves** are present in lead I.

Note: These findings relative to the QRS complexes are significant only in the absence of other causes of right axis deviation:
- **Right ventricular hypertrophy**
- **Pulmonary embolism and/or infarction**
- **Anterolateral myocardial infarction** with Q waves in leads I, aVL, and V_5-V_6
- **Chronic obstructive pulmonary disease (COPD)**

ST Segments: Normal.

T Waves: Normal.

Notes

Left Posterior Fascicular Block

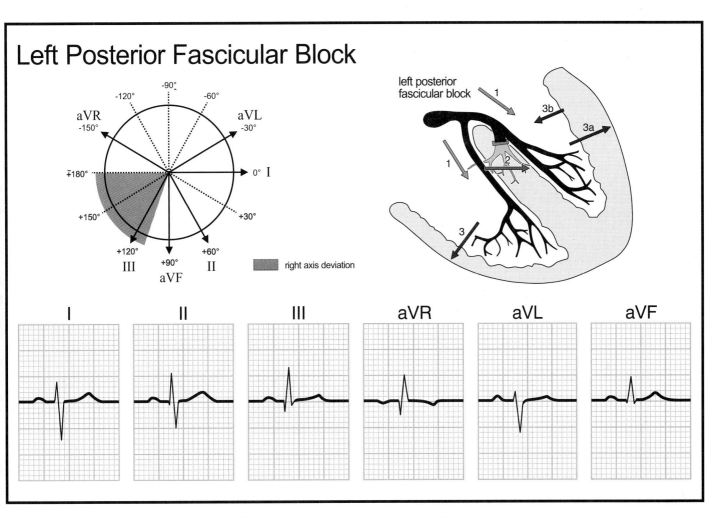

Figure 10-6. Left posterior fascicular block.

1. The time from the onset of the QRS complex to the peak of the R wave in the QRS complex is called:
   A. the ventricular activation time
   B. the preintrinsicoid deflection
   C. all of the above
   D. none of the above

2. The anterior portion of the septum is supplied with blood from the:
   A. posterior descending coronary artery
   B. AV nodal artery
   C. left anterior descending coronary artery
   D. right coronary artery

3. The main blood supply of the AV node and proximal part of the bundle of His is the AV node artery, which arises from the _____ in the majority of hearts.
   A. circumflex coronary artery
   B. right coronary artery
   C. posterior descending coronary artery
   D. none of the above

4. Common causes of bundle branch and fascicular blocks are:
   A. ischemic heart disease
   B. idiopathic degenerative disease of the electrical conduction system
   C. severe left ventricular hypertrophy
   D. all of the above

5. In the setting of an acute MI, a right bundle branch block occurs primarily in a(n):
   A. anteroseptal MI
   B. lateral MI
   C. posterior MI
   D. inferior MI

6. In acute MI patients with a bundle branch block, _____ than in those not complicated by a bundle branch block.
   A. the incidence of pump failure and ventricular arrhythmias is much higher
   B. a temporary transcutaneous pacemaker is less frequently indicated
   C. the incidence of ventricular fibrillation is lower
   D. the incidence of supraventricular tachycardias is higher

7. Common causes of chronic right bundle branch block are:
   A. congestive heart failure, stroke, and seizures
   B. hyperventilation, acute MI, and diabetes
   C. myocarditis, cardiomyopathy, and cardiac surgery
   D. none of the above

8. In a right bundle branch block with an intact interventricular septum, the QRS complex in lead V_1 is:
   A. wide with a tall R wave
   B. wide with a classic triphasic rSR' pattern
   C. narrow with a QRS pattern
   D. none of the above

9. When the electrical impulses are prevented from directly entering the anterior and lateral walls of the left ventricle, the condition is called a:
   A. left anterior fascicular block
   B. left lateral hemiblock
   C. left posterior fascicular block
   D. none of the above

10. The electrical impulses are prevented from entering the interventricular septum and posterior wall of the left ventricle directly when the patient has a:
    A. left anterior fascicular block
    B. right posterior hemiblock
    C. left posterior fascicular block
    D. left inferior hemiblock

CHAPTER 11

Myocardial Ischemia, Injury, and Infarction

Upon completion of all or part of this chapter you should be able to complete the following objectives indicated by your instructor:

☐ 1. Name and identify the right and left coronary arteries and their branches on an anatomical drawing of the coronary circulation.

☐ 2. Given a list of the arteries of the coronary circulation and a list of the regions of the heart, match the arteries with the regions of the heart they supply.

☐ 3. Define myocardial ischemia, myocardial injury, and myocardial infarction and indicate which are reversible and which are not.

☐ 4. List the causes of myocardial ischemia, injury, and infarction.

☐ 5. Describe the process of coronary thrombosis.

☐ 6. On a drawing of an acute myocardial infarction, identify the zones of ischemia, injury, and infarction (necrosis).

☐ 7. Define the following terms:
   ☐ Thrombolysis
   ☐ Transmural infarction
   ☐ Subendocardial infarction

☐ 8. Describe the sequence of changes in the myocardium that occurs during the four phases of evolution of an acute anterior wall transmural myocardial infarction, including the timing and duration of each phase and sequence.

☐ 9. Define "facing" and "opposite" ECG leads.

☐ 10. Describe the changes in the Q, R, and T waves and ST segments in facing and opposite ECG leads in myocardial ischemia, injury, and necrosis and when they appear following the onset of an acute myocardial infarction.

☐ 11. Give the theoretical explanations for the following changes in the T waves associated with an acute myocardial infarction:
   ☐ Inverted T waves over ischemic tissue
   ☐ Inverted T waves over necrotic tissue
   ☐ Tall and peaked T waves over ischemic tissue

☐ 12. Give the measurements characteristic of an abnormally elevated or depressed ST segment.

☐ 13. Explain the theory behind ST segment elevation in acute MI, namely, the current of injury.

☐ 14. Name two cardiac conditions, other than acute myocardial infarction, in which ST segment elevation occurs.

☐ 15. List the three kinds of sloping of the ST segment found in ST depression associated with myocardial ischemia.

☐ 16. Name three cardiac conditions, other than myocardial ischemia, in which ST segment depression occurs.

☐ 17. Define "septal" q and r waves, and indicate in which leads they normally appear.

☐ 18. Discuss the following with regard to abnormal Q waves:
   ☐ Diagnostic characteristics
   ☐ Significance of appearance in the ECG
   ☐ Time of appearance following the onset of an acute myocardial infarction
   ☐ "Window" theory

☐ 19. Describe the following:
   ☐ A Q wave
   ☐ A QS wave; a QS complex
   ☐ A QR complex; a Qr complex

☐ 20. Discuss the significance of abnormal Q waves appearing in the following leads:
   ☐ aVR
   ☐ aVL
   ☐ aVF
   ☐ III
   ☐ V_1

☐ 21. Discuss the significance of abnormal Q waves when they occur in the presence of the following conditions:
   ☐ ST segment elevation and T wave inversion
   ☐ Left or right bundle branch block
   ☐ Left anterior or left posterior fascicular block
   ☐ Left ventricular hypertrophy

☐ 22. Describe the changes in the Q, R, and T waves and ST segments present with each of the four phases in the evolution of the following:
   ☐ Q wave (transmural) infarction
   ☐ Non-Q wave (subendocardial) infarction

23. Review the pathophysiologic changes in the ventricular wall with respect to the associated ECG changes that occur during each of the four phases of a transmural myocardial infarction.

24. Name the coronary artery or arteries occluded and the region of the heart involved in the following acute myocardial infarctions:

☐ Septal MI   ☐ Anterolateral MI
☐ Anterior (local-   ☐ Extensive anterior
   ized) MI   MI
☐ Anteroseptal MI   ☐ Inferior MI
☐ Lateral MI   ☐ Posterior MI

25. List the diagnostic changes in the Q waves, R waves, ST segments, and T waves in the facing and opposite ECG leads (where applicable) during the early and late phases of the following acute myocardial infarctions:

☐ Septal MI   ☐ Anterolateral MI
☐ Anterior (local-   ☐ Extensive anterior
   ized) MI   MI
☐ Anteroseptal MI   ☐ Inferior MI
☐ Lateral MI   ☐ Posterior MI

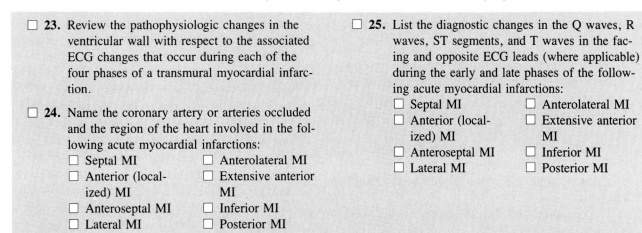

Coronary Circulation

The **coronary circulation** (Table 11-1 and Figure 11-1) consists of the left and right coronary arteries. The **left coronary artery** arises from the base of the aorta just above the left coronary cusp of the aortic valve; and the **right coronary artery,** from above the right aortic coronary cusp.

Left coronary artery. The **left coronary artery** consists of the **left main coronary artery,** a short main stem of about 2 to 10 mm in length that usually divides into two equal major branches, the **left anterior descending coronary artery** and the **left circumflex coronary artery.** Sometimes, a third major branch, the **diagonal (or intermediate) coronary artery,** arises from the left main coronary artery

Table 11-1. The coronary circulation and the regions of the heart it supplies

Left coronary artery		Right coronary artery	
Coronary artery	**Region supplied**	**Coronary artery**	**Region supplied**
Left anterior descending		*Right coronary artery*	
Diagonal	Anterior/lateral wall of the left ventricle	Conus	Upper anterior wall of the right ventricle
Septal perforator	Anterior two thirds of the interventricular septum	Sinoatrial node (50-60%)	SA node
Right ventricular	Anterior wall of the right ventricle	Anterior right ventricular	Anterolateral wall of the right ventricle
Left circumflex		Right atrial	Right atrium
Sinoatrial node (40-60%)	SA node	Acute marginal	Lateral wall of the right ventricle
Left atrial circumflex	Left atrium	Posterior descending (85-90%)	Posterior one third of the interventricular septum
Anterolateral marginal	Anterolateral wall of the left ventricle		
Posterolateral marginal	Posterolateral wall of the left ventricle	AV node (85-90%)	AV node
Distal left circumflex	Posterior wall of the left ventricle	Posterior left ventricular (85-90%)	Proximal bundle of His Inferior wall of the left ventricle
Posterior descending (10-15%)	Posterior one third of the interventricular septum		
AV node (10-15%)	AV node Proximal bundle of His		
Posterior left ventricular (10-15%)	Inferior wall of the left ventricle		

instead of from the left anterior descending coronary artery.

- The **left anterior descending coronary artery (LAD)** travels anteriorly and downward within the interventricular groove over the interventricular septum and circles the apex of the heart to end behind it. The LAD gives rise to at least one and often up to six **diagonal branches,** three to five **septal perforator branches,** and sometimes, one or more **right ventricular branches.**

The **diagonal arteries,** the first of which may originate from the left main coronary artery, course over the anterior and lateral surface of the left ventricle between the left anterior descending coronary artery and the anterolateral marginal branch of the left circumflex coronary artery. The **septal perforator arteries** arise at a right angle from the LAD and run directly into the interventricular septum. The **right ventricular arteries** course over the anterior surface of the right ventricle.

- The **left circumflex coronary artery** arises from the left main coronary artery at an obtuse angle and runs posteriorly along the left atrioventricular groove to end in back of the left ventricle in about 85 to 90 percent of hearts. In the remaining 10 to 15 percent, the left circumflex coronary artery continues along the atrio-ventricular groove to become the **posterior left ventricular arteries.** In the majority of these hearts, the left circumflex continues farther to enter the posterior interventricular groove to become the **posterior descending coronary artery** while giving rise to the **AV node artery.**

The **left circumflex coronary artery** gives rise to the **sinoatrial node artery** in 40 to 50 percent of the hearts, one or two **left atrial circumflex branches,** a large **anterolateral marginal artery** and one or more smaller **posterolateral marginal arteries** (the **left obtuse marginal branches**), and the **distal left circumflex artery.** A left coronary artery with a circumflex coronary artery that gives rise to both the posterior left ventricular arteries and the posterior descending coronary artery is considered to be a **"dominant" left coronary artery.**

The **anterolateral marginal artery** runs over the anterolateral surface of the left ventricular wall toward the apex, lateral to the diagonal branches of the LAD. The **posterolateral marginal arteries** run down the posterolateral wall of the left ventricle, and the **distal left circumflex artery,** down the left atrioventricular groove. When present, the **posterior left ventricular arteries** course over the inferior (or diaphragmatic) wall of the left ventricle; and the **posterior descending coronary artery,** down the posterior interventricular groove.

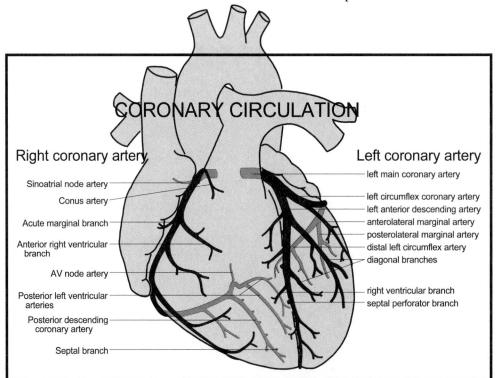

Figure 11-1. The coronary circulation.

Right coronary artery. The **right coronary artery** travels downward and then posteriorly in the right atrioventricular groove, giving off the **conus artery,** the **sinoatrial node artery** in 50 to 60 percent of hearts, several **anterior right ventricular branches,** the **right atrial branch,** and the **acute marginal branch.**

In 85 to 90 percent of hearts, it also gives rise to the **AV node artery** and the **posterior descending coronary artery** (with its **septal branches**) which runs down the posterior interventricular groove, and, then, continuing into the left atrioventricular groove, the right coronary artery terminates as the **posterior left ventricular arteries.** A right coronary artery that gives rise to both the posterior descending coronary artery and the posterior left ventricular arteries is considered to be a **"dominant" right coronary artery.**

Summary. The **left anterior descending coronary artery** supplies the anterior two thirds of the interventricular septum, most of the right and left bundle branches, the anterior (apical) and lateral wall of the left ventricle, and sometimes, the anterior wall of the right ventricle.

The **left circumflex coronary artery** supplies the left atrial wall, the lateral and posterior wall of the left ventricle, and, in 40 to 50 percent of hearts, the SA node. In 10 to 15 percent of hearts, when the posterior left ventricular, AV node, and posterior descending coronary arteries arise from the left circumflex artery, the left circumflex artery also supplies the inferior (diaphragmatic) wall of the left ventricle, the AV node, the proximal bundle of His, and the posterior (inferior) one third of the interventricular septum. When this occurs, the entire interventricular septum is supplied by the left coronary artery.

The **right coronary artery** supplies the right atrial and ventricular wall; the AV node, the proximal bundle of His, the posterior one third of the interventricular septum, and the inferior wall of the left ventricle in 85 to 90 percent of hearts; and the SA node in 50 to 60 percent of hearts.

Pathophysiology and Mechanism of Myocardial Ischemia, Injury, and Infarction

Myocardial ischemia, injury, and infarction results from the failure of local coronary arteries to supply enough oxygenated blood to the myocardial tissue they supply to meet the tissue's need for oxygen. This can result from a variety of causes (Figure 11-2):

- **Occlusion (or obstruction) of an already severely narrowed atherosclerotic coronary artery** by a blood clot (**coronary thrombosis**) following rupture of an atherosclerotic plaque with hemorrhage under or within the plaque. Acute increase in arterial pressure or heart rate, such as that associated with physical exertion or emotional stress, commonly precedes the rupture of an atherosclerotic plaque. Coronary artery spasm and hypercoagulability of the blood predispose to plaque rupture and thrombus formation. Coronary thrombosis is the most common cause of myocardial infarction, occurring in about 90 percent of acute myocardial infarctions.
- **Coronary artery spasm** caused by constriction of smooth muscle in the wall of the coronary artery. Generally, the spasm occurs at the site of narrowing from coronary atherosclerosis. As

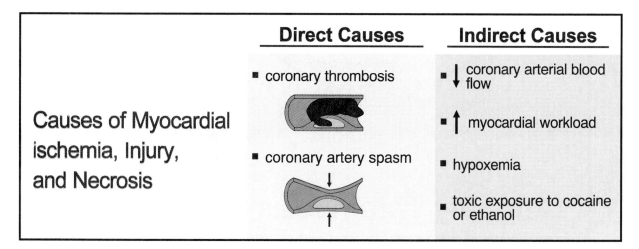

Figure 11-2. Causes of myocardial ischemia, injury, and necrosis.

noted above, coronary artery spasm often accompanies or is the cause of plaque rupture that results in coronary thrombosis.

- **Decreased coronary arterial blood flow** for whatever reason other than coronary artery occlusion or spasm, such as an arrhythmia, pulmonary embolism, or hypotension or shock from any cause (e.g., chest trauma and aortic dissection).
- **Increased myocardial workload** from unaccustomed physical effort, emotional stress, unrelieved fatigue, or increased blood volume (volume overload) imposed on a heart with atherosclerotic coronary arteries.
- **Decreased level of oxygen in the blood delivered to the myocardium** because of hypoxemia from acute respiratory failure.
- **Toxic exposure to cocaine or ethanol.**

Myocardial ischemia is present the moment there is a **decrease** or **complete absence** of the blood supply to myocardial tissue. This immediately results in the lack of oxygen **(anoxia)** within the cardiac cells. Following the onset of anoxia and for a short time after, certain **reversible ischemic changes** usually occur in the internal structure of the affected cells because of the lack of oxygen. These ischemic changes cause a delay in the de-

polarization and repolarization of the cells. Mild or moderate anoxia can be tolerated for a short time by the cardiac cells without greatly affecting their function. There may be some loss in the ability of the myocardial cells to contract and of the specialized cells of the electrical conduction system to generate or conduct electrical impulses. Upon the return of adequate blood flow and reoxygenation, these cells usually return to a normal or near normal condition.

If ischemia is severe or prolonged, the anoxic cardiac cells sustain moderate to severe **myocardial injury** and stop functioning normally, unable to contract or generate or conduct electrical impulses properly. At this stage, the damage to the cells still remains **reversible** so that the injured cells remain viable and salvageable for some time. As in ischemic cells, injured cells may also return to normal or near normal upon the return of adequate blood flow and reoxygenation.

If severe myocardial ischemia continues because of a continued complete absence of the blood supply, the anoxic cardiac cells eventually sustain **irreversible injury** and **die,** becoming electrically inert. At the moment of cellular death, **necrosis** is present, and **myocardial infarction** occurs. Necrotic cells **DO NOT** return to normal upon revascularization or reoxygenation.

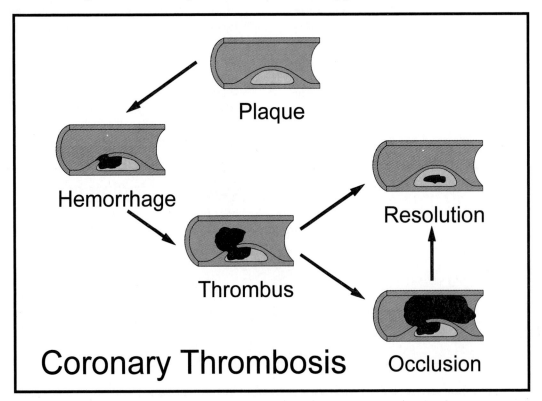

Figure 11-3. Coronary thrombosis.

Acute Myocardial Infarction

Myocardial infarction (MI) usually follows the occlusion of a severely narrowed atherosclerotic epicardial coronary artery by a blood clot—**coronary thrombosis.** This process involves an intricate interaction between the rupture of an atherosclerotic plaque lining the narrowed coronary artery, vasospasm of the coronary artery smooth muscle, platelet activation, and blood clot formation (thrombosis) (Figure 11-3).

Angiographic studies of the coronary arteries performed within the first few hours after the onset of symptoms of acute MI show that about 90 percent of the coronary artery occlusions are the result of blood clots. The incidence of clot-related coronary artery occlusion, as shown by angiographic and autopsy studies, appears to diminish with time, primarily because of recanalization of the occluded coronary artery from spontaneous disintegration of the blood clot **(thrombolysis).**

Following the occlusion of a coronary artery, the myocardium evolves through various stages and degrees of severity of impairment, beginning with **myocardial ischemia,** then progressing through **myocardial injury,** both of which are reversible, and ending with **myocardial infarction,** the stage of tissue **necrosis,** an irreversible condition. Along the way, characteristic changes in the ECG reflect the changes in the myocardium. These will be described later.

Typically, a myocardial infarction at its height consists of a central area of dead, necrotic tissue—the **zone of infarction** (or **necrosis**), surrounded immediately by a layer of injured myocardial tissue—the **zone of injury,** and, then, by an outer layer of ischemic tissue—the **zone of ischemia.**

Myocardial infarction may be either **transmural** or **nontransmural** (Figure 11-4). A **transmural infarction** is one where the zone of infarction involves the entire full thickness of the ventricular wall, from the endocardium to the epicardial surface. A **nontransmural infarction,** on the other hand, is one where the ventricular wall is only partially involved by the infarction. The prime example of a nontransmural myocardial infarction is **subendocardial infarction** where the zone of infarction involves only the inner layer of the ventricular wall closest to the endocardium.

The site of the myocardial infarction depends on which coronary artery is occluded. **Table 11-2** lists

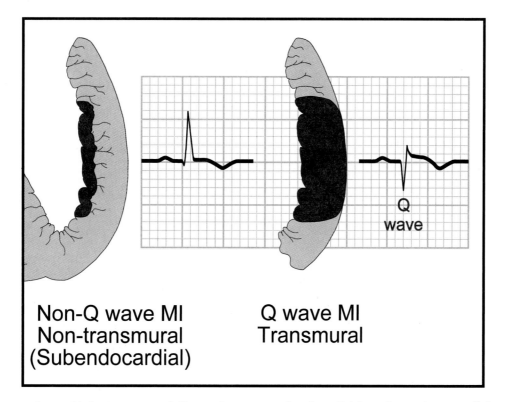

Non-Q wave MI
Non-transmural
(Subendocardial)

Q wave MI
Transmural

Figure 11-4. A transmural (Q wave) versus a subendocardial (non-Q wave) myocardial infarction.

the various types of myocardial infarctions based on their location and the coronary artery or arteries most likely occluded to produce them. Since the distribution of the coronary arteries varies from person to person, the arteries occluded in any specific myocardial infarction may differ from those listed.

The evolution and resolution of a typical transmural myocardial infarction can be divided into four phases, depending on the stage and severity of in-

volvement of the myocardium. The transmural myocardial infarction usually begins in the subendocardium presumably because this area has the highest myocardial oxygen demand and the least supply of blood. The infarct then progresses outward in a wave front pattern until it involves the entire myocardium. While the necrosis is progressing from the endocardium to the epicardium, the acute myocardial infarction is said to be **"evolving."**

Table 11-2. Location of myocardial infarction in relation to the coronary arteries occluded

Location of infarction	Site of coronary artery occlusion
Anterior myocardial infarction	
Septal myocardial infarction (Figure 5A)	**Left anterior descending coronary artery** beyond the first diagonal branch, involving the **septal perforator arteries**
Anterior (localized) myocardial infarction (Figure 5B)	**Diagonal arteries** of the **left anterior descending coronary artery**
Anteroseptal myocardial infarction (Figure 5C)	**Left anterior descending coronary artery** involving both the **septal perforator** and **diagonal arteries**
Lateral myocardial infarction (Figure 5D)	Laterally located **diagonal arteries** of the **left anterior descending coronary artery** and/or the **anterolateral marginal artery** of the **left circumflex coronary artery**
Anterolateral myocardial infarction (Figure 5E)	**Diagonal arteries** of the **left anterior descending coronary artery** alone or in conjunction with the **anterolateral marginal artery** of the **left circumflex coronary artery**
Extensive anterior myocardial infarction (Figure 5F)	**Left anterior descending coronary artery** alone or in conjunction with the **anterolateral marginal artery** of the **left circumflex coronary artery**
Inferior (diaphragmatic) myocardial infarction (Figure 5G)	**Posterior left ventricular arteries** of the **right coronary artery** or, less commonly, of the **left circumflex coronary artery** of the **left coronary artery**
Posterior myocardial infarction (Figure 5H)	**Distal left circumflex artery** and/or **posterolateral artery** of the **circumflex coronary artery**

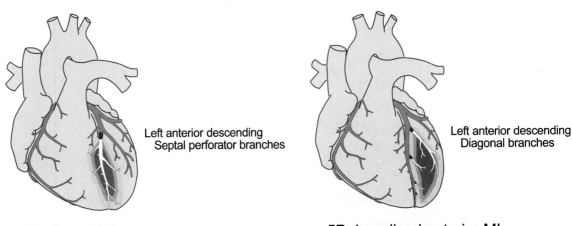

Left anterior descending
Septal perforator branches

Left anterior descending
Diagonal branches

5A. Septal MI   5B. Localized anterior MI

Figure 11-5. Location of myocardial infarction in relation to the coronary arteries occluded.

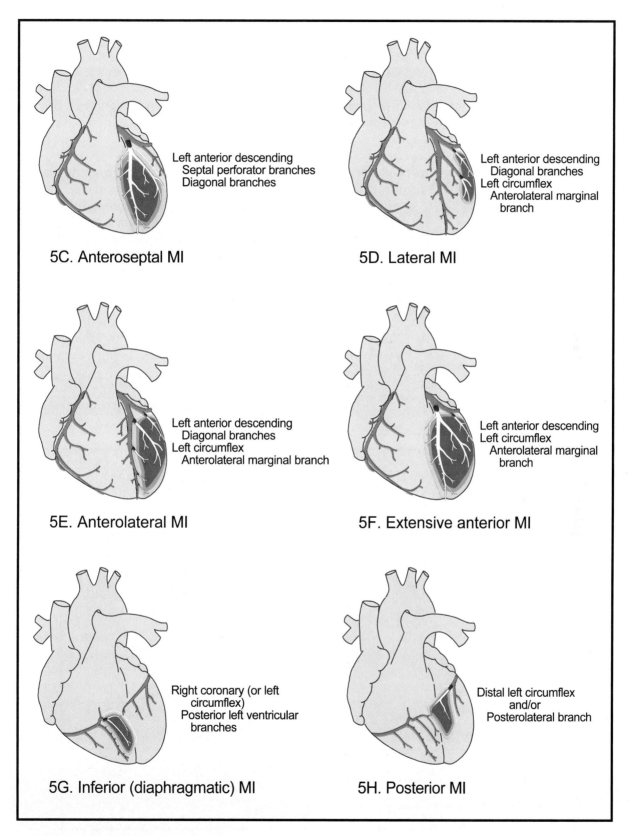

Left anterior descending
  Septal perforator branches
  Diagonal branches

5C. Anteroseptal MI

Left anterior descending
  Diagonal branches
Left circumflex
  Anterolateral marginal
  branch

5D. Lateral MI

Left anterior descending
  Diagonal branches
Left circumflex
  Anterolateral marginal branch

5E. Anterolateral MI

Left anterior descending
Left circumflex
  Anterolateral marginal
  branch

5F. Extensive anterior MI

Right coronary (or left
  circumflex)
Posterior left ventricular
  branches

5G. Inferior (diaphragmatic) MI

Distal left circumflex
  and/or
  Posterolateral branch

5H. Posterior MI

Figure 11-5, cont'd.

Phase 1: Within the first 2 hours after coronary artery occlusion the following sequence of changes occurs in the myocardium supplied by the occluded artery (Figure 11-6, *A*):

A. Within seconds of the coronary artery occlusion, extensive myocardial ischemia occurs.

B. During the first 20 to 40 minutes (average, 30 minutes) following the onset of the myocardial infarction, **reversible myocardial injury** appears in the subendocardium.

C. About 30 minutes after the interruption of blood flow, **irreversible myocardial necrosis (infarction)** occurs in the subendocardium as **myocardial injury** begins to spread toward the epicardium.

D. By 1 hour after the onset, **myocardial necrosis** has spread through over one third of the myocardium.

E. By 2 hours after the onset, **myocardial necrosis** has spread through about half of the myocardium.

Phase 2: Between the second and twenty-fourth hour after the occlusion, the evolution of the myocardial infarction is completed in the following sequence (Figure 11-6, *B*):

A. By 3 hours, about two thirds of the myocardial cells within the affected myocardium become necrotic.

B. By 6 hours, only a small percentage of the cells remain viable. For all practical purposes, the evolution of the transmural myocardial infarction is complete at this point.

C. By 24 hours, the progression of myocardial necrosis to the epicardium is usually complete.

Phase 3: After the first day, during the next 24 to 72 hours, little or no ischemic or injured myocardial cells remain, as all cells have either died or recovered. Acute inflammation with edema and cellular infiltration begins within the necrotic tissue during this phase.

Phase 4: During the second week, inflammation continues, followed by proliferation of connective tissue during the third week. Healing with replacement of the necrotic tissue with fibrous connective tissue is generally complete by the seventh week.

Table 11-3 summarizes the four phases of evolution of an acute transmural myocardial infarction.

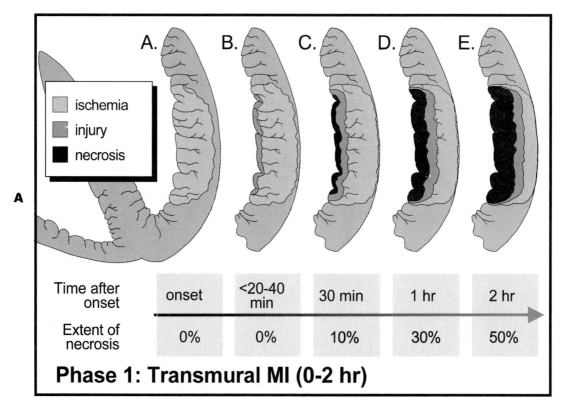

Figure 11-6. The first two early phases of an acute transmural myocardial infarction. **A,** Phase 1.

Table 11-3. The four phases of evolution of an acute transmural myocardial infarction

Phase	Time after onset of acute MI	Pathophysiology
1	**0 to 2 hours** (First few hours)	Extensive myocardial ischemia and injury occur with about 50 percent of the myocardium becoming necrotic.
2	**2 to 24 hours** (First day)	The evolution of the myocardial infarction is complete with about two thirds of the myocardium becoming necrotic by 3 hours and most of the rest becoming necrotic by 6 hours.
3	**24 to 72 hours** (Second to third day)	Little or no ischemic or injured myocardial cells remain, as all cells have either died or recovered. Acute inflammation begins within the necrotic tissue.
4	**2 to 8 weeks**	Fibrous tissue completely replaces the necrotic tissue.

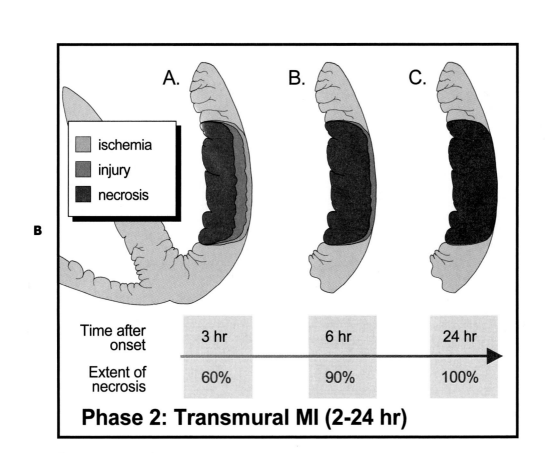

Figure 11-6, cont'd. **B**, Phase 2.

ECG Changes in Acute Myocardial Infarction

The ECG in evolving acute myocardial infarction, with its varying mix of **myocardial ischemia, injury,** and **necrosis,** is characterized by changes in three components of the ECG—the **T wave, ST segment,** and **Q wave.** The changes in the ECG ascribed to myocardial ischemia, injury, and necrosis are:

Myocardial ischemia	=	**Symmetrical T wave inversion** or **elevation**
Myocardial injury	=	**ST segment elevation**
Myocardial necrosis	=	**Abnormal Q waves**

The nature of these ECG changes and the leads in which they appear will depend on (1) the anatomic location of the acute myocardial infarction in the ventricles (**anterior, posterior,** or **inferior**), (2) the extent of the involvement of the myocardial wall (**transmural** or **nontransmural**), and (3) the **time** when the ECG was obtained following the onset of the acute myocardial infarcation. The changes that an acute transmural myocardial infarction produces in the T waves, ST segments, and Q waves are summarized in **Table 11-4** below and described in detail in the following sections.

It is important to note here that the leads that record the electrical forces in acute myocardial infarction through electrodes that view the exterior or epicardial surface of the area of the myocardium involved by myocardial ischemia, injury, and infarction are termed *facing leads* in this book. The leads that record the electrical forces through electrodes that view the epicardial surface of the uninvolved myocardium directly opposite the involved myocardium are termed *opposite* (or *reciprocal*) *leads.*

Table 11-4. ECG changes in acute transmural myocardial infarction

Stage of acute MI	Severity of process	Changes in facing ECG leads	Reciprocal changes in opposite ECG leads	Appearance of ECG changes after onset of acute MI
Ischemia	Reversible	Tall, peaked (a) or inverted (b) T waves	Inverted (a) or tall, peaked (b) T waves	Within seconds of onset
Injury	Reversible	Elevated ST segments	Depressed ST segments	Within 20 to 40 minutes of onset
Necrosis	Irreversible	Abnormal Q waves and QS complexes	Tall R waves	In about 2 hours after onset

Abnormal T Waves

Abnormal T waves indicating myocardial ischemia usually appear within seconds of the onset of an acute myocardial infarction. These **ischemic T waves,** which appear over the **zone of ischemia,** are primarily due to a delay in repolarization of the myocardium because of anoxia (Figure 11-7). They may be **abnormally tall and peaked** or **deeply inverted.** Whether the ischemic T waves are upright or inverted depends on where the ischemia is, **subendocardial** or **subepicardial,** respectively.

In **normal hearts,** repolarization begins at the epicardium and progresses toward the endocardium, producing a positive T wave.

In **subendocardial ischemia,** there is a delay in repolarization of the subendocardial cardiac cells. Repolarization progresses in the normal direction from the epicardium to the endocardium but is slowed when it reaches the ischemic subendocardial area. This produces a **prolonged QT interval** and a **symmetrically positive tall, peaked T wave.**

In **subepicardial ischemia,** on the other hand, there is a delay in the repolarization in the subepicardial cardiac cells. Because of this, repolarization begins at the endocardium and progresses in a reverse direction, from the endocardium to the epicardium, slowing when it reaches the ischemic subepicardial area. This produces a **prolonged QT interval** and a **symmetrically negative deep T wave.**

Abnormal ischemic T waves are often associated with depression of the ST segment, another manifestation of myocardial ischemia. Ischemic T waves and associated ST segment depression revert to normal quickly following an anginal attack. Those present in acute myocardial infarction secondary to myocardial ischemia may disappear more gradually or not at all as healing proceeds.

Abnormal, deeply inverted T waves also appear in association with abnormal Q waves over the zone of necrosis in the later phases of acute myocardial infarction. These T waves are deeply inverted, mirror images of the upright T waves normally generated in the opposite ventricular wall, being produced the same way as abnormal Q waves, described later.

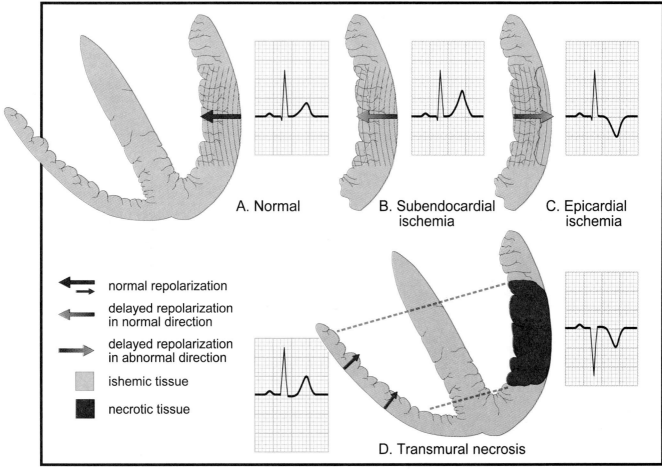

A. Normal

B. Subendocardial ischemia

C. Epicardial ischemia

normal repolarization

delayed repolarization in normal direction

delayed repolarization in abnormal direction

ishemic tissue

necrotic tissue

D. Transmural necrosis

Figure 11-7. The mechanism of formation of abnormal T waves.

Abnormal ST Segments

Abnormal ST segments are present in myocardial infarction indicating **myocardial injury** and in **myocardial ischemia** from whatever cause. The ST segments may be **elevated** or **depressed.**

ST segment elevation. Abnormal ST segment elevation is an ECG sign of severe widespread **myocardial injury** in the evolution of an acute myocardial infarction. It usually indicates a transmural involvement, but it may also be seen in subendocardial infarction. An ST segment is considered to be elevated when it is ≥**1 mm (≥0.1 mV)** above the baseline, measured 0.08 second (2 small boxes) after the J point of the QRS complex.

ST elevation usually appears within 20 to 40 minutes (average, 30 minutes) following the onset of infarction, foreshadowing a progression to myocardial necrosis and development of abnormal Q waves. Such ST segments are **elevated** in the leads facing the zone of injury and **depressed** in the opposite leads (Figure 11-8). ST segment elevation is often accompanied by an increase in the size of the R wave.

The cause of ST segment elevation in acute MI is the **current of injury,** an electrical manifestation of the inability of cardiac cells "injured" by severe ischemia to maintain a normal resting membrane potential during diastole. Following injury, leakage of negative intracellular ions across the cell membrane into the surrounding extracellular fluid occurs during diastole when the cells are in the resting polarized state. The outside of the injured cardiac cells becomes more negative as the inside becomes more positive. As a result, (1) the cells' resting membrane potential drops below its normal level of −90 mV to about −70 mV and (2) the exterior of the injured cardiac cells becomes relatively more negative than that of the surrounding normal cardiac cells.

The difference in potential between the injured and normal cardiac cells causes a downward displacement of the baseline of the ECG in the leads facing the injured cells during electrical diastole. Thus, the T-Q interval in the ECG (the interval between the end of the T wave and the beginning of the QRS complex) shifts downward in the ECG leads facing the zone of injury. The electrical potentials generated by depolarization (the QRS complex) and repolarization (the ST segment and the T wave) of the injured cardiac cells during electrical systole are normal or slightly greater than normal. Since the amplifier circuit of the ECG machine maintains the baseline of each lead at the same level, a false impression is given that the ST segment and T wave, including the R wave, are elevated in the ECG leads facing the zone of injury and depressed in the opposite leads.

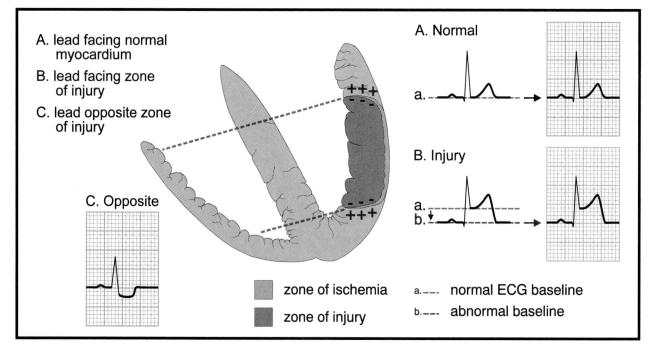

Figure 11-8. The mechanism of ST elevation in acute myocardial infarction.

Following the injury phase, as the myocardial infarction progresses, the injured myocardial tissue turns necrotic and the current of injury disappears as the tissue becomes electrically inert. The ST segments become less elevated in the facing leads and finally return to the baseline. As this is occurring, the R waves begin to become smaller and disappear and significant Q waves and T wave inversion begin to appear in the facing leads.

Other causes of ST segment elevation that can be confused with that of acute myocardial infarction are:

- **Coronary vasospasm.** Intense transmural myocardial ischemia brought on by vasospasm of a major coronary artery, often the left anterior descending coronary artery, **Prinzmetal's angina,** may mimic an acute myocardial infarction electrocardiographically. Clinically, patients with Prinzmetal's angina have recurrent chest pain not related to exercise or other precipitating factors, often several times a day or night, and sometimes associated with significant arrhythmias.
- **Acute pericarditis.** The pain of acute pericarditis may mimic that of acute myocardial infarction, but the younger age of the patient, who usually lacks the coronary risk factors, makes the diagnosis of acute myocardial infarction unlikely. The pain of pericarditis is often pleuritic in nature, made worse on inspiration, and relieved by the patient sitting upright and leaning forward. The pleuritic pain, the presence of a pericardial friction rub, and the appearance of ST segment elevations in practically all the ECG leads support the diagnosis of pericarditis.
- **Ventricular aneurysm**
- **Hyperkalemia**

ST segment depression. ST segment depression is an ECG sign of severe **myocardial ischemia.** Similar to the criteria for ST elevation, an ST segment is considered to be depressed when it is **≥1 mm (≥0.1 mV)** below the baseline, measured 0.08 second (2 small boxes) after the J point of the QRS complex.

ST depression usually appears during the first hour following the onset of subendocardial myocardial infarction, during an anginal attack, or following exercise. The ST segments are **depressed** in the leads facing the ischemic tissue and **elevated** in the opposite leads. Such abnormal ST segments are due to altered repolarization of the myocardium because of anoxia.

The ST segment depressions of myocardial ischemia have been classified according to the nature of the sloping of the segment (i.e., **downsloping, horizontal,** and **upsloping**) (Figure 11-9). The downsloping of an ST segment is most specific for myocardial ischemia, including that present in subendocardial infarction; horizontal, of intermediate specificity; and upsloping, the least. However, no matter what the slope, an ST segment that is depressed ≥1 mm 0.08 second after the end of the QRS complex is significant. ST segment depression is often associated with ischemic T-wave changes, another manifestation of myocardial ischemia.

ST segment depression reverts to normal quickly following an anginal attack or following exercise. When associated with acute subendocardial myocardial infarction, the ST depression may disappear more gradually or not at all as healing proceeds, becoming chronic.

Although ST segment depression is commonly associated with myocardial ischemia, other common causes are:

- Left and right ventricular hypertrophy
- Left and right bundle branch blocks
- Digitalis in therapeutic and toxic doses

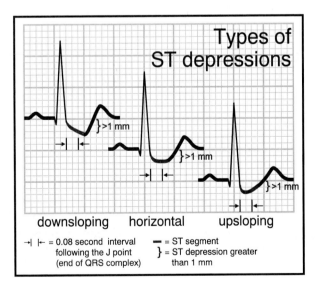

Figure 11-9. Types of ST depression.

Q Waves

A **Q wave** is the first negative deflection of the QRS complex. It may be **normal (insignificant)** or **abnormal (significant)** (Figure 11-10).

Normal Q waves. Normal Q waves result from the normal depolarization of the interventricular septum from left to right. This relatively small electrical force is the first step in the depolarization of the ventricles. The electrical forces responsible for the normal Q wave are negative since they travel away from the leads in which they appear, being opposite in direction to the positive electrical forces producing the R wave. Because the interventricular septum is thin, the electrical forces are small and of short duration—within 0.04 second—and of low amplitude. The resultant **"septal" q wave** is **less than 0.04 second wide** and of a **depth of less than 25% of the height of the succeeding R wave.** Such small normal q waves are commonly present in the QRS complexes in leads I, II, III, aVL, aVF, V_5, and V_6.

Abnormal Q waves. An abnormal Q wave is usually considered an ECG sign of **irreversible myocardial necrosis** in the evolution of an acute myocardial infarction. A Q wave is considered abnormal if it is ≥**0.04 second** wide and has a depth of ≥**25%** of the height of the succeeding R wave.

Abnormal Q waves usually begin to appear about 2 hours after the onset of the myocardial infarction, reaching maximum size in about 24 to 48 hours. They typically appear in the facing leads directly over necrotic, infarcted myocardial tissue—the **zone of infarction.** Abnormal Q waves may persist indefinitely or disappear in months or years.

The cause of abnormal Q waves differs from that of normal Q waves. A popular theory of why Q waves occur is the **"window" theory.** Since infarcted myocardium cannot depolarize or repolarize, no electrical forces are generated, resulting in an electrically inert area. Thus, infarcted myocardium can be considered a **"window"** through which the facing leads actually view the endocardium of the opposite noninfarcted ventricular wall, electrocardiographically speaking. Because depolarization progresses from the endocardium outward, the electrical forces generated by the wall opposite the infarct will be traveling away from the leads facing the infarct. Therefore, these leads will detect the negative electrical forces generated by the opposite, noninfarcted ventricular wall as large negative abnormal Q waves. These abnormal Q waves can be looked upon as mirror images of the R waves produced by the opposite ventricular wall.

The presence and size of the abnormal Q waves and the number of leads in which they occur depend on the size of the infarct, both on its depth (or thickness) and width. The larger the infarct (i.e., the larger the "window"), the larger the Q waves and the greater the number of facing leads in which they appear. In general, the greater the depth of the infarct, the deeper the Q waves; the wider the infarct, the wider the Q waves. A large abnormal Q wave with or without a succeeding R wave is often called a **QS wave.**

In contrast, the smaller the infarct, the smaller the Q waves in both width and depth and the fewer the facing leads with Q waves. If the infarct is relatively small and nontransmural, for example, a subendocardial myocardial infarction, an abnormal Q wave may be completely absent. To complicate matters, an abnormal Q wave may also be completely absent in a significant transmural myocardial infarction.

The thickness of the myocardium of the opposite noninfarcted ventricular wall generally contributes to the size of the abnormal Q waves: the thicker the opposite myocardium, the larger the Q wave; the thinner the myocardium, the smaller the Q wave.

When the infarct is large, transmural, and entirely necrotic, the R waves completely disappear in the facing leads, resulting in a wide and deep **QS complex.** If enough viable cardiac cells capable of generating electrical forces survive within an infarct, if the infarct is nontransmural with viable cardiac cells between it and the epicardium, or if the facing lead overlies the boundary between an infarct and surrounding viable myocardium, an **abnormal Q wave with an R wave** will result. The size of the R wave will depend on the amount of viable cardiac cells lying under the facing electrode. A **QR complex** indicates a greater amount of viable cardiac tissue between the infarct and the facing electrode than does a **Qr complex.**

Another consequence of an electrically inert infarct is that the **R waves in the opposite leads** are larger than normal. The reason for this is that the positive electrical forces generated by the noninfarcted ventricular wall flowing toward the opposite leads are now unopposed by the negative, electrical forces that once were generated by the now infarcted wall and traveled away from the opposite leads.

The abnormal QS waves that occur in the right precordial leads V_1-V_2 within the first few hours of the onset of an acute anterior wall myocardial in-

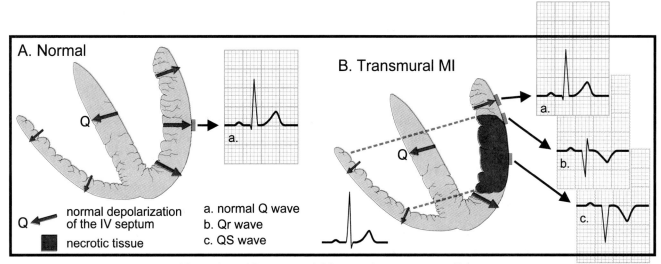

Figure 11-10. The mechanism of formation of Q waves and QS waves in acute myocardial infarction.

farction involving the interventricular septum result from the severe ischemia of the septum. The **"septal" r waves** normally produced by the left to right depolarization of the interventricular septum fail to occur, changing the normal **rS pattern** of the QRS complex in the right precordial leads to a **QS complex.**

Abnormal Q waves are **NOT** present in a 12-lead ECG in a **posterior wall myocardial infarction** since there are no leads facing the infarct.

A myocardial infarction where abnormal Q waves are present in the ECG is called a **Q wave myocardial infarction;** one where abnormal Q waves are absent, a **non-Q wave myocardial infarction.** As noted above, a Q wave myocardial infarction may indicate both a transmural and a nontransmural myocardial infarction. Although abnormal Q waves may be **absent** in both transmural and nontransmural myocardial infarctions, a non-Q wave myocardial infarction will be considered a nontransmural subendocardial myocardial infarction in this book.

Note: Abnormal Q waves may be present in certain leads without being considered significant. An abnormal Q wave is commonly ignored in the following leads, especially if it occurs under certain circumstances.

- **Lead aVR.** An abnormal Q wave in lead aVR is usually ignored since the QRS complex in this lead normally consists of a large S wave.
- **Lead aVL.** A QS or a QR wave in lead aVL alone where the QRS axis is greater than +60 degrees, i.e., an electrically vertical heart, is usually ignored.
- **Lead aVF.** A QS or a QR wave in lead aVF alone is considered insignificant, unless it is accompanied by abnormal Q waves, ST segment elevation, and abnormal T wave changes in one or both of the other inferior leads—leads II and III.
- **Lead III.** An abnormal Q wave in this lead by itself is considered insignificant, unless (1) it is accompanied by abnormal Q waves, ST segment elevation, and abnormal T wave changes in the other inferior leads (lead II or aVF or both) and (2) the abnormal Q wave in **lead III** is wider and deeper than those in leads II and aVF.
- **Lead V$_1$.** An abnormal Q wave in this lead by itself is considered insignificant, unless it is accompanied by abnormal Q waves, ST segment elevation, and abnormal T wave changes in the other precordial leads—leads V$_2$-V$_6$.

Other considerations in determining the significance of abnormal Q waves are:

- **Abnormal Q waves** accompanied by **ST segment elevation** and **T wave inversion** are more significant and more reliable in making a diagnosis of acute myocardial infarction than when the abnormal Q waves occur alone.
- **Abnormal Q waves** in the presence of **left bundle branch block** and **left anterior and posterior fascicular blocks** are usually not considered significant. **Abnormal Q waves** in the presence of **right bundle branch block** are as significant as they are without one.
- **Abnormal Q waves** in the presence of **left ventricular hypertrophy** are not as reliable in making a diagnosis of myocardial infarction as in its absence.

Typical Patterns in Acute Q Wave and Non-Q Wave Myocardial Infarctions

Acute Q wave myocardial infarction occurs in about 50 to 75 percent of patients with acute infarction. In the rest, **non-Q wave myocardial infarction** is present, primarily as a **subendocardial myocardial infarction.**

In **acute Q wave myocardial infarction,** the following typical pattern evolves. In the **facing ECG** leads (Table 11-5), within seconds of the onset of the acute myocardial infarction, the initial ischemic stage produces **symmetrically wide, deeply inverted or tall, peaked T waves.** This is followed within 20 to 40 minutes (average, 30 minutes) by an **elevation of the ST segments** and often an **increase in the size of the R waves** during the injury stage. Then, while the ST segments are still elevated, **abnormal Q waves** and **QS complexes** appear in about 2 hours as necrosis evolves. Finally,

Table 11-5. The changes in the facing ECG leads during the four phases of a transmural, Q wave myocardial infarction

Phase of infarction	Q waves	R waves	ST segments	T waves	ECG
Phase 1 (0 to 2 hours) Onset of extensive ischemia occurs immediately; subendocardial injury, within 20 to 40 minutes; and subendocardial necrosis, in about 30 minutes. Necrosis extends to about half of the myocardial wall by 2 hours.	Unchanged	Unchanged or abnormally tall	Onset of elevation	Amplitude increases; peaking may occur	
Phase 2 (2 to 24 hours) Transmural infarction is considered complete by 6 hours as necrosis involves about 90 percent of the myocardial wall. Rest of the necrosis occurs by the end of phase 2.	Width and depth begin to increase	Amplitude begins to decrease	Maximum elevation	Amplitude and peaking lessen; T waves still positive	
Phase 3 (24 to 72 hours) Little or no ischemia or injury remains as healing begins.	Reach maximum size	Absent	Return to baseline	Become maximally inverted	
Phase 4 (2 to 8 weeks) Replacement of the necrotic tissue by fibrous tissue.	Q waves persist	May return partially	Usually normal	Slight inversion	

as the **R waves become smaller** and the **ST segments return to the baseline, symmetrically deep inverted T waves** appear.

In the **opposite ECG leads,** the ECG changes of evolving acute myocardial infarction differ considerably from those in the facing leads, being, for the most part, opposite in direction. These ECG changes, termed *reciprocal,* include **symmetrically tall, peaked or deeply inverted T waves, depression of the ST segments,** and **abnormally tall R waves.** Generally, **Q waves** do not appear in the opposite leads during an acute myocardial infarction.

In **acute non-Q wave myocardial infarction,** the following typical pattern evolves. In the **facing ECG** leads (Table 11-6), within seconds of the onset of the acute myocardial infarction, the initial ischemic stage produces **symmetrically wide, inverted or tall T waves.** This is followed within about 30 minutes by **elevation** or **depression of the ST segments** during the ischemic/injury stage. Finally, as the **ST segments return to the baseline, symmetrically inverted T waves** appear. Abnormal Q waves do not appear in non-Q wave myocardial infarction.

In the **opposite ECG leads,** the ECG changes of evolving acute myocardial infarction differ considerably from those in the facing leads, being, for the most part, opposite in direction. These ECG changes, termed *reciprocal,* include **symmetrically tall or inverted T waves** and **elevation of the ST segments.**

Table 11-6. The changes in the facing ECG leads during the four phases of a subendocardial, non-Q wave myocardial infarction

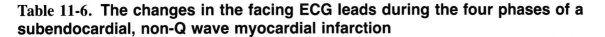

Phase of infarction	Q waves	R waves	ST segments	T waves	ECG
Phase 1 (0 to 2 hours) Onset of localized ischemia occurs immediately; subendocardial injury, within 20 to 40 minutes; and subendocardial necrosis, in about 30 minutes.	Unchanged	Unchanged	Slight elevation **OR** depression	Amplitude may increase slightly	
Phase 2 (2 to 24 hours) Subendocardial infarction is considered complete by 6 hours. Generally, the necrosis involves only the inner parts of the myocardium, usually the subendocardial area, without extending to the epicardial surface.	Unchanged	Amplitude may begin to decrease somewhat	May or may not return to normal	Inversion may occur	
Phase 3 (24 to 72 hours) Little or no ischemia or injury remains as healing begins.	Unchanged	Unchanged	May or may not return to normal	Inversion may occur	
Phase 4 (2 to 8 weeks) Replacement of the infarcted tissue by fibrous tissue.	Unchanged	Unchanged	May or may not return to normal	May or may not return to normal	

The location of an acute Q wave myocardial infarction relates to the leads in which abnormal ST segment elevation and subsequent abnormal Q waves appear (Table 11-7). For example, if **ST segment elevation** and **abnormal Q waves** appear in any or all of the **leads I, aVL, and V$_1$-V$_6$,** the myocardial infarction is "anterior"; and, if **ST segment elevation** and **abnormal Q waves** appear in **leads II, III, and aVF,** the myocardial infarction is **"inferior."** Since there are no facing leads in a posterior myocardial infarction, there are no diagnostic ST segment elevation or abnormal Q waves present in the ECG leads. A posterior myocardial infarction is diagnosed if reciprocal ECG changes of ST segment depression and tall R waves are present in leads **V$_1$-V$_4$.**

Table 11-7. Relationship between the site of an acute Q wave myocardial infarction and the facing leads showing ST segment elevation and abnormal Q waves and the opposite leads showing the reciprocal ECG changes

Site of infarction	Facing leads	Opposite leads
Anterior Wall		
Septal	V$_1$-V$_2$	None
Anterior (Localized)	V$_3$-V$_4$	None
Anteroseptal	V$_1$-V$_4$	None
Lateral	I, aVL, and V$_5$ or V$_6$	II, III, and aVF
Anterolateral	I, aVL, and V$_3$-V$_6$	II, III, and aVF
Extensive Anterior	I, aVL, and V$_1$-V$_6$	II, III, and aVF
Inferior Wall	II, III, and aVF	I and aVL
Posterior Wall	None	V$_1$-V$_4$

Diagnostic Features of Specific Myocardial Infarctions

The diagnostic features of the following specific myocardial infarctions will be presented in this section:

Septal MI	Anterolateral MI
Anterior (localized) MI	Extensive anterior MI
Anteroseptal MI	Inferior MI
Lateral MI	Posterior MI

The diagnostic features of each of the specific myocardial infarctions include the coronary arteries involved, the site of occlusion of the coronary artery, the location of the infarct, and the ECG changes in the facing and opposite leads. It should be noted that if the ECG being analyzed has changes consistent with both an anterolateral and an inferior myocardial infarction, for example, then the patient has both an inferior and an anterolateral myocardial infarction. This would also be true of an anterolateral and a posterior myocardial infarction, an inferior and a posterior myocardial infarction, and so forth.

The changes in the ECG presented for each specific myocardial infarction are based on typical first-time infarcts and may not represent actual changes in a particular patient's ECG. The reasons for this include individual variations in the size, position in the chest, and rotation of the heart and in the distribution of the coronary artery circulation; the presence of bundle branch blocks, ventricular hypertrophy, and previous myocardial infarctions; and co-existing drug- and electrolyte-related ECG changes.

Septal Myocardial Infarction

Coronary Arteries Involved and Site of Occlusion

The major artery involved is the **left coronary artery,** specifically the following branches:

- **Left anterior descending coronary artery** beyond the first diagonal branch, involving the **septal perforator arteries**

Location of Infarct

The myocardial infarction (Figure 11-11 and Table 11-8) involves (1) the **anterior wall of the left ventricle** overlying the interventricular septum and (2) the **anterior two thirds of the interventricular septum.**

Notes

ECG Changes

In **facing leads V_1-V_2:**

Early: Absence of normal **"septal" r waves** in the right precordial leads V_1-V_2, resulting in **QS waves** in these leads. Absence of normal **"septal" q waves** where normally present (i.e., in leads I, II, III, aVF, and V_4-V_6). **ST segment elevation** with **tall T waves** in leads V_1-V_2.

Late: **QS complexes** with **T wave inversion** in leads V_1-V_2.

In **opposite leads II, III,** and **aVF:**

Early: No significant ECG changes.
Late: No significant ECG changes.

Table 11-8. ECG changes in septal MI

	Q waves	R waves	ST segments	T waves
EARLY **Phase 1** **First Few Hours** **(0 to 2 Hours)**	**Absent "septal" q waves** in **I, II, III, aVF,** and V_4-V_6 **QS waves** in V_1-V_2	**Absent "septal" r waves** in V_1-V_2	**Elevated** in V_1-V_2	**Sometimes abnormally tall** with peaking in V_1-V_2
Phase 2 **First Day** **(2 to 24 Hours)**	**Same as in Phase 1**	Same as in **Phase 1**	**Maximally elevated** in V_1-V_2	**Less tall,** but generally still positive, in V_1-V_2
LATE **Phase 3** **Second and Third Day** **(24 to 72 Hours)**	**QS complexes** in V_1-V_2	Same as in **Phase 1**	**Return** of the **ST segments** to the baseline throughout	**T wave inversion** in V_1-V_2

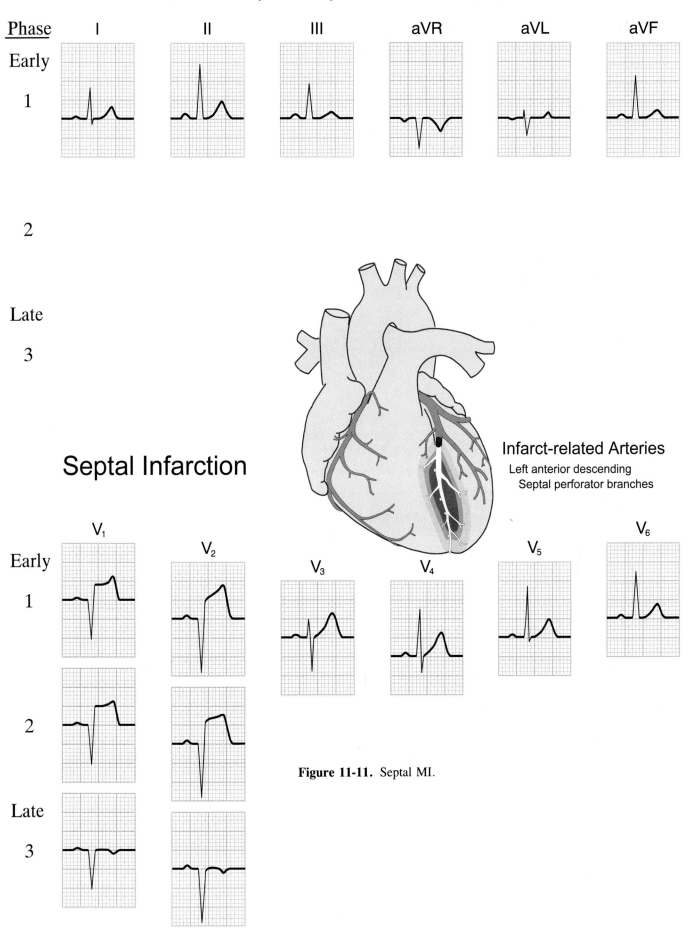

Septal Infarction

Infarct-related Arteries
Left anterior descending
Septal perforator branches

Figure 11-11. Septal MI.

Anterior (Localized) Myocardial Infarction

Coronary Arteries Involved and Site of Occlusion

The major artery involved is the **left coronary artery,** specifically the following branches:

- **Diagonal arteries** of the **left anterior descending coronary artery**

Location of Infarct

The myocardial infarction (Figure 11-12 and Table 11-9) involves an area of the **anterior wall of the left ventricle** immediately to the left of the interventricular septum.

Notes

ECG Changes

In **facing leads V_3-V_4:**

Early: **ST segment elevation** with **tall T waves** and **taller than normal R waves** in the midprecordial leads V_3 and V_4.

Late: **QS complexes** with **T wave inversion** in leads V_3 and V_4.

In **opposite leads II, III,** and **aVF:**

Early: No significant ECG changes.

Late: No significant ECG changes.

Table 11-9. ECG changes in anterior (localized) MI

	Q waves	R waves	ST segments	T waves
EARLY **Phase 1** **First Few Hours** **(0 to 2 Hours)**	**Normal Q waves**	**Normal** or **abnormally tall R waves** in V_3-V_4	**Elevated** in V_3-V_4	**Sometimes abnormally tall** with peaking in V_3-V_4
Phase 2 **First Day** **(2 to 24 Hours)**	**Minimally abnormal** in V_3-V_4	**Minimally decreased** in V_3-V_4	**Maximally elevated** in V_3-V_4	**Less tall,** but generally still positive, in V_3-V_4
LATE **Phase 3** **Second and Third Day** **(24 to 72 Hours)**	**QS complexes** in V_3-V_4	**Absent** in V_3-V_4	**Return** of the **ST segments** to the baseline throughout	**T wave inversion** in V_3-V_4

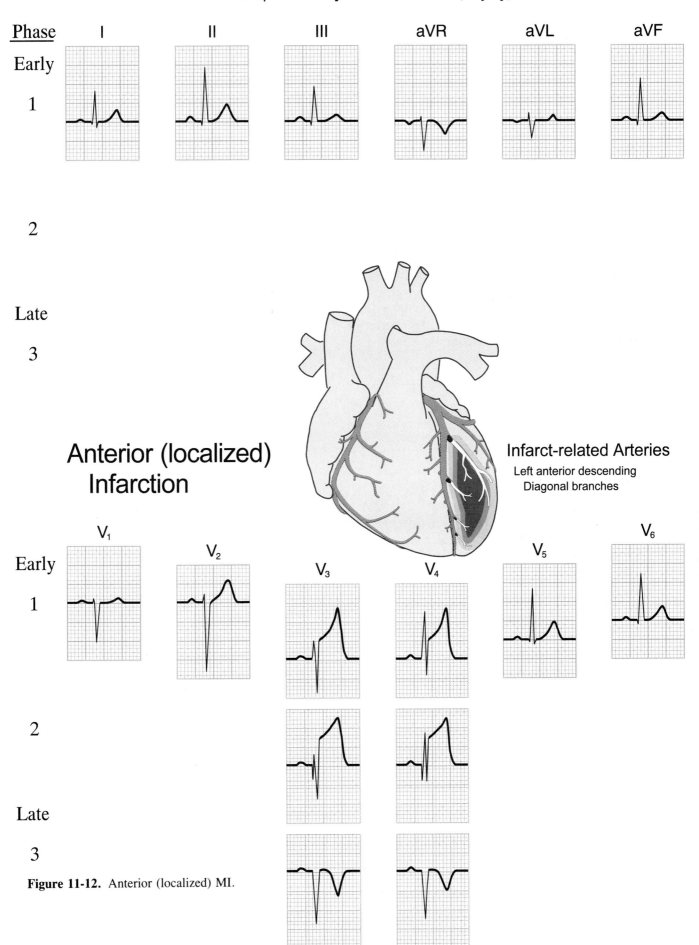

Phase — I — II — III — aVR — aVL — aVF
Early 1

2

Late

3

Anterior (localized) Infarction

Infarct-related Arteries
Left anterior descending
Diagonal branches

Early 1 — V₁ — V₂ — V₃ — V₄ — V₅ — V₆

2

Late

3

Figure 11-12. Anterior (localized) MI.

Anteroseptal Myocardial Infarction

Coronary Arteries Involved and Site of Occlusion

The major artery involved is the **left coronary artery,** specifically the following branches:

- **Left anterior descending coronary artery** involving both the **septal perforator** and **diagonal arteries**

Location of Infarct

The myocardial infarction (Figure 11-13 and Table 11-10) involves (1) the **anterior wall of the left ventricle** overlying the interventricular septum and immediately to the left of it and (2) the **anterior two thirds of the interventricular septum.**

Notes

ECG Changes

In **facing leads V_1-V_4:**

Early: Absence of normal **"septal" r waves** in the right precordial leads V_1-V_2, resulting in **QS waves** in these leads.
Absence of normal **"septal" q waves** where normally present (i.e., in leads I, II, III, aVF, and V_4-V_6).
ST segment elevation with **tall T waves** in leads V_1-V_4 and **taller than normal R waves** in the midprecordial leads V_3-V_4.

Late: **QS complexes** with **T wave inversion** in leads V_1-V_4.

In **opposite leads II, III,** and **aVF:**

Early: No significant ECG changes.
Late: No significant ECG changes.

Table 11-10. ECG changes in anteroseptal MI

	Q waves	R waves	ST segments	T waves
EARLY Phase 1 First Few Hours (0 to 2 Hours)	Absent **"septal" q waves** in I, II, III, aVF, and V_4-V_6 QS waves in V_1-V_2	Absent **"septal" r waves** in V_1-V_2 Normal or abnormally tall R waves in V_3-V_4	**Elevated** in V_1-V_4	Sometimes abnormally tall with peaking in V_1-V_4
Phase 2 First Day (2 to 24 Hours)	QS waves in V_1-V_2 Minimally abnormal in V_3-V_4	Absent **"septal" r waves** in V_1-V_2 Minimally decreased in V_3-V_4	**Maximally elevated** in V_1-V_4	Less tall, but generally still positive, in V_1-V_4
LATE Phase 3 Second and Third Day (24 to 72 Hours)	QS complexes in V_1-V_4	Absent in V_1-V_4	**Return** of the **ST segments** to the baseline throughout	T wave inversion in V_1-V_4

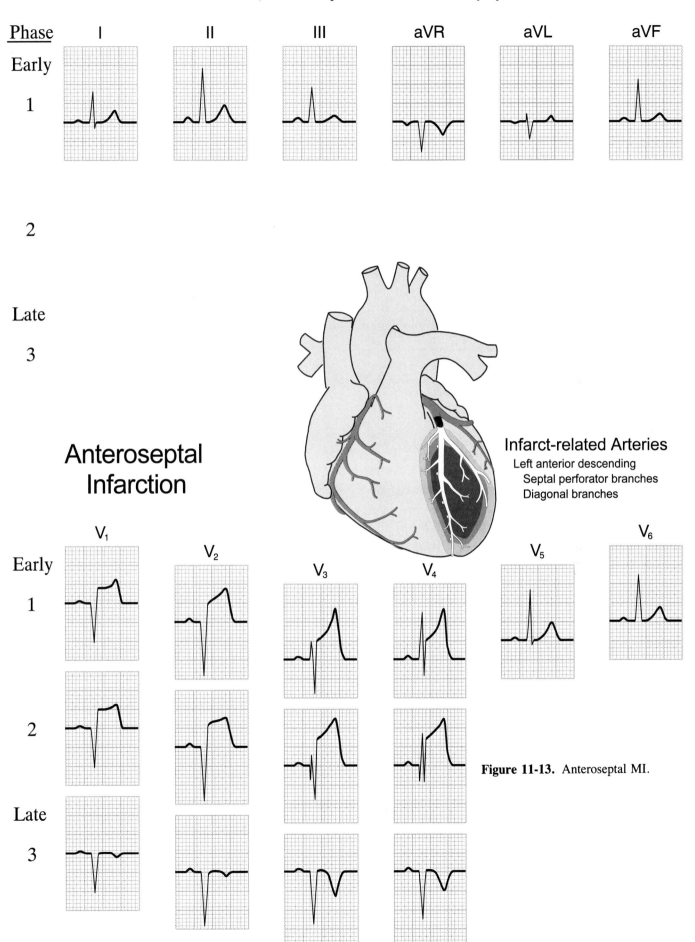

Anteroseptal
Infarction

Infarct-related Arteries
Left anterior descending
Septal perforator branches
Diagonal branches

Figure 11-13. Anteroseptal MI.

Lateral Myocardial Infarction

Coronary Arteries Involved and Site of Occlusion

The major artery involved is the **left coronary artery,** specifically the following branches:

- Laterally located **diagonal arteries** of the **left anterior descending coronary artery** and/or the **anterolateral marginal artery** of the **left circumflex coronary artery**

Location of Infarct

The myocardial infarction (Figure 11-14 and Table 11-11) involves the **lateral wall of the left ventricle.**

Notes

ECG Changes

In **facing leads I, aVL,** and **V₅** or **V₆** or both:

Early:	**ST segment elevation** with **tall T waves** and **taller than normal R waves** in leads I, aVL, and the left precordial lead V_5 or V_6 or both.
Late:	**Abnormal Q waves** and **small R waves** with **T wave inversion** in leads I and aVL. **QS waves** or **complexes** with **T wave inversion** in lead V_5 or V_6 or both.

In **opposite leads II, III,** and **aVF:**

Early:	**ST segment depression** in leads II, III, and aVF.
Late:	**Abnormally tall T waves** in leads II, III, and aVF.

Table 11-11. ECG changes in lateral MI

	Q Waves	R Waves	ST Segments	T Waves
EARLY **Phase 1** **First Few Hours** **(0 to 2 Hours)**	**Normal Q waves**	**Normal** or **abnormally tall R waves** in **I, aVL,** and **V₅** or **V₆** or both	**Elevated** in **I, aVL,** and **V₅** or **V₆** or both **Depressed** in **II, III,** and **aVF**	**Sometimes abnormally tall** with peaking in **I, aVL,** and **V₅** or **V₆** or both
Phase 2 **First Day** **(2 to 24 Hours)**	**Minimally abnormal** in **I, aVL,** and **V₅** or **V₆** or both	**Minimally decreased** in **I, aVL,** and **V₅** or **V₆** or both	**Maximally elevated** in **I, aVL,** and **V₅** or **V₆** or both **Maximally depressed** in **II, III,** and **aVF**	**Less tall,** but generally still positive in **I, aVL,** and **V₅** or **V₆** or both
LATE **Phase 3** **Second and Third Day** **(24 to 72 Hours)**	**QS waves** or **complexes** in **V₅** or **V₆** or both **Significantly abnormal** in **I** and **aVL**	**Decreased** or **absent** in **V₅** or **V₆** or both **Small R waves** in **I** and **aVL**	**Return** of the **ST segments** to the baseline throughout	**T wave inversion** in **I, aVL,** and **V₅** or **V₆** or both **Tall T waves** in **II, III,** and **aVF**

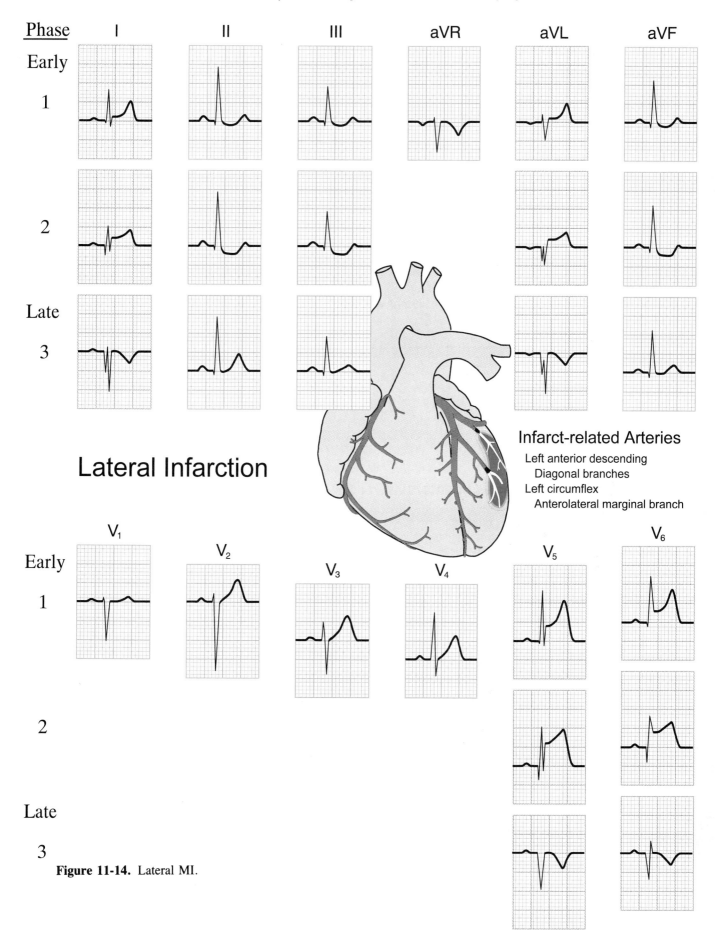

Phase

Early 1, 2   Late 3

I   II   III   aVR   aVL   aVF

Lateral Infarction

Infarct-related Arteries

Left anterior descending
  Diagonal branches
Left circumflex
  Anterolateral marginal branch

V_1 V_2 V_3 V_4 V_5 V_6

Early 1, 2   Late 3

Figure 11-14. Lateral MI.

Anterolateral Myocardial Infarction

Coronary Arteries Involved and Site of Occlusion

The major artery involved is the **left coronary artery,** specifically the following branches:

- **Diagonal arteries** of the **left anterior descending coronary artery** alone or in conjunction with the **anterolateral marginal artery** of the **left circumflex coronary artery**

Location of Infarct

The myocardial infarction (Figure 11-15 and Table 11-12) involves the **anterior and lateral wall of the left ventricle.**

Notes

ECG Changes

In **facing leads I, aVL,** and **V₃-V₆:**

Early: **ST segment elevation** with **tall T waves** and **taller than normal R waves** in leads I, aVL, and the precordial leads V₃-V₆.

Late: **Abnormal Q waves** and **small R waves** with **T wave inversion** in leads I and aVL.
QS waves or complexes with **T wave inversion** in leads V₃-V₆.

In **opposite leads II, III,** and **aVF:**

Early: **ST segment depression** in leads II, III, and aVF.

Late: **Abnormally tall T waves** in leads II, III, and aVF.

Table 11-12. ECG changes in anterolateral MI

	Q Waves	R Waves	ST Segments	T Waves
EARLY **Phase 1** **First Few Hours** **(0 to 2 Hours)**	**Normal Q waves**	**Normal** or **abnormally tall R waves** in **I, aVL,** and **V₃-V₆**	**Elevated** in **I, aVL,** and **V₃-V₆** **Depressed** in **II, III,** and **aVF**	**Sometimes abnormally tall** with peaking in **I, aVL,** and **V₃-V₆**
Phase 2 **First Day** **(2 to 24 Hours)**	**Minimally abnormal** in **I, aVL,** and **V₃-V₆**	**Minimally decreased** in **I, aVL,** and **V₃-V₆**	**Maximally elevated** in **I, aVL,** and **V₃-V₆** **Maximally depressed** in **II, III,** and **aVF**	**Less tall,** but generally still positive in **I, aVL,** and **V₃-V₆**
LATE **Phase 3** **Second and** **Third Day** **(24 to 72 Hours)**	**QS waves** or **complexes** in **V₃-V₆** **Significantly abnormal** in **I** and **aVL**	**Decreased** or **absent** in **V₃-V₆** **Small R waves** in **I** and **aVL**	**Return** of the **ST segments** to the baseline throughout	**T wave inversion** in **I, aVL,** and **V₃-V₆** **Tall T waves** in **II, III,** and **aVF**

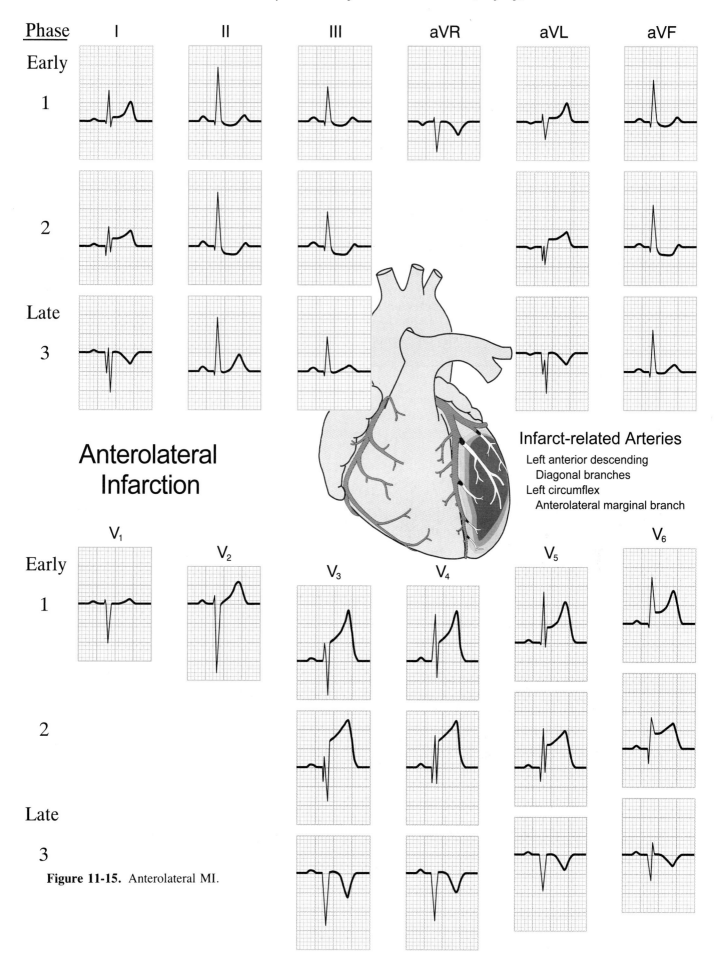

Anterolateral Infarction

Infarct-related Arteries

Left anterior descending
  Diagonal branches
Left circumflex
  Anterolateral marginal branch

Figure 11-15. Anterolateral MI.

Extensive Anterior Myocardial Infarction

Coronary Arteries Involved and Site of Occlusion

The major artery involved is the **left coronary artery,** specifically the following branches:

- **Left anterior descending coronary artery** alone or in conjunction with the **anterolateral marginal artery** of the **left circumflex coronary artery**

Location of Infarct

The myocardial infarction (Figure 11-16 and Table 11-13) involves (1) the entire **anterior and lateral wall of the left ventricle** and (2) the **anterior two thirds of the interventricular septum.**

Notes

ECG Changes

In **facing leads I, aVL,** and **V_1-V_6:**

Early: Absence of normal **"septal" r waves** in the right precordial leads V_1-V_2, resulting in **QS complexes** in these leads. Absence of normal **"septal" q waves** where normally present (i.e., in leads I, II, III, aVF, and V_4-V_6). **ST segment elevation** with **tall T waves** in leads I, aVL, and V_1-V_6 and **taller than normal R waves** in leads I, aVL, and V_3-V_6.

Late: **Abnormal Q waves** and **small R waves** with **T wave inversion** in leads I, aVL, and V_6. **QS waves or complexes** with **T wave inversion** in leads V_1-V_5 and sometimes V_6.

In **opposite leads II, III,** and **aVF:**

Early: **ST segment depression** in leads II, III, and aVF.

Late: **Abnormally tall T waves** in leads II, III, and aVF.

Table 11-13. ECG changes in extensive anterior MI

	Q Waves	R Waves	ST Segments	T Waves
EARLY **Phase 1** **First Few Hours** **(0 to 2 Hours)**	Absent "septal" q waves in I, II, III, aVF, and V_4-V_6 QS waves in V_1-V_2	Absent "septal" r waves in V_1-V_2 Normal or abnormally tall R waves in I, aVL, and V_3-V_6	Elevated in I, aVL, and V_1-V_6 Depressed in II, III, and aVF	Sometimes abnormally tall with peaking in I, aVL, and V_1-V_6
Phase 2 **First Day** **(2 to 24 Hours)**	QS waves in V_1-V_2 Minimally abnormal in I, aVL, and V_3-V_6	Absent in V_1-V_2 Minimally decreased in I, aVL, and V_3-V_6	Maximally elevated in I, aVL, and V_1-V_6 Maximally depressed in II, III, and aVF	Less tall, but generally still positive, in I, aVL, and V_1-V_6
LATE **Phase 3** **Second and Third Day** **(24 to 72 Hours)**	QS waves or complexes in V_1-V_5 and sometimes V_6 Significantly abnormal in I, aVL, and V_6	Absent in V_1-V_2 Decreased or absent in V_3-V_5 and sometimes V_6 Small R waves in I, aVL, and V_6	Return of the ST segments to the baseline throughout	T wave inversion in I, aVL, and V_1-V_6 Tall T waves in II, III, and aVF

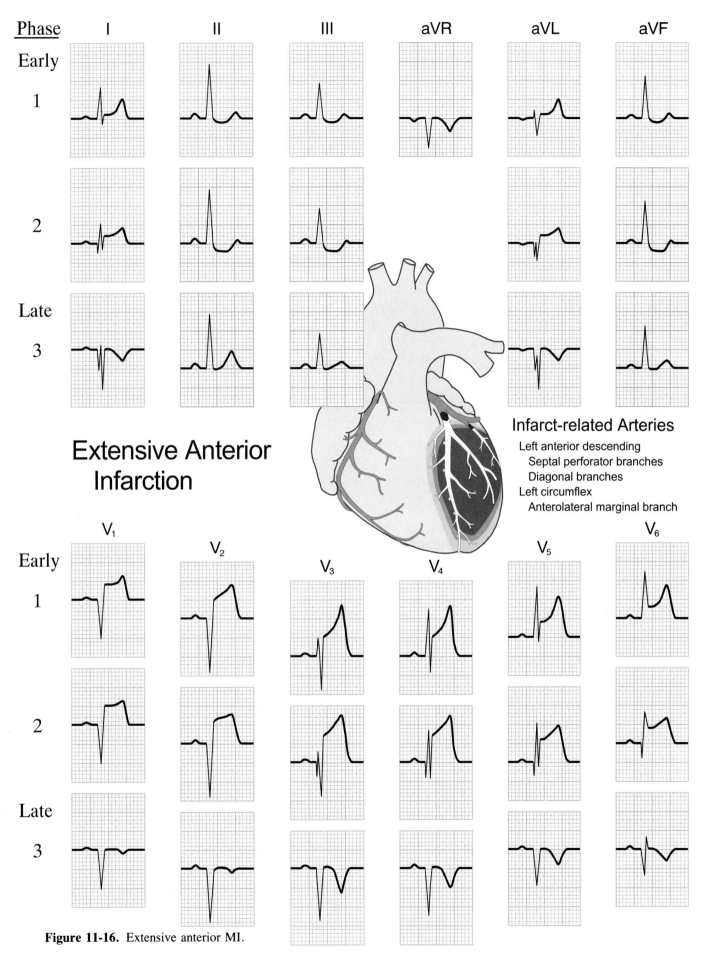

Extensive Anterior Infarction

Infarct-related Arteries

Left anterior descending
  Septal perforator branches
  Diagonal branches
Left circumflex
  Anterolateral marginal branch

Figure 11-16. Extensive anterior MI.

Inferior Myocardial Infarction

Coronary Arteries Involved and Site of Occlusion

The major arteries involved are the **posterior left ventricular arteries,** which commonly arise from the **right coronary artery** or, less commonly, from the **left circumflex coronary artery** of the **left coronary artery.**

Location of Infarct

The myocardial infarction (Figure 11-17 and Table 11-14) involves the **inferior wall of the left ventricle** that rests on the diaphragm. For this reason, inferior myocardial infarction is also termed **diaphragmatic myocardial infarction.**

Notes

ECG Changes

In **facing leads II, III,** and **aVF:**

Early: **ST segment elevation** with **tall T waves** and **taller than normal R waves** in leads II, III, and aVF.

Late: **QS waves or complexes** with **T wave inversion** in leads II, III, and aVF.

In **opposite leads I** and **aVL:**

Early: **ST segment depression** in leads I and aVL.

Late: **Abnormally tall T waves** in leads I and aVL.

Table 11-14. ECG changes in inferior MI

	Q Waves	R Waves	ST Segments	T Waves
EARLY **Phase 1** **First Few Hours** **(0 to 2 Hours)**	**Normal Q waves**	**Normal** or **abnormally tall R waves** in **II, III,** and **aVF**	**Elevated** in **II, III,** and **aVF** **Depressed** in **I** and **aVL**	**Sometimes abnormally tall** with peaking in **II, III,** and **aVF**
Phase 2 **First Day** **(2 to 24 Hours)**	**Minimally abnormal** in **II, III,** and **aVF**	**Minimally decreased** in **II, III,** and **aVF**	**Maximally elevated** in **II, III,** and **aVF** **Maximally depressed** in **I** and **aVL**	**Less tall,** but generally still positive, in **II, III,** and **aVF**
LATE **Phase 3** **Second and Third Day** **(24 to 72 Hours)**	**QS waves** or **complexes** in **II, III,** and **aVF**	**Decreased** or **absent** in **II, III,** and **aVF**	**Return** of the **ST segments** to the baseline throughout	**T wave inversion** in **II, III,** and **aVF** **Tall T waves** in **I** and **aVL**

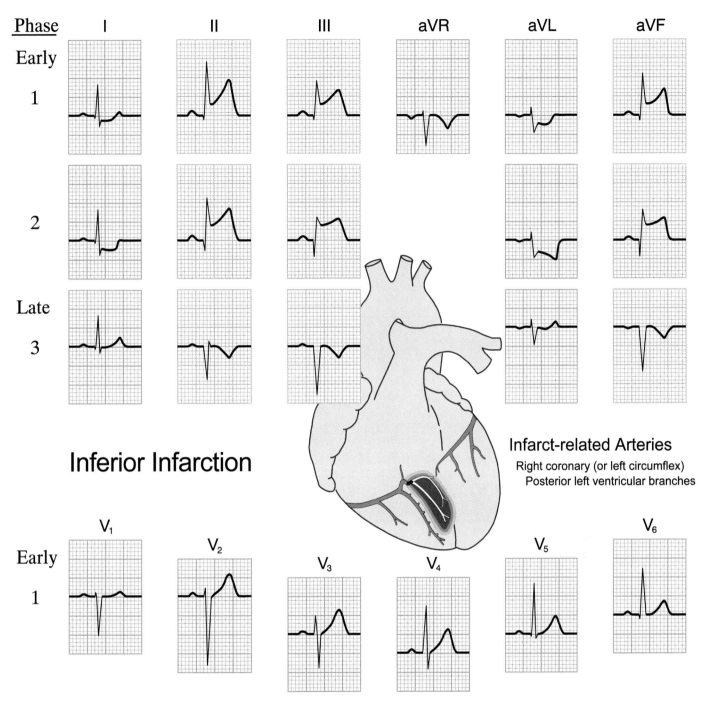

Inferior Infarction

Infarct-related Arteries

Right coronary (or left circumflex)
Posterior left ventricular branches

Figure 11-17. Inferior MI.

Posterior Myocardial Infarction

Coronary Arteries Involved and Site of Occlusion

The major artery(ies) involved are the **distal left circumflex artery** and/or the **posterolateral marginal artery** of the **left circumflex coronary artery.**

Location of Infarct

The myocardial infarction (Figure 11-18 and Table 11-15) involves the **posterior wall of the left ventricle,** located just below the left posterior atrioventricular groove and extending to the inferior wall of the left ventricle.

Notes

ECG Changes

In facing leads: None. There are no facing leads.

In **opposite leads V$_1$-V$_4$:**

Early: **ST segment depression** in leads V$_1$-V$_4$.
Late: **Large R waves** with **tall T waves** in leads V$_1$-V$_4$. The R wave is tall and wide ($\geq$0.04 sec in width) in V$_1$ with slurring and notching. The **S wave** in V$_1$ is decreased, resulting in an **R/S ratio of $\geq$1** in V$_1$.

Table 11-15. ECG changes in posterior MI

	Q waves	R waves	ST segments	T waves
EARLY **Phase 1** **First Few Hours** **(0 to 2 Hours)**	**Normal Q waves**	**Normal R waves**	**Depressed** in V$_1$-V$_4$	**Inverted** in V$_1$-V$_4$
Phase 2 **First Day** **(2 to 24 Hours)**	**Same as in Phase 1**	**Minimally increased** in V$_1$-V$_4$	**Maximally depressed** in V$_1$-V$_4$	**Continuation of inversion** in V$_1$-V$_4$
LATE **Phase 3** **Second and Third Day** **(24 to 72 Hours)**	**Same as in Phase 1**	**Large R waves** in V$_1$-V$_4$ with **slurring and notching** in V$_1$ **S waves** decreased in V$_1$ **Note:** In V$_1$ R/S ratio $\geq$1	**Return** of the **ST segments** to the baseline throughout	**Tall T waves** in V$_1$-V$_4$

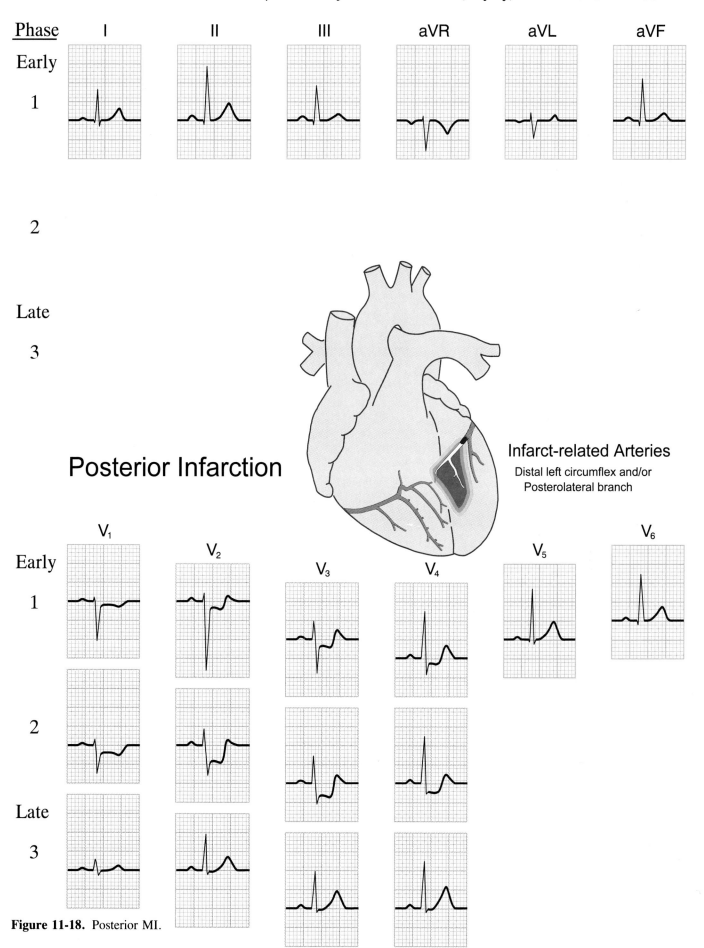

Posterior Infarction

Infarct-related Arteries
Distal left circumflex and/or
Posterolateral branch

Figure 11-18. Posterior MI.

1. The artery that arises from the left main coronary artery at an obtuse angle and runs posteriorly along the left atrioventricular groove to end in back of the left ventricle is called the:
   A. septal perforator artery
   B. left circumflex coronary artery
   C. right ventricular artery
   D. left anterior descending coronary artery

2. The SA node is supplied with blood from:
   A. the left circumflex coronary artery
   B. the right coronary artery
   C. either of the above
   D. none of the above

3. Myocardial ischemia or infarction may be caused by:
   A. occlusion of an atherosclerotic coronary artery
   B. coronary artery spasm
   C. increased myocardial workload
   D. all of the above

4. The most common cause of acute MI is a(n):
   A. coronary thrombosis
   B. coronary artery spasm
   C. air embolism
   D. none of the above

5. Upon revascularization or reoxygenation, necrotic cells:
   A. return to normal or near normal function
   B. do not return to normal function
   C. usually take 24 hours to return to normal function
   D. Revert to a previous state of injury

6. A myocardial infarction in which the zone of infarction involves the entire full thickness of the ventricular wall, from the endocardium to the epicardial surface, is called a:
   A. nontransmural infarction
   B. necrotic infarction
   C. transmural infarction
   D. subendocardial infarction

7. By six hours following an acute transmural MI, the following can be said of the involved myocardium:
   A. only a small percentage of cells remain viable
   B. a large area of reversible myocardial injury is still present
   C. progression of the acute MI continues at a rapid pace
   D. none of the above

8. Inverted or tall peaked T waves in a facing lead during the early phase of an acute MI are an indication of:
   A. necrosis
   B. injury
   C. ischemia
   D. none of the above

9. The most likely cause of an inferior myocardial infarction is an occlusion of the:
   A. left anterior descending artery
   B. anterolateral marginal artery
   C. posterior descending artery
   D. posterior left ventricular arteries

10. The ECG in an acute anteroseptal MI is characterized by ST segment elevation in the following facing leads:
    A. leads II, III, and aVF
    B. leads V_1-V_4
    C. leads I, aVL, and V_1-V_6
    D. leads V_5-V_6

CHAPTER
12

Miscellaneous ECG Changes

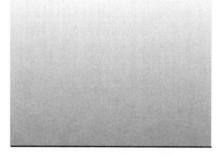

Chamber Enlargement

Pericarditis

Electrolyte Imbalance

Drug Effect

Pulmonary Disease

◁ OBJECTIVES ▷

Upon completion of all or part of this chapter you should be able to complete the following objectives indicated by your instructor:

☐ **1.** Discuss the pathophysiology of atrial and ventricular dilatation and hypertrophy and list four examples of atrial and ventricular dilatation and four examples of atrial and ventricular hypertrophy or enlargement.

☐ **2.** Discuss the pathophysiology of enlargement or hypertrophy of the following heart chambers and list the ECG abnormalities characteristic of each:
  ☐ Right atrial enlargement
  ☐ Left atrial enlargement
  ☐ Right ventricular hypertrophy
  ☐ Left ventricular hypertrophy

☐ **3.** Discuss the effect each of the following conditions has on the heart and list the ECG changes characteristic of each:
  ☐ Pericarditis
  ☐ Chronic obstructive pulmonary disease (COPD)
  ☐ Cor pulmonale
  ☐ Pulmonary embolism

☐ **4.** List the characteristic ECG changes in the following serum electrolyte imbalances according to the serum levels where applicable:
  ☐ Hyperkalemia   ☐ Hypercalcemia
  ☐ Hypokalemia   ☐ Hypocalcemia

☐ **5.** List the excitatory and inhibitory effects of the following drugs on the heart and its electrical conduction system and the characteristic ECG changes that occur with each:
  ☐ Digitalis   ☐ Quinidine
  ☐ Procainamide

Chamber Enlargement

Pathophysiology

Enlargement of the atria and ventricles often occurs because of heart disease where they must accommodate greater pressure and/or volume than they normally do. The term *enlargement* includes **dilatation** and **hypertrophy.**

Dilatation means the distension of an individual heart chamber; it may be acute or chronic. Acute dilatation is usually not associated with hypertrophy of the chamber wall, whereas chronic dilatation commonly is. Examples of acute chamber dilatation are:
- **Left atrial dilatation** in acute left heart failure.
- **Right atrial and ventricular dilatation** in acute pulmonary edema and acute pulmonary embolism.

Examples of chronic chamber dilatation are:
- **Left ventricular dilatation** in severe aortic valve stenosis or insufficiency.
- **Left atrial dilatation** in severe mitral valve stenosis or insufficiency.

Hypertrophy is a chronic condition of the heart characterized by an increase in the thickness of a chamber's myocardial wall secondary to the increase in the size of the muscle fibers. This is the usual response of the myocardium to an increase in its workload over a period of time. Commonly, dilatation of the chamber accompanies hypertrophy; to what extent depends on the heart disease causing the hypertrophy. Examples of chamber hypertrophy are:

- **Left ventricular hypertrophy** in aortic valve stenosis or insufficiency and systemic hypertension.
- **Right ventricular hypertrophy** in pulmonary valve stenosis and chronic obstructive pulmonary disease (COPD).
- **Left atrial enlargement** in mitral valve stenosis and insufficiency and left ventricular hypertrophy from whatever cause.
- **Right atrial enlargement** in tricuspid valve stenosis and insufficiency and right ventricular hypertrophy from whatever cause.

Notes

Right Atrial Enlargement

Pathophysiology

Right atrial enlargement (right atrial dilatation and hypertrophy) (Figure 12-1) is usually caused by increased pressure and/or volume in the right atrium—**right atrial overload.** It is found in pulmonary valve stenosis, tricuspid valve stenosis and insufficiency (relatively rare), and pulmonary hypertension from various causes. These include chronic obstructive pulmonary disease (COPD), status asthmaticus, pulmonary embolism, pulmonary edema, mitral valve stenosis or insufficiency, and congenital heart disease. The result of right atrial enlargement is, typically, a tall, symmetrically peaked P wave—the **P pulmonale.**

ECG Characteristics

P waves:

Duration: The duration of the P waves is usually normal (0.10 second or less).

P wave shape: P waves characteristic of right atrial enlargement include:

- A typically **tall and symmetrically peaked P wave**—the **P pulmonale,** present in leads II, III, and aVF.
- A **sharply peaked biphasic P wave** in lead V_1.

Direction: The direction of the P waves is positive (upright) in leads II, III, and aVF and biphasic in V_1 with the initial deflection greater than the terminal deflection.

Amplitude: The amplitude of the P waves is 2.5 mm or greater in leads II, III, and aVF.

Notes

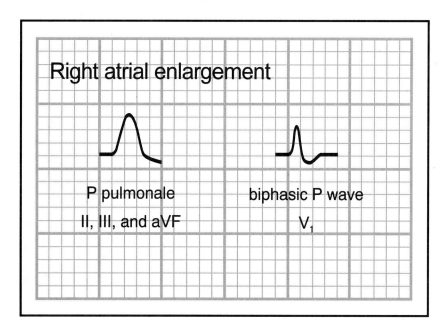

Figure 12-1. Right atrial enlargement.

Left Atrial Enlargement

Pathophysiology

Left atrial enlargement (left atrial dilatation and hypertrophy) (Figure 12-2) is usually caused by increased pressure and/or volume in the left atrium—**left atrial overload.** It is found in mitral valve stenosis and insufficiency, acute myocardial infarction, left heart failure, and left ventricular hypertrophy from various causes, such as aortic stenosis or insufficiency, systemic hypertension, and hypertrophic cardiomyopathy. The result of left atrial enlargement is, typically, a wide, notched P wave—the **P mitrale.** Such P waves may also result from a delay or block of the progression of the electrical impulses through the interatrial conduction tract between the right and left atria.

ECG Characteristics

P waves:

Duration: The duration of the P waves is usually greater than 0.10 second.

P wave shape: P waves characteristic of left atrial enlargement include:

- A **broad positive (upright) P wave,** 0.12 second or greater in duration, in any lead.

- A **wide, notched P wave** with two "humps" 0.04 second or more apart—the **P mitrale.** The first hump represents the depolarization of the right atrium, the second hump, the depolarization of the enlarged left atrium. **The P mitrale is usually present in leads I, II, and V$_4$-V$_6$.**

- A **biphasic P wave,** greater than 0.10 second in total duration, with the terminal, negative component 1 mm (0.1 mV) or more deep and 1 mm (0.04 second) or more in duration, i.e., **1 small square** or **greater.** The initial, positive (upright) component of the P wave represents the depolarization of the right atrium; the terminal, negative component, the depolarization of the enlarged left atrium. **Such biphasic P waves are commonly present in leads V$_1$-V$_2$.**

Direction: The direction of the P waves is positive (upright) in leads I, II, and V$_4$-V$_6$ and biphasic in leads V$_1$-V$_2$. The P wave may be negative in leads III and aVF.

Amplitude: The amplitude of the P waves is usually normal (0.5 to 2.5 mm).

Notes

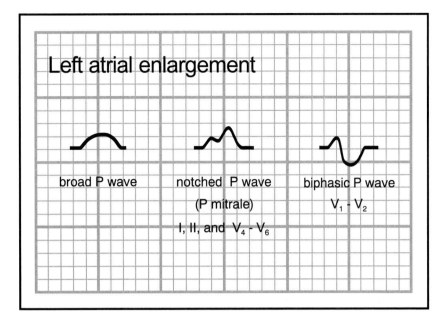

Figure 12-2. Left atrial enlargement.

Right Ventricular Hypertrophy

Pathophysiology

Right ventricular hypertrophy (Figure 12-3) is usually caused by increased pressure and/or volume in the right ventricle—**right ventricular overload.** It is found in pulmonary valve stenosis and other congenital heart defects (e.g., atrial and ventricular septal defects), tricuspid valve insufficiency (relatively rare), and pulmonary hypertension from various causes. These include chronic obstructive pulmonary disease (COPD), status asthmaticus, pulmonary embolism, pulmonary edema, and mitral valve stenosis or insufficiency.

Right ventricular hypertrophy produces abnormally large rightward electrical forces that travel toward lead V_1 and away from the left precordial leads V_5-V_6. The sequence of depolarization of the ventricles, however, remains normal.

ECG Characteristics

P waves: Changes indicative of right atrial enlargement are present.

QRS complexes:

Duration: The duration of the QRS complexes is 0.10 second or less.

QRS axis: A right axis deviation of $+90°$ or more is usually present: $\geq +110°$ in adults; $\geq +120°$ in the young.

Ventricular activation time (VAT): The ventricular activation time is prolonged beyond the upper normal limit of 0.03 second in the right precordial leads V_1 and V_2.

QRS pattern:

Q waves: Q waves may be present in leads II, III, and aVF.

R waves: Tall R waves are present in leads II, III, and V_1. The R waves are usually 7 mm or more (≥ 0.7 mV) in height in lead V_1. They are equal to or greater than the S waves in depth in this lead. Relatively tall R waves are also present in the other right precordial leads V_2-V_3.

Note: Tall R waves equal to or greater than the S waves in lead V_1 may also be present in acute posterior myocardial infarction and in counterclockwise rotation of the heart.

S waves: Relatively deeper than normal S waves are present in lead I and the left precordial leads V_4-V_6. In lead V_6, the depth of the S waves may be greater than the height of the R waves.

ST segments: **"Downsloping" ST segment depression** of 1 mm or more may be present in leads II, III, aVF, and V_1 and sometimes in leads V_2 and V_3.

T waves: T wave inversion is often present in leads II, III, aVF, and V_1 and sometimes in leads V_2 and V_3.

Note: The downsloping ST segment depression and the T wave inversion together form the **"strain" pattern** characteristic of long-standing right ventricular hypertrophy. This pattern gives the so-called **"hockey stick"** appearance to the QRS-ST-T complex.

Notes

Right Ventricular Hypertrophy

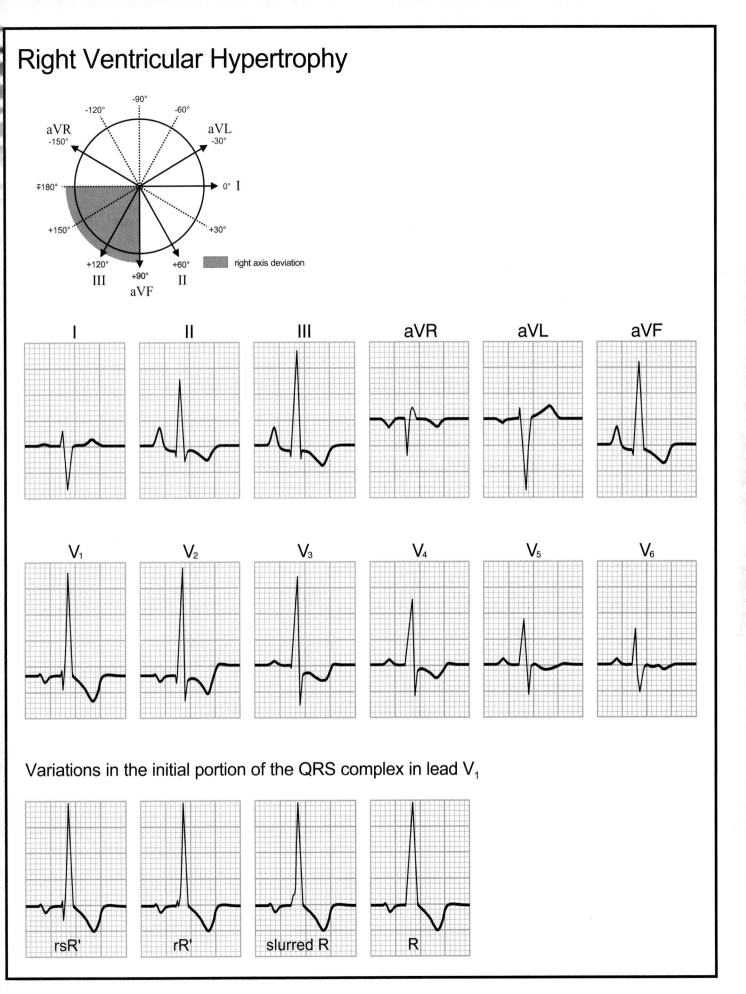

Figure 12-3. Right ventricular hypertrophy.

Left Ventricular Hypertrophy

Pathophysiology

Left ventricular hypertrophy (Figure 12-4) is usually caused by increased pressure and/or volume in the left ventricle—**left ventricular overload.** It is found in mitral insufficiency, aortic stenosis or insufficiency, systemic hypertension, acute myocardial infarction, and hypertrophic cardiomyopathy.

Left ventricular hypertrophy produces abnormally large leftward electrical forces that travel toward the left precordial leads V_5-V_6 and away from lead V_1. The sequence of depolarization of the ventricles, however, remains normal.

ECG Characteristics

P waves: Changes indicative of left atrial enlargement are present.

QRS complexes:

Duration: The duration of the QRS complexes is 0.10 second or less.

QRS axis: The QRS axis is usually normal, but it may be deviated to the left (i.e., left axis deviation: $> -30°$).

Ventricular activation time (VAT): The ventricular activation time is prolonged beyond the upper normal limit to 0.05 second or more in the left precordial leads V_5 and V_6.

QRS pattern:

R waves: Tall R waves are present in leads I and aVL and the left precordial leads V_5-V_6. The following criteria concerning the amplitude (or voltage) of the R wave in various leads are often used to diagnose left ventricular hypertrophy:

- An **R wave** of **20 mm (2.0 mV)** or more in **lead I.**
- An **R wave** of **11 mm (1.1 mV)** or more in **lead aVL.**
- An **R wave** of **30 mm (3.0 mV)** or more in **lead V_5 or V_6.**

S waves: Deep S waves are present in lead III and the right precordial lead V_1. The following criteria

concerning the depth (or voltage) of the S wave in various leads are often used to diagnose left ventricular hypertrophy:

- An **S wave** of **20 mm (2.0 mV)** or more in **lead III.**
- An **S wave** of **30 mm (3.0 mV)** or more in **lead V_1 or V_2.**

Sum of R and S waves: The sum of the height of the R waves and the depth of the S waves (in mm or mV) in leads in which these two waves are most prominent is often used to determine the presence of left ventricular hypertrophy. Left ventricular hypertrophy is considered to be present if any one of the following summations is exceeded:

- The sum of any R wave and any S wave in any of the limb leads I, II, or III is 20 mm (2.0 mV) or more.

R (I, II, or III) + S (I, II, or III) = $\geq$20 mm ($\geq$2.0 mV)

- The sum of the R wave in lead I and the S wave in lead III is 25 mm (2.5 mV) or more.

R I + S III = $\geq$25 mm ($\geq$2.5 mV)

- The sum of the S wave in lead V_1 or V_2 and the R wave in lead V_5 or V_6 is 35 mm (3.5 mV) or more.

S V_1 (or V_2) + R V_5 (or V_6) = $\geq$35 mm ($\geq$3.5 mV)

ST segments: "**Downsloping**" **ST segment depression** of 1 mm or more is present in leads I, aVL, and V_5-V_6.

T waves: T wave inversion is present in leads I, aVL, and V_5-V_6.

Note: the downsloping ST segment depression and the T wave inversion together form the **"strain" pattern** characteristic of long-standing left ventricular hypertrophy. This pattern gives the so-called **"hockey stick"** appearance to the QRS-ST-T complex. The strain pattern is less significant if the patient is taking digitalis, as this medication can also cause ST segment depression and T wave flattening and inversion.

Notes

Left Ventricular Hypertrophy

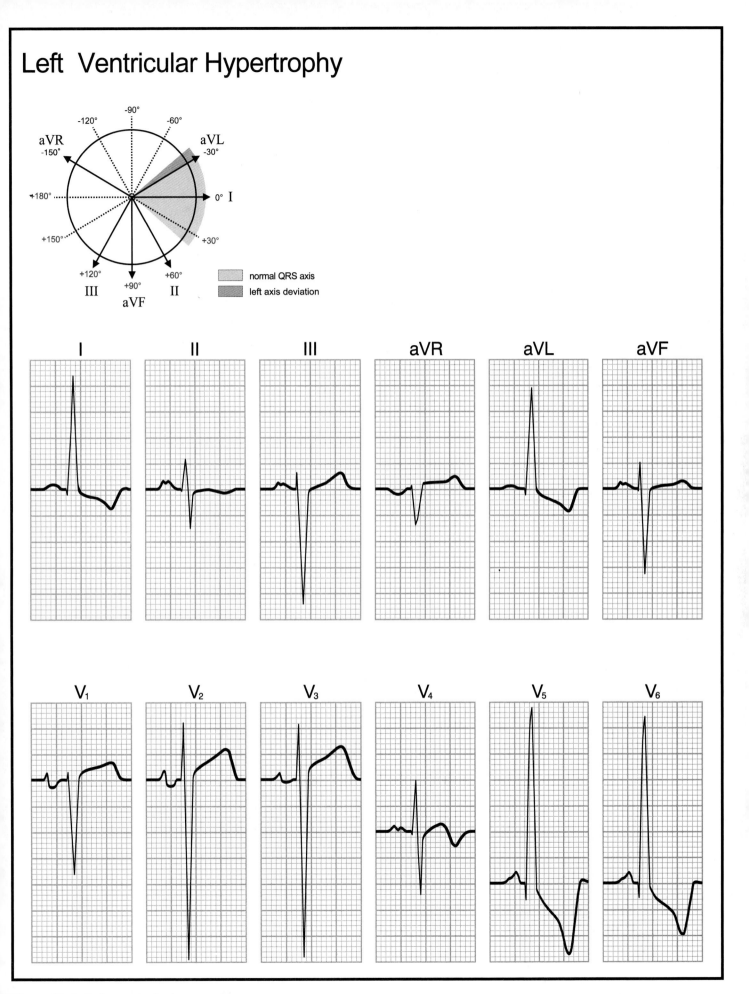

Figure 12-4. Left ventricular hypertrophy.

Diagnosis of Left Ventricular Hypertrophy:

Many criteria for the diagnosis of left ventricular hypertrophy exist. All are based on the three major ECG characteristics of left ventricular hypertrophy:
- **Increased amplitude or depth of the R and S waves in specific limb and precordial leads**
- **QRS axis greater than** $-15°$
- **ST segment depression**

An acceptable set of criteria for diagnosing left ventricular hypertrophy might include:
- **Increased amplitude or depth of the R and S waves in any appropriate lead(s) satisfying the amplitude (or voltage) criteria of left ven-** tricular hypertrophy, expressed in mm or mV (Table 12-1):

  The amplitude or depth of an R or S wave in lead I or III of 20 mm (2.0 mV) or greater,
  OR
  The sum of the S wave in lead V_1 or V_2 and the R wave in V_5 or V_6 of greater than 35 mm (3.5 mV),
- **AND,** one of the following:
  QRS axis between $-15°$ and $-30°$ or greater than $-30°$ (left axis deviation),
  OR
  ST segment depression of ≥ 1 mm in leads with an R wave having the amplitude (or voltage) criteria of left ventricular hypertrophy.

Table 12-1. Criteria for height or depth of R and S waves used to diagnose left ventricular hypertrophy

			Lead		
Wave	**I**	**III**	**aVL**	**V_1 or V_2**	**V_5 or V_6**
R Wave	$\geq$20 mm		$\geq$11 mm		$\geq$30 mm
S Wave		$\geq$20 mm		$\geq$30 mm	
Summation	R (I, II, or III) + S (I, II, or III) = $\geq$20 mm ($\geq$2.0 mV)				
	R I + S III = $\geq$25 mm ($\geq$2.5 mV)				
	S V_1 (or V_2) + R V_5 (or V_6) = $\geq$35 mm ($\geq$3.5 mV)				

Pericarditis

Pathophysiology

Pericarditis (Figure 12-5) is an inflammatory disease of the pericardium, directly involving the epicardium with deposition of inflammatory cells and a variable amount of serous, fibrous, purulent, or hemorrhagic exudate within the pericardial sac. Depending on the nature of the exudate, acute fibrinous pericarditis, pericardial effusion, cardiac tamponade, or constrictive pericarditis may develop. A variety of agents and conditions can cause acute pericarditis, including infectious agents (bacteria, viruses, tubercle bacilli, and mycotic agents), acute myocardial infarction, trauma, connective tissue disorders, allergic and hypersensitivity diseases, and metabolic disorders. Unlike acute myocardial infarction, which pericarditis may mimic, pericarditis usually occurs in younger patients without cardiac risk factors who are not suspected of having coronary artery disease.

The signs and symptoms of acute pericarditis are chest pain, dyspnea, tachycardia, fever, malaise, weakness, and chills. The chest pain, which can mimic that of acute myocardial infarction, is sharp and severe, with radiation to the neck, back, left shoulder, and, rarely, the arm. Characteristically, it is present along the sternum, made worse by lying flat, and relieved by sitting or leaning forward. Often, the pain is pleuritic, made worse by breathing, especially during inspiration. Unlike the pain of acute MI, the pain may last for hours or even days. A pericardial friction rub, resulting from the inflammation of the pericardial surface, is heard, and even palpated, along the lower left sternal border. Characteristic ECG findings are present in 90 percent of the patients with acute pericarditis.

ECG Characteristics

QRS complexes: Abnormal Q waves and QS complexes are absent. In pericarditis with pleural effusion, the QRS complexes are of low voltage. When pleural effusion becomes severe, cardiac tamponade may occur, causing the QRS complexes to alternate between normal and low voltage, coincident with respiration (**electrical alternans**).

ST segments: ST segment elevation is the primary ECG abnormality in acute pericarditis. The ST segments are somewhat concave, in contrast to the convex ST segment elevation in acute myocardial infarction.

The ST segments are usually elevated in most, if not all, leads except leads aVR and V_1, because pericarditis usually affects the entire myocardial surface of the heart. In lead aVR, the ST segment is either normal or slightly depressed. Occasionally, pericarditis will be localized and therefore the ST segment elevation will only be seen in the leads reflecting the involved area. In this case, differentiating between pericarditis and an acute anterior- or posterior-wall myocardial infarction may be difficult. Reciprocal ST segment depression except in lead aVR is usually not present. As the pericarditis resolves, the ST segments return to the baseline.

Location of pericarditis	Leads with ST segment elevation
Anterior	I, V_2-V_4
Lateral	I, aVL, V_5-V_6
Inferior	II, III, aVL
Generalized	I, II, III, aVL, aVF, V_2-V_6

T waves: The T waves remain elevated during the acute phase of pericarditis. As the pericarditis resolves, the T waves become inverted in the leads that had the ST segment elevation.

QT intervals: The QT intervals are normal.

Notes

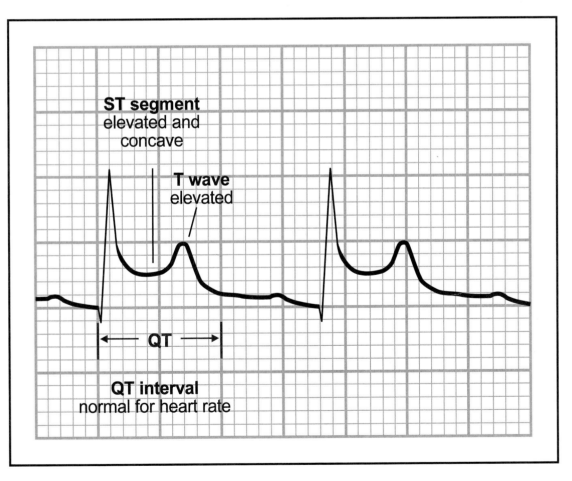

Figure 12-5. Pericarditis.

Electrolyte Imbalance:
Hyperkalemia

Pathophysiology

Hyperkalemia (Figure 12-6) is the excess of serum potassium above the normal levels of 3.5-5.0 milliequivalents per liter (mEq/L), The most common causes of hyperkalemia are kidney failure and certain diuretics (e.g., triamterene). Characteristic ECG changes occur at various levels of hyperkalemia. Sinus arrest may occur when the serum potassium level reaches about 7.5 mEq/L, and cardiac standstill or ventricular fibrillation, at about 10 to 12 mEq/L.

ECG Characteristics

P waves: The P waves begin to flatten out and become wider when the serum potassium level reaches about 6.5 mEq/L and disappear at 7.0-9.0 mEq/L.

PR intervals: The PR intervals may be normal or prolonged, greater than 0.20 second. The PR interval is absent when the P waves disappear.

QRS complexes: The QRS complexes begin to widen when the serum potassium level reaches about 6.0-6.5 mEq/L, becoming markedly slurred and abnormally widened beyond 0.12 second at 10 mEq/L. The QRS complexes may widen so that they "merge" with the following T waves, resulting in a **"sine wave"** QRS-ST-T pattern.

ST segments: The ST segments disappear when the serum potassium level reaches about 6 mEq/L.

T waves: The T waves become typically tall and peaked when the serum potassium level reaches about 5.5-6.5 mEq/L.

Notes

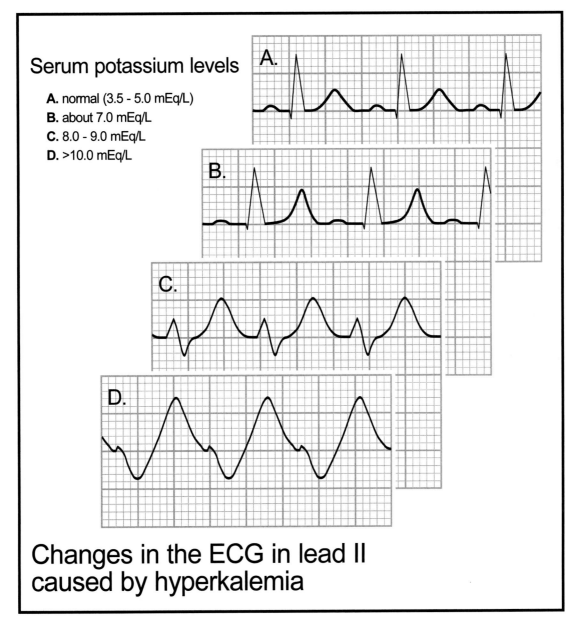

Serum potassium levels

A. normal (3.5 - 5.0 mEq/L)
B. about 7.0 mEq/L
C. 8.0 - 9.0 mEq/L
D. >10.0 mEq/L

Changes in the ECG in lead II caused by hyperkalemia

Figure 12-6. Hyperkalemia.

Electrolyte Imbalance: Hypokalemia

Pathophysiology

Hypokalemia (Figure 12-7) is the deficiency of serum potassium below the normal levels of 3.5-5.0 milliequivalents per liter (mEq/L). The most common cause of hypokalemia is loss of potassium in body fluids through vomiting, gastric suction, and excessive use of diuretics. Hypokalemia may also result from low serum magnesium levels (hypomagnesemia). The ECG characteristics of hypomagnesemia, incidentally, resemble those of hypokalemia.

Symptoms of hypokalemia are polyuria in mild cases and muscle weakness in more severely affected patients. Digitalis in the presence of hypokalemia may precipitate serious ventricular arrhythmias, including the torsade de pointes form of ventricular tachycardia. The diagnosis of hypokalemia is often made by the characteristic ECG changes caused by low serum potassium. Characteristic ECG changes occur at various levels of hypokalemia.

ECG Characteristics

QRS complexes: The QRS complexes begin to widen when the serum potassium level drops to about 3.0 mEq/L.

ST segments: The ST segments may become depressed by 1 mm or more.

T waves: The T waves begin to flatten when the serum potassium level drops to about 3.0 mEq/L and continue to become smaller as the **U waves** increase in size. The T waves may either merge with the U waves or become inverted.

U waves: The U waves begin to increase in size, becoming as tall as the T waves, when the serum potassium level drops to about 3.0 mEq/L, becoming taller than the T waves at about 2 mEq/L. The U waves reach "giant" size and fuse with the T waves at 1 mEq/L.

QT intervals: the QT intervals may appear to be prolonged when the U waves become prominent and fuse with the T waves.

Notes

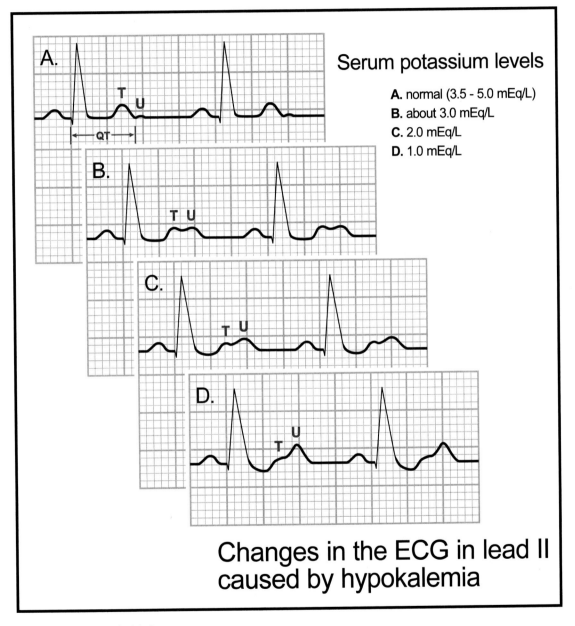

Serum potassium levels

A. normal (3.5 - 5.0 mEq/L)
B. about 3.0 mEq/L
C. 2.0 mEq/L
D. 1.0 mEq/L

Changes in the ECG in lead II
caused by hypokalemia

Figure 12-7. Hypokalemia.

Electrolyte Imbalance: Hypercalcemia

Pathophysiology

Hypercalcemia (Figure 12-8 *A, B*) is the excess of serum calcium above the normal levels of 2.1-2.6 milliequivalents per liter (mEq/L) (or 4.25-5.25 mg/100 ml). Common causes of hypercalcemia include adrenal insufficiency, hyperparathyroidism, immobilization, kidney failure, malignancy, sarcoidosis, thyrotoxicosis, and vitamin A and D intoxication. Severe hypercalcemia is life threatening.

Digitalis in the presence of hypercalcemia may precipitate serious arrhythmias.

ECG Characteristics

QT intervals: The QT intervals are shorter than normal for the heart rate.

Notes

Electrolyte Imbalance: Hypocalcemia

Pathophysiology

Hypocalcemia (Figure 12-8 *A, C*) is the shortage of serum calcium below the normal levels of 2.1-2.6 milliequivalents per liter (mEq/L) (or 4.25-5.25 mg/100 ml). Common causes of hypocalcemia include chronic steatorrhea, diuretics (such as furosemide or ethacrynic acid), hypomagnesemia (possibly because of release of parathyroid hormone), hypomalacia in adults and rickets in children, hypoparathyroidism, pregnancy, and respiratory alkalosis and hyperventilation.

ECG Characteristics

ST segments: The ST segments are prolonged.

QT intervals: The QT intervals are prolonged beyond the normal limits for the heart rate because of the prolongation of the ST segments.

Notes

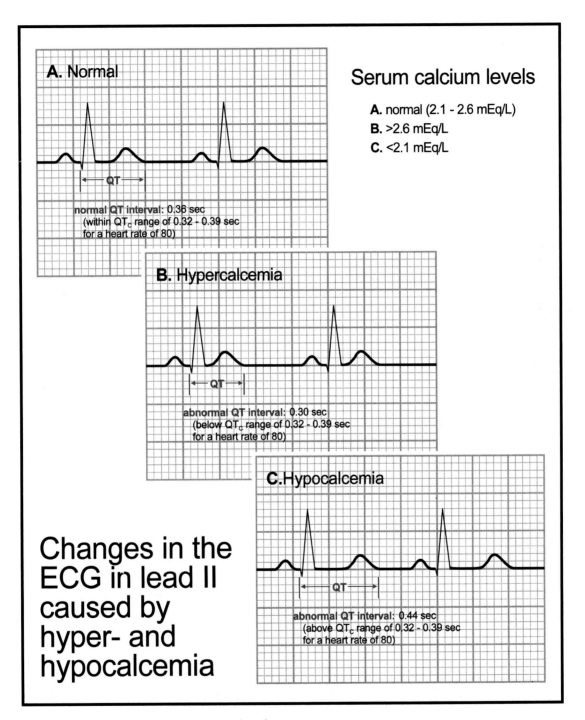

A. Normal

QT

normal QT interval: 0.36 sec
(within QT_c range of 0.32 - 0.39 sec
for a heart rate of 80)

Serum calcium levels

A. normal (2.1 - 2.6 mEq/L)
B. >2.6 mEq/L
C. <2.1 mEq/L

B. Hypercalcemia

QT

abnormal QT interval: 0.30 sec
(below QT_c range of 0.32 - 0.39 sec
for a heart rate of 80)

C.Hypocalcemia

QT

abnormal QT interval: 0.44 sec
(above QT_c range of 0.32 - 0.39 sec
for a heart rate of 80)

Changes in the ECG in lead II caused by hyper- and hypocalcemia

Figure 12-8. Hypercalcemia and hypocalcemia.

Drug Effect:
Digitalis

Pathophysiology

Digitalis (Figure 12-9) administered within therapeutic range produces characteristic changes in the ECG. In addition, when given in excess, digitalis toxicity occurs, causing **excitatory** or **inhibitory effects** on the heart and its electrical conduction system.

Excitatory effects include:
- **Premature atrial contractions**
- **Paroxysmal atrial tachycardia with block**
- **Paroxysmal junctional tachycardia**
- **Premature ventricular contractions**
- **Ventricular tachycardia**
- **Ventricular fibrillation**

Inhibitory effects include:
- **Sinus bradycardia**
- **Sinoatrial (SA) exit block**
- **Atrioventricular (AV) block**

ECG Characteristics

The ECG changes characteristic of a **"digitalis effect"** are as follows:

PR intervals: The PR intervals are prolonged over 0.2 second.

ST segments: The ST segments are depressed 1 mm or more in many of the leads, with a characteristic "scooped-out" appearance.

T waves: The T waves may be flattened, inverted, or biphasic.

QT intervals: The QT intervals are shorter than normal for the heart rate.

Notes

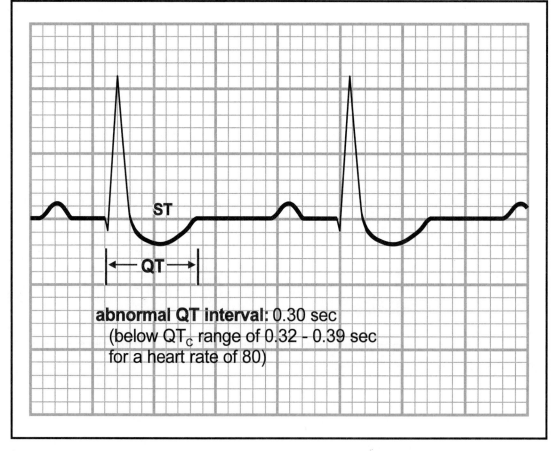

ST

QT

abnormal QT interval: 0.30 sec
(below QT$_C$ range of 0.32 - 0.39 sec
for a heart rate of 80)

Figure 12-9. Digitalis effect.

Drug Effect:
Procainamide

Pathophysiology

Procainamide (Figure 12-10) administered within therapeutic range produces characteristic changes in the ECG. In addition, when given in excess, procainamide toxicity occurs, causing **excitatory** or **inhibitory effects** on the heart and its electrical conduction system.

Excitatory effects include:
- **Premature ventricular contractions**
- **Ventricular tachycardia in the form of torsade de pointes** (occurrence less common than in quinidine administration)
- **Ventricular fibrillation**

Inhibitory effects include:
- **Depression of myocardial contractility,** which may cause **hypotension** and **congestive heart failure**
- **Atrioventricular (AV) block**
- **Ventricular asystole**

ECG Characteristics

QRS complexes: The duration of the QRS complexes may be increased beyond 0.12 second. QRS complex widening is a sign of toxicity. The R waves may be decreased in amplitude.

T waves: The T waves may be decreased in amplitude. Occasionally the T waves may be widened and notched because of the appearance of a **U wave.**

PR intervals: The PR intervals may be prolonged.

ST segments: The ST segments may be depressed 1 mm or more.

QT intervals: The QT intervals may occasionally be prolonged beyond the normal limits for the heart rate. Prolongation of the QT intervals is a sign of procainamide toxicity.

Notes

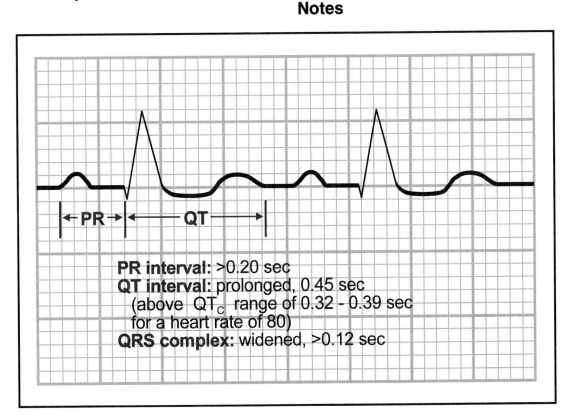

PR interval: >0.20 sec
QT interval: prolonged, 0.45 sec
    (above QT$_C$ range of 0.32 - 0.39 sec
    for a heart rate of 80)
QRS complex: widened, >0.12 sec

Figure 12-10. Procainamide toxicity.

Drug Effect: Quinidine

Pathophysiology

Quinidine (Figure 12-11) administered within therapeutic range produces characteristic changes in the ECG. In addition, when given in excess, quinidine toxicity occurs, causing **excitatory** or **inhibitory effects** on the heart and its electrical conduction system.

Excitatory effects include:
- **Premature ventricular contractions**
- **Ventricular tachycardia in the form of torsade de pointes** (occurrence more common than in procainamide administration)
- **Ventricular fibrillation**

Inhibitory effects include:
- **Depression of myocardial contractility,** which may cause **hypotension** and **congestive heart failure**
- **Sinoatrial (SA) exit block**
- **Atrioventricular (AV) block**
- **Ventricular asystole**

ECG Characteristics

P waves: The P waves may be wide, often notched.

QRS complexes: The duration of the QRS complexes may be increased beyond 0.12 second. QRS complex widening is a sign of toxicity.

T waves: The T waves may be decreased in amplitude, wide, and notched, or they may be inverted. The notching is caused by the appearance of a **U wave** as the T wave widens.

PR intervals: The PR intervals may be prolonged beyond normal.

ST segments: The ST segments may be depressed 1 mm or more.

QT intervals: The QT intervals may be prolonged beyond the normal limits for the heart rate. Prolongation of the QT intervals is a sign of quinidine toxicity.

Notes

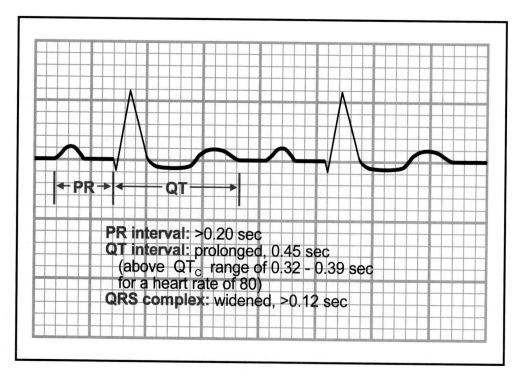

PR interval: >0.20 sec
QT interval: prolonged, 0.45 sec
 (above QT$_c$ range of 0.32 – 0.39 sec
 for a heart rate of 80)
QRS complex: widened, >0.12 sec

Figure 12-11. Quinidine toxicity.

Pulmonary Disease:
Chronic Obstructive Pulmonary Disease (COPD)

Pathophysiology

The following atrial arrhythmias frequently occur in **chronic obstructive pulmonary disease (COPD)**:

- **Premature atrial contractions (PACs)**
- **Wandering atrial pacemaker (WAP)**
- **Multifocal atrial tachycardia (MAT)**
- **Atrial flutter**
- **Atrial fibrillation**

ECG Characteristics

P waves: Changes indicative of **right atrial enlargement** may be present (Figure 12-12).

QRS complexes: The QRS complexes are usually of low voltage. **Poor R-wave progression** across the precordium is usually present.

QRS axis: The QRS axis may be **greater than +90°.**

Notes

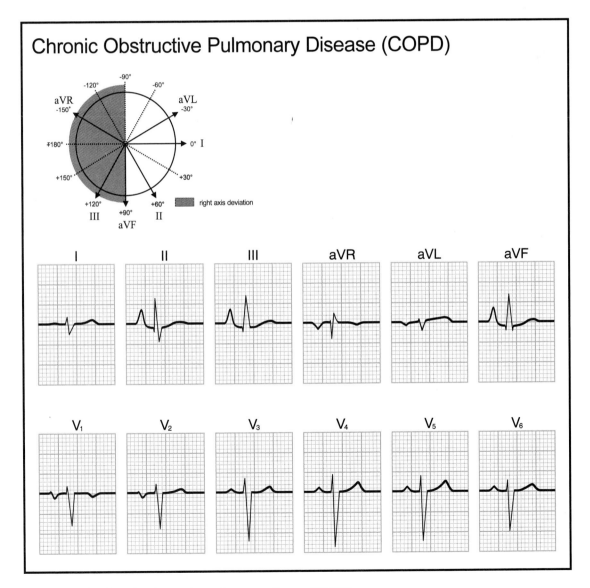

Figure 12-12. Chronic obstructive pulmonary disease (COPD).

Pulmonary Disease: Cor Pulmonale

Pathophysiology

Cor pulmonale is often associated with atrial arrhythmias, including:

- **Premature atrial contractions (PACs)**
- **Wandering atrial pacemaker (WAP)**
- **Multifocal atrial tachycardia (MAT)**
- **Atrial flutter**
- **Atrial fibrillation**

ECG Characteristics

P waves: Changes indicative of **right atrial enlargement** are present (Figure 12-13).

QRS complexes: **Right ventricular hypertrophy** is present.

QRS axis: The QRS axis is **greater than +90°**.

ST segments/T waves: A **right ventricular "strain" pattern** is present in leads V_1-V_2.

Notes

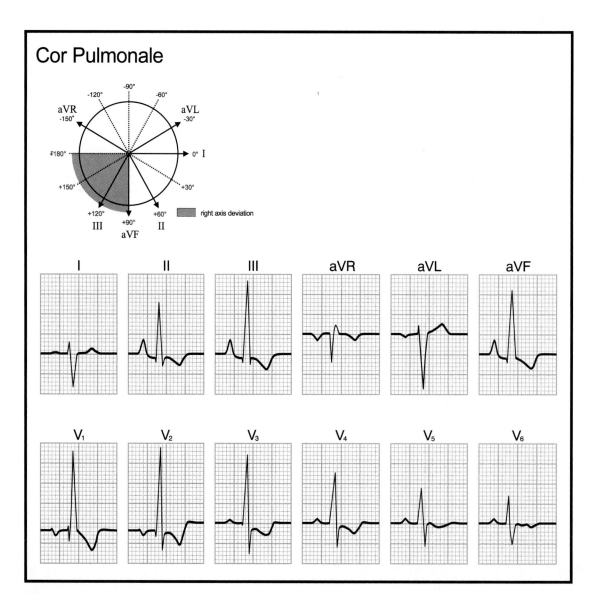

Figure 12-13. Cor pulmonale.

Pulmonary Disease:
Pulmonary Embolism

Pathophysiology

Sinus tachycardia is commonly present in **acute pulmonary embolism.** The ECG may be normal, but often, characteristic changes in the ECG occur.

ECG Characteristics

P waves: Changes of **right atrial enlargement** may be present (Figure 12-14).

QRS complexes: An **S** wave in lead I, a **Q wave** in lead III, and an **inverted T wave** in lead III (the $S_1Q_3T_3$ pattern) may occur acutely. In addition, a **right bundle branch block** may also occur.

QRS axis: A QRS axis of **greater than +90°.**

ST segments/T waves: A **right ventricular "strain" pattern** may be present in leads V_1-V_2.

Notes

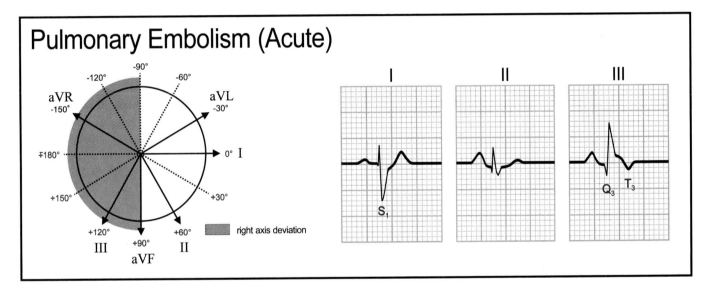

Figure 12-14. Pulmonary embolism.

1. A chronic condition of the heart characterized by an increase in the thickness of a chamber's myocardial wall secondary to the increase in the size of the muscle fibers is called:
   A. stenosis
   B. dilatation
   C. hypertrophy
   D. none of the above

2. A patient who has mitral valve insufficiency or left heart failure may have:
   A. right atrial and ventricular enlargement
   B. left atrial and ventricular enlargement
   C. right ventricular enlargement alone
   D. left ventricular enlargement alone

3. Left ventricular hypertrophy, a condition usually caused by increased pressure or volume in the left ventricle, is often found in:
   A. systemic hypertension and acute MI
   B. mitral insufficiency and hypertrophic cardiomyopathy
   C. aortic stenosis or insufficiency
   D. all of the above

4. The diagnosis of left ventricular hypertrophy is based on the ECG characteristics of increased amplitude or depth of the R and S waves in specific limb and precordial leads and:
   A. a QRS axis greater than $-15°$
   B. ST segment elevation
   C. all of the above
   D. none of the above

5. An inflammatory disease directly involving the epicardium with deposition of inflammatory cells and a variable amount of serous, fibrous, purulent, or hemorrhagic exudate within the sac surrounding the heart is called:
   A. pericarditis
   B. myocarditis
   C. cardiac tamponade
   D. none of the above

6. Signs and symptoms of the acute medical problem described in question number 5 include:
   A. chest pain and dyspnea
   B. chills and weakness
   C. fever and malaise
   D. all of the above

7. In a diffuse pericarditis (i.e., one that is not localized), the ST segments are elevated in:
   A. the precordial leads V_1 through V_4
   B. leads aVR, aVL, and aVF
   C. all leads except aVR and V_1
   D. the biphasic leads only

8. An excess serum potassium above the normal levels of 3.5 to 5.0 milliequivalents per liter (mEq/L) is called:
   A. hypernatremia
   B. hypercalcemia
   C. hypercarbia
   D. hyperkalemia

9. The ECG changes that occur at various levels of excess serum potassium are:
   A. the QRS complexes widen and the T waves become tall
   B. The ST segments disappear and the T waves become peaked
   C. the PR intervals become prolonged and a "sine wave" QRS-ST-T pattern appears
   D. all of the above may occur

10. A medication normally prescribed to heart patients, which when taken in excess causes depression of myocardial contractility, AV block, ventricular asystole, and PVCs, is:
   A. digitalis
   B. procainamide
   C. Lasix
   D. verapamil

Clinical Significance and Treatment of Arrhythmias

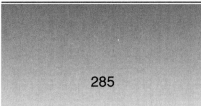

▽ OBJECTIVES ◁

Upon completion of all or part of this chapter you should be able to complete the following objectives indicated by your instructor:

☐ **1.** Discuss the clinical significance of the following bradycardias, the indications for their treatment, and their treatment:

- ☐ Sinus bradycardia
- ☐ Sinus arrest/sino-atrial (SA) exit block
- ☐ Junctional escape rhythm
- ☐ Ventricular escape rhythm
- ☐ Second-degree, Type I AV block (Wenckebach)
- ☐ Second-degree, Type II AV block
- ☐ Second-degree, 2:1 and high-degree (advanced) AV block
  - ☐ With narrow QRS complexes
  - ☐ With wide QRS complexes
- ☐ Third-degree AV block
  - ☐ With narrow QRS complexes
  - ☐ With wide QRS complexes

☐ **2.** Discuss the clinical significance of the following tachycardias, the indications for their treatment, and their treatment:

- ☐ Sinus tachycardia
- ☐ Nonparoxysmal atrial tachycardia without block
- ☐ Wide-QRS-complex tachycardia of unknown origin (with pulse)
  - ☐ Patient hemodynamically stable
- ☐ Paroxysmal supraventricular tachycardia (PSVT) with narrow QRS complexes
  - ☐ Paroxysmal atrial tachycardia (PAT)
  - ☐ Patient hemodynamically stable
- ☐ Atrial tachycardia with block
- ☐ Atrial flutter (AF)
- ☐ Atrial fibrillation
- ☐ Junctional tachycardia
  - ☐ Paroxysmal junctional tachycardia (PJT)
  - ☐ Patient hemodynamically unstable

☐ **3.** Discuss the clinical significance of ventricular tachycardia, the indications for its treatment, and its treatment under the following circumstances:

- ☐ Ventricular tachycardia (VT) with pulse
  - ☐ Patient hemodynamically stable
  - ☐ Patient hemodynamically unstable
- ☐ Torsade de pointes with pulse

☐ **4.** Discuss the clinical significance of the following premature ectopic beats, the indications for their treatment, and their treatment:

- ☐ Premature atrial contractions (PACs)
- ☐ Premature junctional contractions (PJCs)
- ☐ Premature ventricular contractions (PVCs)

☐ **5.** Discuss the clinical significance of ventricular fibrillation/pulseless ventricular tachycardia (VF/VT), the indications for their treatment, and their treatment under the following circumstances:

- ☐ Unmonitored cardiac arrest
- ☐ Monitored cardiac arrest

☐ **6.** Discuss the clinical significance of ventricular asystole, indications for its treatment, and its treatment under the following circumstances:

- ☐ Unmonitored cardiac arrest
- ☐ Monitored cardiac arrest

☐ **7.** Discuss the clinical significance of pulseless electrical activity, indications for its treatment, and its treatment under the following circumstances:

- ☐ Unmonitored cardiac arrest
- ☐ Monitored cardiac arrest

Introduction to This Chapter

The arrhythmia treatment protocols presented in this chapter are based on the recommendations of the 1992 National Conference on Standards and Guidelines for Cardiopulmonary Resuscitation (CPR) and Emergency Cardiac Care (ECC) sponsored by the American College of Cardiology, the American Heart Association, the American Red Cross, and the National Heart, Lung and Blood Institute.

These treatment protocols may be used as guidelines for the development of local or regional protocols for the management of arrhythmias during the prehospital and in-hospital phase of emergency cardiac care. Management may deviate from these treatment protocols or include additional treatment modalities when the physician in charge of the patients determines if such a deviation or addition is in the best interests of the patients.

The treatment sections have been color-coded to differentiate between prehospital and in-hospital emergency cardiac care. The drugs and techniques authorized for both prehospital and in-hospital emergency cardiac care are printed in black; those for in-hospital care only are in dark red. However, the scheme of authorization may be changed at the discretion of the medical control of the prehospital advanced life support system.

Part I includes the arrhythmias present in noncardiac-arrest situations: hemodynamically stable and unstable bradycardias and tachycardias and premature ectopic beats. **Part II** includes arrhythmias present in cardiac arrest situations: ventricular fibrillation / pulseless ventricular tachycardia, ventricular asystole, and pulseless electrical activity.

Part I

Bradycardias

Sinus Bradycardia
Sinus Arrest / Sinoatrial (SA) Exit Block
Junctional Escape Rhythm
Ventricular Escape Rhythm
Second-degree, Type I AV Block (Wenckebach)
Second-degree, Type II AV Block
Second-degree, 2:1 and High-degree (Advanced) AV Block
Third-degree AV Block (Complete AV Block)

Clinical Significance of Bradycardias

A **bradycardia** with a heart rate between 50 to 59 beats per minute **(mild bradycardia)** usually does not produce symptoms by itself. If the heart rate slows to 30 to 45 beats per minute or less **(marked bradycardia),** the cardiac output may drop significantly, causing the systolic blood pressure to fall to 80 to 90 mm Hg or less and signs and symptoms of decreased perfusion of the body, especially of the vital organs, to appear. The skin may become pale, cold, and clammy; the pulse, weak or absent; and the patient, agitated, lightheaded, confused, or unconscious. The patient may experience chest pain and also become dyspneic.

In the presence of acute myocardial infarction, **mild bradycardia** may actually be beneficial in some patients because of the decrease in the workload of the heart, which reduces the oxygen requirements of the myocardium, minimizes the extension of the infarction, and lessens the predisposition to certain arrhythmias. **Marked bradycardia,** however, may result in hypotension with a marked reduction of cardiac output leading to congestive heart failure, loss of consciousness, and shock and predispose the patient to more serious arrhythmias (i.e., premature ventricular contractions, ventricular tachycardia or fibrillation, or ventricular asystole).

If sinus arrest or sinoatrial (SA) exit block is prolonged or second-degree AV block suddenly progresses to a third-degree AV block and if an escape pacemaker in the AV junction (junctional escape rhythm) or ventricles (ventricular escape rhythm) does not take over, ventricular asystole will follow.

Indications for Treatment of Bradycardias

Treatment as outlined below is usually not indicated if the heart rate is 60 beats per minute or less and the signs and symptoms listed below are not present.

Treatment of bradycardia, whatever its cause, is indicated immediately if the heart rate is less than 60 beats per minute and one or more of the following signs or symptoms are present (such a bradycardia is considered a **symptomatic bradycardia**):

- **Hypotension (systolic blood pressure, 80 to 90 mm Hg or less)**
- **Congestive heart failure**
- **Chest pain or dyspnea**
- **Signs and symptoms of decreased cardiac output (e.g., decreased level of consciousness)**
- **Premature ventricular contractions, particularly in the setting of an acute MI.**

Treatment to increase the heart rate may also be indicated if the heart rate is somewhat above 60 beats per minute and one or more of the above signs and symptoms are present. This may result if the heart rate is too slow relative to the existing metabolic needs. Such a slow heart rate is called a **symptomatic "relative" bradycardia** and requires treatment immediately.

Treatment may not be indicated even if the heart rate falls below 50 beats per minute if the systolic blood pressure remains greater than 80 mm Hg and stable; if congestive heart failure, chest pain, and dyspnea are not present; if agitation, lightheadedness, confusion, and loss of consciousness are absent; and if premature ventricular contractions do not occur. Such a bradycardia is considered to be an **asymptomatic bradycardia.**

In certain bradycardias associated with acute anteroseptal myocardial infarction, such as **(1) second-degree, type II and 2:1 and high-degree (advanced) AV blocks, with wide QRS complexes** (because of their propensity to progress rapidly to complete third-degree AV block without warning), and **(2) third-degree AV block with wide QRS complexes,** a temporary transcutaneous pacemaker is indicated immediately, whether or not the bradycardia is symptomatic.

Atropine sulfate should be used with caution in patients with acute myocardial infarction because of the possibility of an excessive increase in the heart rate with the potential of increasing myocardial ischemia and precipitating ventricular tachycardia or ventricular fibrillation. Transcutaneous pacing is preferred in such patients and in those where an IV access is difficult or delayed, or where thrombolytic therapy is anticipated. In addition to use in treatment of symptomatic bradycardias, atropine is also indicated for nausea and vomiting associated with administration of morphine sulfate.

Sinus Bradycardia
Sinus Arrest/Sinoatrial (SA) Exit Block
Second-degree, Type I AV Block (Wenckebach)
Second-degree, 2:1 and High-degree (Advanced) AV Block
with Narrow QRS Complexes
Third-degree AV Block with Narrow QRS Complexes

Treatment

If the **bradycardia is symptomatic:**

1. Administer **high concentration oxygen**.

2. Establish an **IV line.**

3. Administer a 0.5- to 1-mg **bolus of atropine sulfate** IV rapidly. Repeat every 3 to 5 minutes until the heart rate increases to 60 to 100 beats per minute or the maximum dose of 3.0 mg (0.04 mg/kg) of atropine has been administered.

AND/OR

4. Initiate **transcutaneous pacing.** If the **patient is conscious and not hypotensive,** administer 5 to 15 mg of **diazepam** or 2 to 5 mg of **morphine sulfate** IV slowly to produce amnesia/analgesia after onset of pacing, if necessary.

If the **bradycardia, hypotension, or both persist:**

5. Start an **infusion of dopamine hydrochloride** (400 mg of dopamine in 250 mL of 5 percent dextrose in water [D_5W] [1600 μg/mL]) at an initial rate of 2.5 to 5 μg/kg per minute, and adjust the infusion rate up to 20 μg/kg per minute to increase the heart rate to 60 to 100 beats per minute and the systolic blood pressure to 90 to 100 mm Hg.

OR

Start an **infusion of epinephrine** (1 mg [1 mL of a 1:1000 solution] of epinephrine in 500 mL of D_5W [2 μg/mL]) at an initial rate of 1 to 2 μg per minute (0.5 to 1 mL of the diluted epinephrine solution per minute), and adjust the infusion rate up to 10 μg per minute to increase the heart rate to 60 to 100 beats per minute and the systolic blood pressure to 90 to 100 mm Hg.

6. Insert a **temporary transvenous pacemaker** immediately.

Notes

Second-degree, Type II AV Block
Second-degree, 2:1 and High-degree (Advanced) AV Block
with Wide QRS Complexes
Third-degree AV Block with Wide QRS Complexes

Treatment

If the **bradycardia is asymptomatic and the cause of the second- or third-degree AV block with wide QRS complexes is an acute anteroseptal MI:**

1. Administer **high concentration oxygen.**

2. Establish an **IV line.**

3. Attach a **transcutaneous pacemaker,** test for ventricular capture and patient tolerance, and put on standby.

If the **bradycardia is or becomes symptomatic:**

4. Initiate **transcutaneous pacing.** If the **patient is conscious and not hypotensive,** administer 5 to 15 mg of **diazepam** or 2 to 5 mg of **morphine** IV slowly to produce amnesia/analgesia after onset of pacing, if necessary.

If the **bradycardia, hypotension, or both persist:**

5. Start an **infusion of dopamine** (400 mg of dopamine in 250 mL of D_5W [1600 μg/mL]) at an initial rate 2.5 to 5 μg/kg per minute, and adjust the infusion rate up to 20 μg/kg per minute to increase the heart rate to 60 to 100 beats per minute and the systolic blood pressure to 90 to 100 mm Hg.

OR

Start an **infusion of epinephrine** (1 mg [1 mL of a 1:1000 solution] of epinephrine in 500 mL of D_5W [2 μg/mL]) at an initial rate of 1 to 2 μg per minute (0.5 to 1 mL of the diluted epinephrine solution per minute), and adjust the infusion rate up to 10 μg per minute to increase the heart rate to 60 to 100 beats per minute and the systolic blood pressure to 90 to 100 mm Hg.

6. Insert a **temporary transvenous pacemaker** immediately.

Notes

Junctional Escape Rhythm
Ventricular Escape Rhythm

Treatment

If the **bradycardia is symptomatic:**

1. Administer **high concentration oxygen.**

2. Establish an **IV line.**

3. Initiate **transcutaneous pacing.** If the **patient is conscious and not hypotensive,** administer 5 to 15 mg of **diazepam** or 2 to 5 mg of **morphine** IV slowly to produce amnesia/analgesia after onset of pacing, if necessary.

If the **bradycardia, hypotension, or both persist:**

4. Start an **infusion of dopamine** (400 mg of dopamine in 250 mL of D_5W [1600 μg/mL]) at an initial rate 2.5 to 5 μg/kg per minute, and adjust the infusion rate up to 20 μg/kg per minute to increase the heart rate to 60 to 100 beats per minute and the systolic blood pressure to 90 to 100 mm Hg.

OR

Start an **infusion of epinephrine** (1 mg [1 mL of a 1:1000 solution] of epinephrine in 500 mL of D_5W [2 μg/mL]) at an initial rate of 1 to 2 μg per minute (0.5 to 1 mL of the diluted epinephrine solution per minute), and adjust the infusion rate up to 10 μg per minute to increase the heart rate to 60 to 100 beats per minute and the systolic blood pressure to 90 to 100 mm Hg.

5. Insert a **temporary transvenous pacemaker** immediately.

Notes

Tachycardias

Sinus Tachycardia
Atrial Tachycardia
(Nonparoxysmal Atrial Tachycardia without Block
Paroxysmal Atrial Tachycardia (PAT)
Atrial Tachycardia with Block)
Atrial Flutter (AF)
Atrial Fibrillation
Junctional Tachycardia
Paroxysmal Junctional Tachycardia (PJT)
Paroxysmal Supraventricular Tachycardia (PSVT)
Ventricular Tachycardia (VT, V-TACH)

Clinical Significance of Tachycardias

The signs and symptoms in a **tachycardia** depend upon the presence or absence of heart disease, the nature of the heart disease, the ventricular rate, and the duration of the tachycardia. Frequently, a tachycardia is accompanied by feelings of palpitations, nervousness, or anxiety.

A tachycardia with a heart rate over 120 to 140 beats per minute may cause the cardiac output to drop significantly because of the inability of the ventricles to fill completely during the extremely short diastole that results from the very rapid beating of the heart. Consequently, the systolic blood pressure may fall to 80 to 90 mm Hg or less, and signs and symptoms of decreased perfusion of the body, especially of the brain and other vital organs, may occur. The skin may become pale, cold, and clammy; the pulse may become weak or disappear; and the patient may become agitated, confused, lightheaded, or unconscious or may experience chest pain and also become dyspneic.

In addition, since a rapid heart rate increases the workload of the heart, the oxygen requirements of the myocardium are usually increased in a tachycardia. Thus, in addition to the consequences of decreased cardiac output, a tachycardia in acute myocardial infarction may increase myocardial ischemia and the frequency and severity of chest pain, bring about the extension of the infarct, cause congestive heart failure, hypotension or cardiogenic shock, or predispose the patient to serious ventricular arrhythmias.

Another reason for low cardiac output in certain tachycardias (atrial flutter, atrial fibrillation, and junctional and ventricular tachycardias) is that because an atrial contraction does not precede each ventricular contraction, the so-called "atrial kick," as it normally does, the ventricles do not fill completely during diastole. Consequently, the cardiac output may drop by as much as 25 percent.

Indications for Treatment of Tachycardias

Specific treatment of **nonparoxysmal atrial tachycardia without block, atrial flutter, atrial fibrillation,** and **paroxysmal supraventricular tachycardia** (including **paroxysmal atrial** and **junctional tachycardia**) is indicated if the heart rate is greater than 120 to 140 beats per minute (or even as low as 100 to 120 beats per minute) and, particularly, if signs and symptoms of decreased cardiac output or increased workload of the heart are associated with the tachycardia.

Treatment of **ventricular tachycardia,** however, is indicated immediately, whether or not signs and symptoms of decreased cardiac output are present, because of its potential of initiating or degenerating into ventricular fibrillation.

No specific treatment of **sinus tachycardia, nonparoxysmal** and **paroxysmal atrial tachycardia with block,** and **junctional tachycardia** is indicated.

Sinus Tachycardia

Treatment

No specific treatment of **sinus tachycardia** is indicated.

1. Treat the underlying cause of the tachycardia (anxiety, exercise, pain, fever, congestive heart failure, hypoxemia, hypovolemia, hypotension, or shock).

If excessive amounts of drugs, such as **atropine, epinephrine,** or a **vasopressor,** have been administered:

2. Discontinue such drugs.

Notes

Atrial Tachycardia with Block
Junctional Tachycardia

Treatment

No specific treatment of **atrial tachycardia with block** or **junctional tachycardia** is indicated.

1. Treat the underlying cause of the tachycardia.

If an excessive dose of **digitalis** is suspected:

2. Discontinue **digitalis.**

> **CAUTION!**
> Do not attempt vagal maneuvers or cardioversion!

Notes

Paroxysmal Supraventricular Tachycardia (PSVT)
with Narrow QRS Complexes
Paroxysmal Atrial Tachycardia (PAT)
Paroxysmal Junctional Tachycardia (PJT)

(Patient Hemodynamically Stable)

Treatment

If the **patient's condition is stable,** that is, the patient is normotensive, without chest pain or congestive heart failure and not having an acute myocardial infarction or ischemic episode:

1. Administer **high concentration oxygen.**

2. Establish an **IV line.**

3. Attempt **vagal maneuvers,** such as **unilateral carotid sinus massage,** or have the patient perform the **Valsalva maneuver** or **take a deep breath while in a head-down tilt po-** sition. ECG monitoring and an IV line must be in place and atropine and lidocaine immediately available before vagal maneuvers are performed. The technique of immersing the patient's face in ice water (**"diving reflex"**) may also be tried but only if ischemic heart disease is not present or suspected.

> **CAUTION!**
> Verify the absence of known carotid artery disease or carotid bruits before attempting carotid sinus massage!

If the **vagal maneuvers are unsuccessful** and the **patient remains stable:**

4. Administer a 6-mg **bolus of adenosine** IV rapidly over 1 to 3 seconds followed by a 20-ml flush of IV fluid.

AND

If the initial dose is not immediately effective, administer, in 1 to 2 minutes, a 12-mg **bolus of adenosine** IV rapidly over 1 to 3 seconds followed by a 20-ml flush of IV fluid. Repeat the 12-mg **bolus of adenosine** a second time, in 1 to 2 minutes, if needed.

If **adenosine is not effective** and the **patient continues to be stable:**

5. Administer a 20-mg (0.25-mg/kg) **bolus of diltiazem hydrochloride** IV slowly over 2 minutes. If the initial dose is not effective in 15 minutes, repeat a second 25-mg (0.35-mg/kg) **bolus of diltiazem** IV slowly over 2 minutes.

AND

Start a **maintenance infusion of diltiazem** (125 mg diltiazem in 125 mL [1 mg/mL]) at 5 to 15 mg per hour (5 to 15 mL per hour) to control the ventricular rate.

CAUTION!

Diltiazem is contraindicated:

- **If hypotension, cardiogenic shock, second-or third-degree AV block, sick sinus syndrome, or a preexcitation syndrome is present,**
- **If beta blockers are being administered intravenously, or**
- **If there is a history of bradycardia.**

Ditiazem should be used cautiously in congestive heart failure and patients receiving oral beta blockers.

The patient's blood pressure and pulse must be monitored frequently during and after the administration of diltiazem.

If hypotension occurs with diltiazem, place the patient in a Trendelenburg's position and administer 1.0 g of calcium chloride IV slowly, IV fluids, and a vasopressor.

If bradycardia, AV block, or asystole occurs, refer to the appropriate treatment protocol.

If the **vagal maneuvers, adenosine, and diltiazem** are unsuccessful and if an **excessive dose of digitalis** is not suspected and the **patient remains stable:**

6. Deliver a **synchronized countershock (50 joules*).** If the **patient is conscious,** administer 5 to 15 mg of **diazepam** or 2 to 5 mg of **morphine** IV slowly to produce amnesia/analgesia before cardioversion.

CAUTION!

Do not attempt cardioversion if paroxysmal supraventricular tachycardia recurs after initial conversion to a sinus rhythm and any underlying causes of the arrhythmia (e.g., electrolyte and acid-base abnormalities) have not been corrected!

If the **paroxysmal supraventricular tachycardia, including paroxysmal atrial and junctional tachycardia,** persists:

7. Consider **transcutaneous overdrive pacing.** If the **patient is conscious,** administer 5 to 15 mg of **diazepam** or 2 to 5 mg of **morphine** IV slowly to produce amnesia/analgesia before pacing the patient.

If an **excessive dose of digitalis** is suspected:

8. Withhold digitalis, and administer 40 mEq of **potassium chloride** in 500 mL of 0.9% saline IV at a rate of 10 to 15 mEq/hr (125 to 188 mL of the diluted potassium chloride solution per hour).

*The energy delivered in countershock is indicated as joules (watt/seconds) of delivered energy. Generally, delivered energy is approximately 80% of the energy stored in the defibrillator.

Notes

Paroxysmal Supraventricular Tachycardia (PSVT) with Narrow QRS Complexes
Paroxysmal Atrial Tachycardia (PAT)
Paroxysmal Junctional Tachycardia (PJT)
(Patient Hemodynamically Unstable)

Treatment

If the **patient's condition is unstable,** that is, the patient is hypotensive with evidence of poor peripheral perfusion, has chest pain or congestive heart failure, or is having an acute myocardial infarction or ischemic episode:

1. Administer **high concentration oxygen.**

2. Establish an **IV line.**

3. Deliver a **synchronized countershock** (50 joules). If the **patient is conscious and not hypotensive,** consider the administration of 5 to 15 mg of **diazepam** or 2 to 5 mg of **morphine** IV slowly to produce amnesia/analgesia before cardioversion.

   ADMINISTRATION OF DIAZEPAM OR MORPHINE SHOULD NOT DELAY CARDIOVERSION IF IT IS INDICATED IMMEDIATELY BY THE PATIENT'S CONDITION!

CAUTION!

Do not attempt cardioversion if an excessive dose of digitalis is suspected as the cause of the paroxysmal supraventricular tachycardia or if the tachycardia recurs after initial conversion to a sinus rhythm and any underlying causes of the arrhythmia (e.g., electrolyte and acid-base abnormalities) have not been corrected!

If the **first countershock** is unsuccessful:

4. Deliver a **second synchronized countershock** (100 joules).

If the **second countershock** is unsuccessful:

5. Deliver a **third synchronized countershock** (200 joules).

If the **third countershock** is unsuccessful:

6. Consider **transcutaneous overdrive pacing.** If the **patient is conscious and not hypotensive,** administer 5 to 15 mg of **diazepam** or 2 to 5 mg of **morphine** IV slowly to produce amnesia/analgesia after onset of pacing, if necessary.

If the **paroxysmal supraventricular tachycardia, including paroxysmal atrial and junctional tachycardia,** persists:

7. Correct any underlying causes of paroxysmal supraventricular tachycardia (e.g., electrolyte and acid-base abnormalities).

8. Consider the treatment protocol for **Hemodynamically Stable Paroxysmal Supraventricular Tachycardia (PSVT) with Narrow QRS Complexes.**

Notes

Atrial Flutter (AF)
Nonparoxysmal Atrial Tachycardia without Block

Treatment

If the **heart rate is over 150 beats per minute.**
AND
The **patient's condition is hemodynamically stable**—that is, the patient is conscious and has a pulse, the systolic blood pressure is greater than 80 mm Hg, and pulmonary edema and signs and symptoms of decreased cardiac output are absent:

1. Administer **high concentration oxygen.**

2. Establish an **IV line.**

3. Deliver a **synchronized, low-energy, countershock** (50 joules). Administer 5 to 15 mg of **diazepam** or 2 to 5 mg of **morphine** IV slowly to produce amnesia/analgesia before cardioversion.
OR
4. Administer a 20-mg (0.25-mg/kg) **bolus of diltiazem** IV slowly over 2 minutes. If the initial dose is not effective in 15 minutes, repeat a second 25-mg (0.35-mg/kg) **bolus of diltiazem** IV slowly over 2 minutes.
AND
Start a **maintenance infusion of diltiazem** (125 mg diltiazem in 125 mL [1 mg/mL]) at 5 to 15 mg per hour (5 to 15 mL per hour) to control the ventricular rate.

If **cardioversion is unsuccessful** in cardioverting the arrhythmia to normal sinus rhythm or diltiazem is unsuccessful in slowing the ventricular rate:

5. Repeat the **synchronized countershock** (100 joules or more) or administer **diltiazem** if cardioversion attempted initially.
OR
Deliver an initial **synchronized countershock** (50 joules) if diltiazem administered initially.

If the **heart rate is over 150 beats per minute.**
AND
The **patient is hemodynamically unstable**—that is, the patient is hypotensive (systolic blood pressure of 80 to 90 mm Hg or less) with evidence of poor peripheral perfusion, has congestive heart failure or symptoms (e.g., chest pain or dyspnea), or is having an acute myocardial infarction or ischemic episode:

1. Administer **high concentration oxygen.**

2. Establish an **IV line.**

3. Deliver a **synchronized, low-energy, countershock** (50 joules). If the **patient is conscious and not hypotensive,** administer 5 to 15 mg of **diazepam** or 2 to 5 mg of **morphine** IV slowly to produce amnesia/analgesia before cardioversion.

If **cardioversion is unsuccessful** and the indications for treatment of **atrial flutter** or **nonparoxysmal atrial tachycardia without block** are still present:

4. Repeat the **synchronized countershock** (100 joules or more).

Notes

CAUTION!

Diltiazem is contraindicated:

- **If hypotension, cardiogenic shock, second-or third-degree AV block, sick sinus syndrome, or a preexcitation syndrome is present,**
- **If beta blockers are being administered intravenously, or**
- **If there is a history of bradycardia.**

Diltiazem should be used cautiously in congestive heart failure and patients receiving oral beta blockers.

The patient's blood pressure and pulse must be monitored frequently during and after the administration of diltiazem.

If hypotension occurs with diltiazem, place the patient in a Trendelenburg position and administer 1.0 g of calcium chloride IV slowly, IV fluids, and a vasopressor.

If bradycardia, AV block, or asystole occurs, refer to the appropriate treatment protocol.

Atrial Fibrillation

Treatment

If the **heart rate is over 150 beats per minute.**
AND
The **patient's condition is hemodynamically stable**—that is, the **patient is conscious** and has a pulse, the systolic blood pressure is greater than 80 mm Hg, and pulmonary edema and signs and symptoms of decreased cardiac output are absent:

1. Administer **high concentration oxygen.**

2. Establish an **IV line.**

3. Administer a 20-mg (0.25-mg/kg) **bolus of diltiazem** IV slowly over 2 minutes. If the initial dose is not effective in 15 minutes, repeat a second 25-mg (0.35-mg/kg) **bolus of diltiazem** IV slowly over 2 minutes.
AND
Start a **maintenance infusion of diltiazem** (125 mg diltiazem in 125 mL [1 mg/mL]) at 5 to 15 mg per hour (5 to 15 mL per hour) to control the ventricular rate.

CAUTION!
Diltiazem is contraindicated:

- **If hypotension, cardiogenic shock, second- or third-degree AV block, sick sinus syndrome, or a preexcitation syndrome is present,**
- **If beta blockers are being administered intravenously, or**
- **If there is a history of bradycardia.**

Diltiazem should be used cautiously in congestive heart failure and patients receiving oral beta blockers.

The patient's blood pressure and pulse must be monitored frequently during and after the administration of diltiazem.

If hypotension occurs with diltiazem, place the patient in a Trendelenburg position and administer 1.0 g of calcium chloride IV slowly, IV fluids, and a vasopressor.

If bradycardia, AV block, or asystole occurs, refer to the appropriate treatment protocol.

If the **heart rate is over 150 beats per minute.**
AND
The **patient is hemodynamically unstable**—that is, the patient is hypotensive (systolic blood pressure of 80 to 90 mm Hg or less) with evidence of poor peripheral perfusion, has congestive heart failure or symptoms (e.g., chest pain or dyspnea), or is having an acute myocardial infarction or ischemic episode.
AND
The atrial fibrillation is of recent origin, that is, of less than a day or so:

1. Administer **high concentration oxygen.**

2. Establish an **IV line.**

3. Deliver a **synchronized countershock** (100 joules). If the **patient is conscious and not hypotensive,** administer 5 to 15 mg of **diazepam** or 2 to 5 mg of **morphine** IV slowly to produce amnesia/analgesia before cardioversion.

If **cardioversion is unsuccessful** and the indications for treatment of **atrial fibrillation** are still present:

4. Repeat the **synchronized countershock** (200 joules or more).

Notes

Wide-QRS-Complex Tachycardia of Unknown Origin (with Pulse)

(Patient Hemodynamically Stable)

Treatment

If the **patient's condition is hemodynamically stable**—that is, the patient is conscious and has a pulse, the systolic blood pressure is greater than 80 mm Hg, and pulmonary edema and signs and symptoms of decreased cardiac output are absent:

1. Administer **high concentration oxygen.**

2. Establish an **IV line.**

3. Administer a 1- to 1.5-mg/kg **bolus of lidocaine** IV slowly.

4. Repeat administration of a 0.5- to 0.75-mg/kg **bolus of lidocaine** IV slowly every 5 to 10 minutes until the wide-QRS-complex tachycardia is suppressed or a total dose of 3 mg/kg of lidocaine has been administered.

If **lidocaine is successful** in suppressing the **wide-QRS-complex tachycardia:**

5. Start a **maintenance infusion of lidocaine** (1 g of lidocaine in 500 mL of D₅W [2 mg/mL]) at a rate of 2 mg of lidocaine per minute (1 mL of the diluted lidocaine solution per minute) to prevent the recurrence of the wide-QRS-complex tachycardia. If additional boluses of lidocaine were administered initially, increase the rate of the lidocaine infusion by 1-mg increments for each additional 1-mg/kg dose of lidocaine to a maximum rate of 4 mg of lidocaine per minute.

Initial dose of lidocaine	Rate of lidocaine infusion
1 mg/kg	2 mg/min
1-2 mg/kg	3 mg/min
2-3 mg/kg	4 mg/min

If **lidocaine is unsuccessful** in suppressing the **wide-QRS-complex tachycardia** and the **patient remains stable:**

6. Discontinue the lidocaine infusion if it has been started.

7. Administer a 6-mg **bolus of adenosine** IV rapidly over 1 to 3 seconds followed by a 20-ml flush of IV fluid.

AND

If the initial dose is not immediately effective, administer, in 1 to 2 minutes, a 12-mg **bolus of adenosine** IV rapidly over 1 to 3 seconds followed by a 20-ml flush of IV fluid. Repeat the 12-mg **bolus of adenosine** a second time, in 1 to 2 minutes, if needed.

If **lidocaine and adenosine are unsuccessful** in suppressing the **wide-QRS-complex tachycardia** and the **patient remains stable:**

8. Consider **transcutaneous overdrive pacing.** If the **patient is conscious,** administer 5 to 15 mg of **diazepam** or 2 to 5 mg of **morphine** IV slowly to produce amnesia/analgesia before pacing the patient.

If the **wide-QRS-complex tachycardia** persists and the **patient remains hemodynamically stable and has a pulse:**

9. Continue with **Step 7** in **Ventricular Tachycardia (with Pulse) (Patient Hemodynamically Stable).**

If the **wide-QRS-complex tachycardia** persists and the **patient is or becomes hemodynamically unstable and has a pulse:**

10. Continue with **Step 3** in **Ventricular Tachycardia (with Pulse) (Patient Hemodynamically Unstable).**

If the **wide-QRS-complex tachycardia** persists and the **patient becomes pulseless:**

11. Continue with **Step 4** in **Ventricular Fibrillation/Pulseless Tachycardia (VF/VT).**

Notes

Ventricular Tachycardia (with Pulse)
(Patient Hemodynamically Stable)

Treatment

If the **patient's condition is hemodynamically stable**—that is, the patient is conscious and has a pulse, the systolic blood pressure is greater than 80 mm Hg, and pulmonary edema and signs and symptoms of decreased cardiac output are absent:

1. Administer **high concentration oxygen.**

2. Establish an **IV line.**

3. Administer a 1- to 1.5-mg/kg **bolus of lidocaine** IV slowly.

4. Repeat administration of a 0.5- to 0.75-mg/kg **bolus of lidocaine** IV slowly every 5 to 10 minutes until the ventricular tachycardia is suppressed or a total dose of 3 mg/kg of lidocaine has been administered.

If **lidocaine is successful** in suppressing the **ventricular tachycardia:**

5. Start a **maintenance infusion of lidocaine** (1 g of lidocaine in 500 mL of D_5W [2 mg/mL]) at a rate of 2 mg of lidocaine per minute (1 mL of the diluted lidocaine solution per minute) to prevent the recurrence of the ventricular tachycardia. If additional

Initial dose of lidocaine	Rate of lidocaine infusion
1 mg/kg	2 mg/min
1-2 mg/kg	3 mg/min
2-3 mg/kg	4 mg/min

boluses of lidocaine were administered initially, increase the rate of the lidocaine infusion by 1-mg increments for each additional 1-mg/kg dose of lidocaine to a maximum rate of 4 mg of lidocaine per minute.

If **lidocaine is unsuccessful** in suppressing the **ventricular tachycardia** and the **patient remains stable:**

6. Discontinue the lidocaine infusion if it has been started.

7. Start an **infusion of procainamide hydrochloride** (1 g of procainamide in 50 mL of D_5W [20 mg/mL]) at a rate of 20 to 30 mg/minute (1 to 1.5 mL of the diluted procainamide solution per minute).

8. Continue the **infusion of procainamide** until:

   • The ventricular tachycardia is suppressed,
   • A total dose of 17 mg/kg of procainamide has been administered (1.2 g of procainamide for a 70-kg patient),
   • Side effects from the procainamide appear (such as hypotension), or
   • The QRS complex widens by 50% of its original width.

9. Start a **maintenance infusion of procainamide** (1 g of procainamide in 500 mL of D_5W [2 mg/mL]) if indicated, at a rate of 1 to 4 mg per minute (0.5 to 2 mL of the diluted procainamide solution per minute).

If **lidocaine and procainamide are unsuccessful** in suppressing the **ventricular tachycardia** and the **patient remains stable:**

10. Administer a dose of 5 to 10 mg/kg of **bretylium tosylate** diluted to 50 mL with D_5W, IV slowly over 8 to 10 minutes.

11. Start a **maintenance infusion of bretylium** (1 g of bretylium in 500 mL of D_5W [2 mg/mL]) at a rate of 1 to 2 mg per minute (0.5 to 1 mL of the diluted bretylium solution per minute).

If **lidocaine, procainamide, and bretylium are unsuccessful** in suppressing the **ventricular tachycardia** and the **patient remains stable:**

12. Deliver a **synchronized countershock** (100 joules). In the conscious patient, consider the administration of 5 to 15 mg of **diazepam** or 2 to 5 mg of **morphine** IV slowly to produce amnesia/analgesia before cardioversion.

If the **first countershock** is unsuccessful:

13. Deliver a **second synchronized countershock** (200 joules).

If the **second countershock** is unsuccessful:

14. Deliver a **third synchronized countershock** (300 joules).

If the **third countershock** is unsuccessful:

15. Deliver a **fourth synchronized countershock** (up to 360 joules).

If the patient with **ventricular tachycardia** becomes **hemodynamically unstable** (e.g., drowsy, stuporous, unconscious, or hypotensive [systolic blood pressure of 80 to 90 mm Hg or less]) or if signs and symptoms of decreased cardiac output (e.g., chest pain or dyspnea) appear:

16. Deliver an **unsynchronized shock** (100 joules or the energy level at which termination of ventricular tachycardia was previously effective). If the patient is still conscious, consider the administration of 5 to 15 mg of **diazepam** or 2 to 5 mg of **morphine** IV slowly to produce amnesia/analgesia before delivering the shock.

ADMINISTRATION OF DIAZEPAM OR MORPHINE SHOULD NOT DELAY THE DELIVERY OF SHOCKS IF THEY ARE INDICATED IMMEDIATELY BY THE PATIENT'S CONDITION!

17. Consider **transcutaneous overdrive pacing.** If the **patient is conscious and not hypotensive,** administer 5 to 15 mg of **diazepam** or 2 to 5 mg of **morphine** IV slowly to produce amnesia/analgesia after onset of pacing, if necessary.

If the **shocks are successful** in terminating the **ventricular tachycardia:**

18. Administer a 1-mg/kg **bolus of lidocaine** IV slowly.

19. Start a **maintenance infusion of lidocaine,** if one has not already been started (1 g of lidocaine in 500 mL of D_5W [2 mg/mL]) at a rate of 2 mg of lidocaine per minute (1 mL of the diluted lidocaine solution per minute) to prevent the recurrence of the ventricular tachycardia.

Notes

Ventricular Tachycardia (with Pulse)
(Patient Hemodynamically Unstable)

Treatment

If the patient is conscious (or unconscious) and has a pulse, but with a hemodynamically unstable condition—that is, the patient is hypotensive (systolic blood pressure of 80 to 90 mm Hg or less) with evidence of poor peripheral perfusion, has congestive heart failure or symptoms (e.g., chest pain or dyspnea), or is having an acute myocardial infarction or ischemic episode:

1. Administer **high concentration oxygen.**

2. Establish an **IV line.**

3. Deliver an **unsynchronized shock** (100 joules). If the **patient is conscious and not hypotensive,** consider the administration of 5 to 15 mg of **diazepam** or 2 to 5 mg of **morphine** IV slowly to produce amnesia/analgesia before delivering the shock.

   ADMINISTRATION OF DIAZEPAM OR MORPHINE SHOULD NOT DELAY THE DELIVERY OF SHOCKS IF THEY ARE INDICATED IMMEDIATELY BY THE PATIENT'S CONDITION!

If the **first shock** is unsuccessful:

4. Deliver a **second unsynchronized shock** (200 joules).

If the **second shock** is unsuccessful:

5. Deliver a **third unsynchronized shock** (300 joules).

If the **third shock** is unsuccessful:

6. Deliver a **fourth unsynchronized shock** (360 joules).

If the **shocks are successful** in terminating the **ventricular tachycardia:**

7. Administer a 1- to 1.5-mg/kg **bolus of lidocaine** IV slowly.

8. Start a **maintenance infusion of lidocaine** (1 g of lidocaine in 500 mL of D_5W [2 mg/mL]) at a rate of 2 mg of lidocaine per minute (1 mL of the diluted lidocaine solution per minute) to prevent the recurrence of the ventricular tachycardia.

If **ventricular tachycardia** persists (or recurs):

9. Administer a 1- to 1.5-mg/kg **bolus of lidocaine** IV slowly.

10. Repeat administration of a 0.5- to 0.75-mg/kg **bolus of lidocaine** IV slowly every 5 to 10 minutes until the ventricular tachycardia is suppressed or a total dose of 3 mg/kg of lidocaine has been administered.

If **lidocaine is successful** in suppressing the **ventricular tachycardia:**

11. Start a **maintenance infusion of lidocaine** (1 g of lidocaine in 500 mL of D_5W [2 mg/mL]) at a rate of 2 mg of lidocaine per minute (1 mL of the diluted lidocaine solution per minute) to prevent the recurrence of the ventricular tachycardia. If additional boluses of lidocaine were administered initially, increase the rate of the lidocaine infusion by 1-mg increments for each additional 1-mg/kg dose of lidocaine to a maximum rate of 4 mg of lidocaine per minute.

Initial dose of lidocaine	Rate of lidocaine infusion
1 mg/kg	**2 mg/min**
1-2 mg/kg	**3 mg/min**
2-3 mg/kg	**4 mg/min**

If **ventricular tachycardia** persists:

12. Deliver an **unsynchronized shock** at the energy level at which the shocks were previously effective, and repeat the **unsynchronized shock** at progressively increasing energy levels if needed.

If **lidocaine and shock are unsuccessful** in suppressing the **ventricular tachycardia** and the **patient remains unstable:**

13. Discontinue the **lidocaine infusion** if it has been started.

14. Start an **infusion of procainamide** (1 g of procainamide in 50 mL of D_5W [20 mg/mL]) at a rate of 20 to 30 mg/minute (1 to 1.5 mL of the diluted procainamide solution per minute).

> ### CAUTION!
> **Do not administer procainamide if hypotension or pulmonary edema is present or if the patient is unconscious. Administer, instead, bretylium as in step 18 opposite.**

15. Continue the **infusion of procainamide** until:

    • The ventricular tachycardia is suppressed,
    • A total dose of 17 mg/kg of procainamide has been administered (1.2 g of procainamide for a 70-kg patient),
    • Side effects from the procainamide appear (such as hypotension), or
    • The QRS complex widens by 50% of its original width.

16. Start a **maintenance infusion of procainamide** (1 g of procainamide in 500 mL of D_5W [2 mg/mL]) if indicated, at a rate of 1 to 4 mg per minute (0.5 to 2 mL of the diluted procainamide solution per minute).

If **ventricular tachycardia** persists:

17. Deliver an **unsynchronized shock** at the energy level at which termination of ventricular tachycardia was previously effective, and repeat the **unsynchronized shock** at progressively increasing energy levels if needed.

If **lidocaine, procainamide and shock are unsuccessful** in suppressing the **ventricular tachycardia** and the **patient remains unstable:**

18. Administer a dose of 5- to 10-mg/kg of **bretylium,** diluted to 50 mL with D_5W, IV slowly over 8 to 10 minutes.

19. Start a **maintenance infusion of bretylium** (1 g of bretylium in 500 mL of D_5W [2 mg/mL]) at a rate of 1 to 2 mg per minute (0.5 to 1 mL of the diluted bretylium solution per minute).

If **ventricular tachycardia** persists:

20. Consider **transcutaneous overdrive pacing.** If the **patient is conscious and not hypotensive,** administer 5 to 15 mg of **diazepam** or 2 to 5 mg of **morphine** IV slowly to produce amnesia/analgesia after onset of pacing, if necessary.

If **ventricular tachycardia** recurs:

21. Deliver an **unsynchronized shock** at the energy level at which termination of ventricular tachycardia was previously effective, and repeat the **unsynchronized shock** at progressively increasing energy levels if needed, until the ventricular tachycardia is terminated.

___

Notes

Torsade de Pointe (with Pulse)
(Patient Hemodynamically Stable or Unstable)

Treatment

1. Administer **high concentration oxygen.**

2. Establish an **IV line.**

3. Initiate **transcutaneous overdrive pacing.** If the **patient is conscious,** administer 5 to 15 mg of **diazepam** or 2 to 5 mg of **morphine** IV slowly to produce amnesia/analgesia before pacing the patient.

If **torsade de pointes** persists and the **patient is not hypotensive:**

4. Administer a dose of 1 to 2 g (8 to 16 mEq) of **magnesium sulfate,** diluted to 100 mL with D_5W, IV over 1 to 2 minutes.

5. Start a **maintenance infusion of magnesium sulfate** (1 to 2 g [8 to 16 mEq] of magnesium sulfate in 100 mL) to run for 1 hour.

If **torsade de pointes** persists:

6. Deliver an **unsynchronized shock** (200 joules), and repeat the **unsynchronized shock** at progressively increasing energy levels if needed. If the **patient is conscious and not hypotensive,** consider the administration of 5 to 15 mg of **diazepam** or 2 to 5 mg of **morphine** IV slowly to produce amnesia/analgesia before delivering the first shock.

ADMINISTRATION OF DIAZEPAM OR MORPHINE SHOULD NOT DELAY THE DELIVERY OF SHOCKS IF THEY ARE INDICATED IMMEDIATELY BY THE PATIENT'S CONDITION!

Notes

Premature Ectopic Beats

Premature Atrial Contractions (PACs)
Premature Junctional Contractions (PJCs)
Premature Ventricular Contractions (PVCs)

Premature Atrial Contractions (PACs)

Clinical Significance of Premature Atrial Contractions

Single, isolated premature atrial contractions are not significant. Frequent PACs may indicate the presence of enhanced atrial automaticity, an atrial reentry mechanism, or both, and herald impending atrial arrhythmias (such as atrial tachycardia, atrial flutter, and atrial fibrillation) and paroxysmal supraventricular tachycardia.

Indications for Treatment of Premature Atrial Contractions

Treatment may be indicated if the premature atrial contractions are frequent (eight to ten per minute), occur in groups of two or more, or alternate with the QRS complexes of the underlying rhythm (bigeminy).

Treatment

If stimulants (such as caffeine, tobacco, or alcohol) or excessive amounts of sympathomimetic drugs (such as epinephrine or dopamine) have been administered:

1. Discontinue the stimulants and sympathomimetic drugs.

If the **premature atrial contractions** continue and the indication for treatment is still present:

2. Administer 200 mg of **quinidine sulfate** by mouth.

If an **excessive dose of digitalis** is suspected:

3. Withhold **digitalis.**

Notes

Premature Junctional Contractions (PJCs)

Clinical Significance of Premature Junctional Contractions

Single, isolated premature junctional contractions are not significant. Frequent PJCs may indicate the presence of enhanced AV junctional automaticity, an AV junctional reentry mechanism, or both, and herald an impending junctional tachycardia.

Indications for Treatment of Premature Junctional Contractions

Treatment is indicated if the premature junctional contractions are frequent (four to six per minute), occur in groups of two or more, or alternate with the QRS complexes of the underlying rhythm (bigeminy).

Treatment

Treatment of premature junctional contractions is the same as that of premature atrial contractions indicated above.

Notes

Premature Ventricular Contractions (PVCs)

Clinical Significance of Premature Ventricular Contractions

Single premature ventricular contractions, especially in patients who have no heart disease, are generally not significant. In patients with acute myocardial infarction or an ischemic episode, PVCs may indicate the presence of enhanced ventricular automaticity, a ventricular reentry mechanism, or both, or herald the appearance of life-threatening arrhythmias, such as ventricular tachycardia, flutter, or fibrillation. Although these lethal arrhythmias may occur without warning, they are often initiated by premature ventricular contractions, especially if the PVCs:

- Are frequent (six or more per minute),
- Occur in groups of two or more (group beats),
- Have different QRS configurations (multiform),
- Arise from different ventricular ectopic pacemakers (multifocal),
- Are close coupled, or
- Fall on the T wave (R-on-T phenomenon).

Indications for Treatment of Premature Ventricular Contractions

Treatment is indicated for all premature ventricular contractions in patients suspected of acute myocardial infarction or ischemic episode **except for those that occur in conjunction with bradycardias.** In such circumstances, the underlying bradycardia is treated first. Refer to page 288 for the treatment of bradycardias. If feasible, identify and correct any underlying causes of premature ventricular contractions (e.g., low serum potassium [hypokalemia], low serum magnesium [hypomagnesemia], excessive administration of digitalis or sympathomimetic drugs [e.g., epinephrine and dopamine], hypoxia, acidosis, and congestive heart failure).

Treatment

1. Administer **high concentration oxygen.**

2. Establish an **IV line.**

3. Administer a 1- to 1.5-mg/kg **bolus of lidocaine** IV slowly.

4. Repeat administration of a 0.5- to 0.75-mg/kg **bolus of lidocaine** IV slowly every 5 to 10 minutes until the premature ventricular contractions are suppressed or a total dose of 3 mg/kg of lidocaine has been administered.

5. Start a **maintenance infusion of lidocaine** (1 g of lidocaine in 500 mL of D_5W [2 mg/mL]) at a rate of 2 mg of lidocaine per minute (1 mL of the diluted lidocaine solution per minute) to prevent the recurrence of the premature ventricular contractions. If additional boluses of lidocaine were administered initially, increase the rate of the lidocaine infusion by 1-mg increments for each additional 1-mg/kg dose of lidocaine to a maximum rate of 4 mg of lidocaine per minute.

Initial dose of lidocaine	Rate of lidocaine infusion
1 mg/kg	**2 mg/min**
1-2 mg/kg	**3 mg/min**
2-3 mg/kg	**4 mg/min**

If **lidocaine is unsuccessful** in suppressing the **premature ventricular contractions** and the **patient remains stable:**

6. Discontinue the lidocaine infusion if it has been started.

7. Start an **infusion of procainamide** (1 g of procainamide in 50 mL of D₅W [20 mg/mL]) at a rate of 20 to 30 mg/minute (1 to 1.5 mL of the diluted procainamide solution per minute).

> **CAUTION!**
>
> **Do not administer procainamide if hypotension or pulmonary edema is present or if the patient is unconscious. Administer, instead, bretylium as in step 10 farther on.**

8. Continue the **infusion of procainamide** until:

   - The premature ventricular contractions are suppressed,
   - A total dose of 17 mg/kg of procainamide has been administered (1.2 g of procainamide for a 70-kg patient),

- Side effects from the procainamide appear (such as hypotension), or
- The QRS complex widens by 50% of its original width.

9. Start a **maintenance infusion of procainamide** (1 g of procainamide in 500 mL of D₅W [2 mg/mL]) if indicated, at a rate of 1 to 4 mg per minute (0.5 to 2 mL of the diluted procainamide solution per minute) to prevent the recurrence of premature ventricular contractions.

If **lidocaine and procainamide are unsuccessful** in suppressing the **premature ventricular contractions** and the **patient remains stable:**

10. Administer a dose of 5 to 10 mg/kg of **bretylium** diluted to 50 mL with D₅W, IV slowly over 8 to 10 minutes.

11. Start a **maintenance infusion of bretylium** (1 g of bretylium in 500 mL of D₅W [2 mg/mL]) at a rate of 1 to 2 mg per minute (0.5 to 1 mL of the diluted bretylium solution per minute) to prevent the recurrence of the premature ventricular contractions.

If **lidocaine, procainamide, and bretylium are unsuccessful** in suppressing the **premature ventricular contractions** and the patient remains stable:

12. Consider **transcutaneous overdrive pacing.** If the **patient is conscious,** administer 5 to 15 mg of **diazepam** or 2 to 5 mg of **morphine** IV slowly to produce amnesia/analgesia before pacing the patient.

Notes

Part II

Ventricular Fibrillation/Pulseless Ventricular Tachycardia (VF/VT)

Clinical Significance of Ventricular Fibrillation/Pulseless Ventricular Tachycardia

Ventricular fibrillation is a life-threatening arrhythmia resulting in chaotic beating of the heart and the immediate end of organized ventricular contractions, cardiac output, and pulse.

Pulseless ventricular tachycardia, like ventricular fibrillation, becomes a life-threatening arrhythmia when the ventricular contractions are unable to maintain an adequate cardiac output and a pulse.

At the moment ventricular fibrillation or pulseless ventricular tachycardia occurs and cardiac output stops, **clinical death** is present. **Biological death** occurs within 10 minutes unless cardiopulmonary resuscitation (CPR), defibrillation shocks, or both are administered within minutes.

Indications for Treatment of Ventricular Fibrillation/Pulseless Ventricular Tachycardia

Treatment of ventricular fibrillation and pulseless ventricular tachycardia is indicated immediately.

Treatment

A. Unmonitored Cardiac Arrest

If the cardiac arrest is witnessed by the resuscitation team or if cardiac arrest occurred before the arrival of the team and the patient is not being monitored:

Rescuer One:

1. Assess the **patient's unresponsiveness.**
2. Check the **patient's ABCs.**
3. Perform **CPR** until the defibrillator paddles or defibrillation pads are applied.

Rescuer Two:

1. Apply the **defibrillator paddles** or **defibrillation pads** to the patient.
2. Determine the ECG rhythm on the **ECG monitor.**
3. Verify cardiac arrest by checking the **patient's pulse.**

If **ventricular fibrillation/pulseless ventricular tachycardia** is present:

4. Deliver a **defibrillation shock** (200 joules) immediately, and check the patient's ECG rhythm on the **ECG monitor.**

If **ventricular fibrillation/pulseless ventricular tachycardia** persists:

5. Deliver a **second defibrillation shock** (200 to 300 joules) immediately after the first shock, and check the patient's ECG rhythm on the **ECG monitor.**

If **ventricular fibrillation/pulseless ventricular tachycardia** persists:

6. Deliver a **third defibrillation shock** (up to 360 joules) immediately after the second shock, and check the patient's ECG rhythm on the **ECG monitor.**

If **ventricular fibrillation/pulseless ventricular tachycardia** persists:

7. Resume **CPR.**
8. **Intubate** the patient.
9. Ventilate with **high concentration oxygen.**
10. Establish an **IV line.**
11. Administer 1.0 mg of **epinephrine** (10 mL of a 1:10,000 solution of epinephrine) IV followed by a 20-mL flush of IV fluid; repeat every 3 to 5 minutes during resuscitation.

EPINEPHRINE OPTIONS

- **Epinephrine infusion:**

  Infusion of epinephrine (30 mg epinephrine [30 mL of a 1:1000 solution] in 250 mL of NS or D₅W) administered at a rate of 100 mL per hour and titrated as necessary. Administration through a central venous line is the preferred route.

- **Intermediate dose of epinephrine by bolus:**

  2- to 5-mg bolus every 3 to 5 minutes.

- **Escalating dose of epinephrine by bolus:**

  A 1-mg bolus followed by a 3-mg bolus followed by a 5-mg bolus every 3 minutes.

- **High dose of epinephrine by bolus:**

  0.1-mg/kg bolus every 3 to 5 minutes.

Note: If an IV line cannot be established, administer **2 to 2.5 times the proposed peripheral IV dose of epinephrine** via the endotracheal tube, if one is in place. If *both* an IV line and an endotracheal tube *are not* in place, consider administration of 0.5 mg of epinephrine (5 mL of a 1:10,000 solution of epinephrine) by intracardiac injection and repeat if needed.

12. Continue **CPR** for 30 to 60 seconds to circulate the drug.
13. Determine the ECG rhythm on the **ECG monitor.**
14. Verify cardiac arrest by checking the **patient's pulse.**

If **ventricular fibrillation/pulseless ventricular tachycardia** persists:

15. Deliver a **fourth defibrillation shock** (up to 360 joules), and check the patient's ECG rhythm and pulse.

If **ventricular fibrillation/pulseless ventricular tachycardia** persists:

16. Administer a 1.5-mg/kg **bolus of lidocaine** IV followed by a 20-mL flush of IV fluid.
17. Continue **CPR** for 30 to 60 seconds to circulate the drug.
18. Deliver a **fifth defibrillation shock** (360 joules), and check the patient's ECG rhythm and pulse.

If **ventricular fibrillation/pulseless ventricular tachycardia** persists:

19. Administer a second 1.5-mg/kg **bolus of lidocaine** IV in 3 to 5 minutes, followed by a 20-mL flush of IV fluid, for a total dose of 3 mg/kg of lidocaine.
20. Continue **CPR** for 30 to 60 seconds to circulate the drug.
21. Deliver a **sixth defibrillation shock** (360 joules), and check the patient's ECG rhythm and pulse.

If **ventricular fibrillation/pulseless ventricular tachycardia** persists:

22. Administer a 5-mg/kg **bolus of bretylium** IV followed by a 20-mL flush of IV fluid.
23. Continue **CPR** for 1 to 2 minutes to circulate the drug.
24. Deliver a **seventh defibrillation shock** (360 joules), and check the patient's ECG rhythm and pulse.

If **ventricular fibrillation/pulseless ventricular tachycardia** persists:

25. Administer a second 10-mg/kg **bolus of bretylium** IV followed by a 20-mL flush of IV fluid, in 5 minutes.
26. Continue **CPR** for 1 to 2 minutes to circulate the drug.
27. Deliver an **eighth defibrillation shock** (360 joules), and check the patient's ECG rhythm and pulse.

If **ventricular fibrillation/pulseless ventricular tachycardia** persists:

28. Administer additional 10-mg/kg boluses of **bretylium** IV, each followed by a 20-mL flush of IV fluid, every 5 minutes up to a total dose of 30 to 35 mg/kg. After each dose continue **CPR** for 1 to 2 minutes to circulate the drug and then deliver a **defibrillation shock** (360 joules) and check the patient's ECG rhythm and pulse.

If **ventricular fibrillation/pulseless ventricular tachycardia** is terminated:

29. Perform **CPR** until the patient's pulse is palpable and the systolic blood pressure is 90 to 100 mm Hg or greater.

IF LIDOCAINE HAS NOT BEEN ADMINISTERED PREVIOUSLY:

30. Administer a 1-mg/kg **bolus of lidocaine** IV slowly.
31. Start a **maintenance infusion of lidocaine** (1 g of lidocaine in 500 mL of D_5W [2 mg/mL]) at a rate of 2 mg of lidocaine per minute (1 mL of the diluted lidocaine solution per minute) to prevent the recurrence of ventricular fibrillation/pulseless ventricular tachycardia.

If a **symptomatic post-defibrillation bradycardia or tachycardia** is present:

32. Refer to the **appropriate symptomatic bradycardia or tachycardia treatment protocol.**

If **hypotension** is present (**systolic blood pressure, 80 to 90 mm Hg or less**) in the **absence of pulmonary edema:**

33. Elevate the **patient's legs 18 inches above the level of the heart.**

34. Consider the rapid administration of **fluid boluses of 250 to 500 mL of 0.9% saline or Ringer's lactate solution** while monitoring the pulse and blood pressure and auscultating the lungs for pulmonary edema. Repeat the **fluid boluses** if a hemodynamic response is observed.

If **hypotension** persists (**systolic blood pressure, 80 to 90 mm Hg or less**):
If the **systolic blood pressure is less than 70 mm Hg**:

35. Start an **infusion of norepinephrine** (4 mg base of norepinephrine [1 4-mL ampul] in 250 mL of D_5W [16 μg/mL]) at an initial rate of 0.5 to 1 μg per minute, and adjust the infusion rate up to 8 to 30 μg per minute to increase the systolic blood pressure to 70 to 100 mm Hg. **Note:** The **infusion of norepinephrine** may be replaced by an **infusion of dopamine** at this point.

OR

If the **systolic blood pressure is greater than 70 mm Hg**:

Start an **infusion of dopamine** (400 mg of dopamine in 250 mL of D_5W [1600 μg/mL]) at an initial rate of 2.5 to 5 μg/kg per minute, and adjust the infusion rate up to 20 μg/kg per minute to increase the systolic blood pressure to 90 to 100 mm Hg.

If **severe pulmonary edema** is present and the **patient is not hypotensive** (**systolic blood pressure greater than 100 mm Hg**):

36. Place the patient in a **semireclining or full upright position with the legs dependent,** if possible.

37. Administer a 0.4-mg **nitroglycerin tablet** sublingually, and repeat every 5 to 10 minutes as needed.

AND/OR

38. Administer 1 to 3 mg of **morphine** IV slowly.

39. Administer a dose of 40 to 80 mg (0.5 to 1.0 mg/kg) of **furosemide** IV slowly over 4 to 5 minutes.

If **ventricular fibrillation/pulseless ventricular tachycardia** recurs:

40. Deliver a **defibrillation shock** immediately at the energy level at which termination of **ventricular fibrillation/pulseless ventricular tachycardia** was previously effective, and check the patient's ECG rhythm and pulse.

Treatment
B. Monitored Cardiac Arrest

If the patient is being monitored and **ventricular fibrillation/pulseless ventricular tachycardia** occurs:

1. Verify cardiac arrest by checking the **patient's pulse** while checking the patient's ECG rhythm on the **ECG monitor.**

If **ventricular fibrillation/pulseless ventricular tachycardia** is present:

2. Consider the administration of a **precordial thump** immediately, and check the patient's ECG rhythm on the **ECG monitor.**

If **ventricular fibrillation/pulseless ventricular tachycardia** persists:

3. Apply the **defibrillator paddles** or **defibrillation pads** to the patient.

4. Deliver a **defibrillation shock** (200 joules) immediately, and check the patient's ECG rhythm on the **ECG monitor.**

If **ventricular fibrillation/pulseless ventricular tachycardia** persists:

5. Deliver a **second defibrillation shock** (200 to 300 joules) immediately after the first shock, and check the patient's ECG rhythm on the **ECG monitor.**

If **ventricular fibrillation/pulseless ventricular tachycardia** persists:

6. Deliver a **third defibrillation shock** (up to 360 joules) immediately after the second shock, and check the patient's ECG rhythm on the **ECG monitor.**

If **ventricular fibrillation/pulseless ventricular tachycardia persists:**

7. Perform **CPR.**

8. Continue with **Step 8** in **A. Unmonitored Cardiac Arrest** under **Ventricular Fibrillation/Pulseless Ventricular Tachycardia VF/VT.**

Notes

Notes

Ventricular Asystole

Clinical Significance of Ventricular Asystole

Ventricular asystole is a life-threatening arrhythmia resulting in the absence of ventricular contractions, cardiac output, and a pulse. At the moment ventricular asystole occurs in a person with an adequate circulation, cardiac output stops and **clinical death** occurs. **Biological death** follows within 10 minutes unless ventricular asystole is reversed.

Indications for Treatment of Ventricular Asystole

Treatment of ventricular asystole is indicated immediately.

Treatment

A. Unmonitored Cardiac Arrest

If the cardiac arrest is witnessed by the resuscitation team or if cardiac arrest occurred before the arrival of the team and the patient is not being monitored:

Rescuer One:

1. Assess the **patient's unresponsiveness.**
2. Check the **patient's ABCs.**
3. Perform **CPR** until the defibrillator paddles or defibrillation pads are applied.

Rescuer Two:

1. Apply the **defibrillator paddles** or **defibrillation pads** to the patient.
2. Determine the ECG rhythm on the **ECG monitor.**
3. Verify cardiac arrest by checking the **patient's pulse.**

If **ventricular asystole** is present:

CONFIRM VENTRICULAR ASYSTOLE IN TWO ECG LEADS IF POSSIBLE OR BY 90°-ROTATED DEFIBRILLATOR PADDLES AS FINE VENTRICULAR FIBRILLATION MAY MIMIC VENTRICULAR ASYSTOLE.

4. Consider the treatment protocol for **A. Unmonitored Cardiac Arrest** under **Ventricular Fibrillation/Pulseless Ventricular Tachycardia** (VF/VT), page 306, and deliver **three defibrillation shocks** if ventricular asystole cannot be definitely confirmed.

5. Consider **transcutaneous pacing** if the cardiac arrest was witnessed or of short duration.
6. Continue **CPR.**
7. **Intubate** the patient.
8. Ventilate with **high concentration oxygen.**
9. Establish an **IV line.**
10. Administer 1.0 mg of **epinephrine** (10 mL of a 1:10,000 solution of epinephrine) IV followed by a 20-mL flush of IV fluid, and repeat every 3 to 5 minutes during resuscitation.

EPINEPHRINE OPTIONS

- **Epinephrine infusion:**

  Infusion of epinephrine (30 mg epinephrine [30 mL of a 1:1000 solution] in 250 mL of NS or D$_5$W) administered at a rate of 100 mL per hour and titrated as necessary. Administration through a central venous line is the preferred route.

- **Intermediate dose of epinephrine by bolus:**

  2- to 5-mg bolus every 3 to 5 minutes.

- **Escalating dose of epinephrine by bolus:**

  A 1-mg bolus followed by a 3-mg bolus followed by a 5-mg bolus every 3 minutes.

- **High dose of epinephrine by bolus:**

  0.1-mg/kg bolus every 3 to 5 minutes.

Note: If an IV line cannot be established, administer **2 to 2.5 times the proposed peripheral IV dose of epinephrine** via the endotracheal tube, if one is in place. If *both* an IV line and an endotracheal tube *are not* in place, consider administration of 0.5 mg of epinephrine (5 mL of a 1:10,000 solution of epinephrine) by intracardiac injection and repeat if needed.

11. Continue **CPR** for 30 to 60 seconds to circulate the drug.
12. Determine the ECG rhythm on the **ECG monitor.**
13. Verify cardiac arrest by checking the **patient's pulse.**

If **ventricular asystole** persists:

14. Administer a 1-mg **bolus of atropine** IV rapidly followed by a 20-mL flush of IV fluid. Repeat every 3 to 5 minutes up to a total dose of 3.0 mg (0.04 mg/kg) of atropine.

15. Continue **CPR.**

If **ventricular asystole** persists:

16. Continue administration of **epinephrine, atropine,** and **CPR** until ventricular asystole is terminated or a physician orders an end to the resuscitative efforts.

Notes

Treatment

B. Monitored Cardiac Arrest

If the patient is being monitored and **ventricular asystole** occurs:

1. Verify cardiac arrest by checking the **patient's pulse** while checking the patient's ECG rhythm on the **ECG monitor.**

If **ventricular asystole** is present:

CONFIRM VENTRICULAR ASYSTOLE IN TWO ECG LEADS IF POSSIBLE OR BY 90°-ROTATED DEFIBRILLATOR PADDLES AS FINE VENTRICULAR FIBRILLATION MAY MIMIC VENTRICULAR ASYSTOLE.

2. Consider the treatment protocol for **A. Unmonitored Cardiac Arrest** under **Ventricular Fibrillation/Pulseless Ventricular Tachycardia** (VF/VT), page 306, and deliver **three defibrillation shocks** if ventricular asystole cannot be definitely confirmed.

3. Consider **transcutaneous pacing.**

4. Continue **CPR.**

5. Continue with **Step 7** in **A. Unmonitored Cardiac Arrest** under **Ventricular Asystole.**

Notes

Pulseless Electrical Activity (PEA)

Clinical Significance of Pulseless Electrical Activity

Pulseless electrical activity—the absence of a detectable pulse and blood pressure in the presence of electrical activity of the heart as evidenced by some type of an ECG rhythm other than ventricular fibrillation or ventricular tachycardia—is a life-threatening condition. At the moment pulseless electrical activity occurs in a person with an adequate circulation, cardiac output ceases and **clinical death** occurs. **Biological death** follows within 10 minutes unless pulseless electrical activity is reversed.

Pulseless electrical activity is commonly the result of either (1) complete absence of ventricular contractions (**electromechanical dissociation [EMD]**) or (2) a marked decrease in cardiac output because of (a) hypovolemia or (b) failure of the myocardium or electrical conduction system or both from a variety of causes, resulting in ventricular contractions too weak to produce a detectable pulse and blood pressure (**pseudo-electromechanical dissociation**). The ECG rhythms encountered in pulseless electrical activity include (1) organized electrical activity with narrow QRS complexes as typically seen with electromechanical dissociation, (2) marked bradyarrhythmias, and (3) wide-QRS-complex arrhythmias,

such as idioventricular rhythms and ventricular escape rhythms, which are more commonly seen in pseudo-electromechanical dissociation.

Pulseless electrical activity can occur in the following conditions:

- **Hypovolemia** from acute blood loss (hemorrhagic shock secondary to trauma or other causes, such as ruptured abdominal aortic aneurysm or gastrointestinal hemorrhage)
- **Hypoxemia**
- **Massive acute myocardial infarction**
- **Excessive vagal tone or loss of sympathetic tone**
- **Obstruction of blood flow to or from the heart (tension pneumothorax or severe pulmonary embolization)**
- **Pericardial tamponade**
- **Myocardial rupture**
- **Hypothermia**
- **Severe acidosis**
- **Drug overdose from tricyclics, β blockers, calcium channel blockers, and digitalis**
- **Hyperkalemia**

Whenever CPR is unsuccessful in producing a palpable peripheral or carotid pulse or evidence of perfusion, pulseless electrical activity must be suspected.

Indications for Treatment of Pulseless Electrical Activity

Treatment of pulseless electrical activity is indicated immediately.

Treatment

A. Unmonitored Cardiac Arrest

If the cardiac arrest is witnessed by the resuscitation team or if cardiac arrest occurred before the arrival of the team and the patient is not being monitored:

Rescuer One:

1. Assess the **patient's unresponsiveness.**
2. Check the **patient's ABCs.**
3. Perform **CPR** until the defibrillator paddles or defibrillation pads are applied.

Rescuer Two:

1. Apply the **defibrillator paddles** or **defibrillation pads** to the patient.
2. Determine the ECG rhythm on the **ECG monitor.**
3. Verify cardiac arrest by checking the **patient's pulse.**

If **pulseless electrical activity** is present:

4. Continue **CPR.**
5. **Intubate** the patient.
6. Ventilate with **high concentration oxygen.**
7. Establish an **IV line.**
8. Administer 1 mg of **epinephrine** (10 mL of a 1:10,000 solution of epinephrine) IV followed by a 20-mL flush of IV fluid, and repeat every 3 to 5 minutes during resuscitation.

Note: If an IV line cannot be established, administer **2 to 2.5 times the proposed peripheral IV dose**

EPINEPHRINE OPTIONS

- **Epinephrine infusion:**

  Infusion of epinephrine (30 mg epinephrine [30 mL of a 1:1000 solution] in 250 mL of NS or D₅W) administered at a rate of 100 mL per hour and titrated as necessary. Administration through a central venous line is the preferred route.

- **Intermediate dose of epinephrine by bolus:**

  2- to 5-mg bolus every 3 to 5 minutes.

- **Escalating dose of epinephrine by bolus:**

  A 1-mg bolus followed by a 3-mg bolus followed by a 5-mg bolus every 3 minutes.

- **High dose of epinephrine by bolus:**

  0.1-mg/kg bolus every 3 to 5 minutes.

---

of epinephrine via the endotracheal tube, if one is in place. If both an IV line and an ET tube are not in place, consider administration of 0.5 mg of epinephrine (5 mL of a 1:10,000 solution of epinephrine) by intracardiac injection and repeat if needed.

9. Continue **CPR** for 30 to 60 seconds to circulate the drug.
10. Determine the ECG rhythm on the **ECG monitor.**
11. Verify cardiac arrest by checking the **patient's pulse.**

If **pulseless electrical activity** persists and the **rate of the QRS complexes is about 80 per minute or less:**

12. Administer a 1-mg **bolus of atropine** IV rapidly followed by a 20-mL flush of IV fluid. Repeat every 3 to 5 minutes up to a total dose of 3.0 mg (0.04 mg/kg) of atropine.
13. Continue **CPR.**

If **pulseless electrical activity** persists and **hypovolemia** is suspected:

14. Elevate the **patient's legs 18 inches above the level of the heart.**
15. Consider the administration of **fluid boluses of 250 to 500 mL of 0.9% saline or Ringer's lactate solution** while monitoring the patient's pulse.
16. Continue **CPR.**

If **pulseless electrical activity** persists:

17. Consider the presence of hypoxemia, tension pneumothorax, severe pulmonary embolization, cardiac tamponade, myocardial rupture, hypothermia, severe acidosis, hyperkalemia, or drug overdose from tricyclics, β blockers, calcium channel blockers, or digitalis. Treat the underlying condition.
18. Continue CPR.

Notes

Treatment

B. Monitored Cardiac Arrest

If the patient is being monitored and **pulseless electrical activity** occurs:

1. Verify cardiac arrest by checking the **patient's pulse** while checking the patient's ECG rhythm on the **ECG monitor.**

If **pulseless electrical activity** is present:

2. Consider **transcutaneous pacing.**
3. Continue **CPR.**
4. Continue with **Step 5** in **A. Unmonitored Cardiac Arrest** under **Pulseless Electrical Activity (PEA).**

Notes

1. In a patient with symptomatic bradycardia and an ECG showing a second-degree, type II AV block, you should administer oxygen, start an IV line, and administer or begin:
   A. an isoproterenol drip
   B. atropine
   C. transcutaneous pacing
   D. lidocaine

2. Patients with symptomatic sinus tachycardia should be treated with:
   A. diltiazem
   B. epinephrine
   C. dopamine
   D. appropriate treatment for the underlying cause of the tachycardia

3. If a patient is stable with an ECG showing PSVT after administering oxygen and starting an IV line, you should:
   A. attempt vagal maneuvers
   B. administer diltiazem
   C. administer adenosine
   D. administer Valium

4. Your patient presents with chest pain and signs and symptoms of an acute MI. His ECG shows PAT. After administering oxygen and starting an IV line you should immediately consider:
   A. transcutaneous pacing
   B. a lidocaine drip
   C. a synchronized countershock of 50 joules
   D. an adenosine bolus

5. Your patient is conscious and hemodynamically stable with an ECG showing ventricular tachycardia. After administering oxygen and starting an IV you should:
   A. start an infusion of procainamide
   B. administer a 1- to 1.5- mg/kg bolus of lidocaine
   C. deliver a synchronized countershock of 100 joules
   D. administer a 2-mg/minute lidocaine drip

6. If your patient in question number 5 begins to complain of chest pain and his blood pressure has fallen to 70/50 mm Hg, you should immediately:
   A. deliver an unsynchronized shock of 100 joules
   B. administer a lidocaine bolus
   C. deliver a synchronized shock of 200 joules
   D. begin transcutaneous pacing

7. Pulseless electrical activity (PEA) may result from:
   A. electromechanical dissociation (EMD)
   B. hypovolemia
   C. cardiac rupture
   D. all of the above

8. PVCs should be treated if they occur in a patient with chest pain or if they:
   A. are frequent (six or more per minute)
   B. occur in groups of two or more (group beats)
   C. have different QRS configurations (multiform)
   D. all of the above

9. In a cardiac arrest when you are having difficulty starting a peripheral IV line and your patient has just been defibrillated three times, you should:
   A. attempt a central IV line
   B. terminate the arrest
   C. administer epinephrine at 2 to 2.5 times the normal dose down the ET tube
   D. attempt an intraosseous line

10. If you suspect asystole, you should:
    A. confirm the arrhythmia in two ECG leads
    B. consider delivering three defibrillation shocks if asystole cannot be definitely confirmed
    C. consider transcutaneous pacing after confirming the presence of asystole
    D. all of the above

CHAPTER
14

Arrhythmia Interpretation: Self-Assessment

I. Arrhythmias

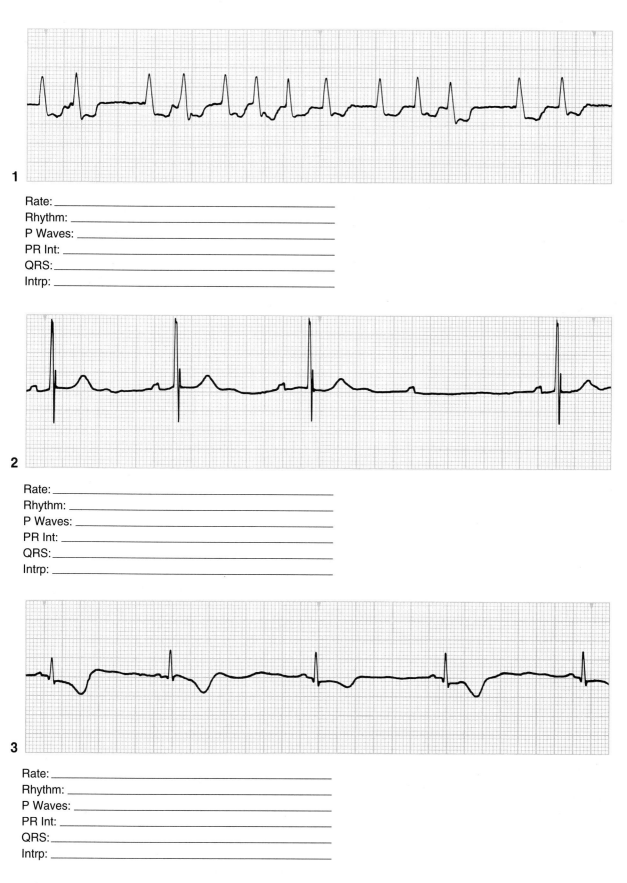

1

Rate: _____

Rhythm: _____

P Waves: _____

PR Int: _____

QRS: _____

Intrp: _____

2

Rate: _____

Rhythm: _____

P Waves: _____

PR Int: _____

QRS: _____

Intrp: _____

3

Rate: _____

Rhythm: _____

P Waves: _____

PR Int: _____

QRS: _____

Intrp: _____

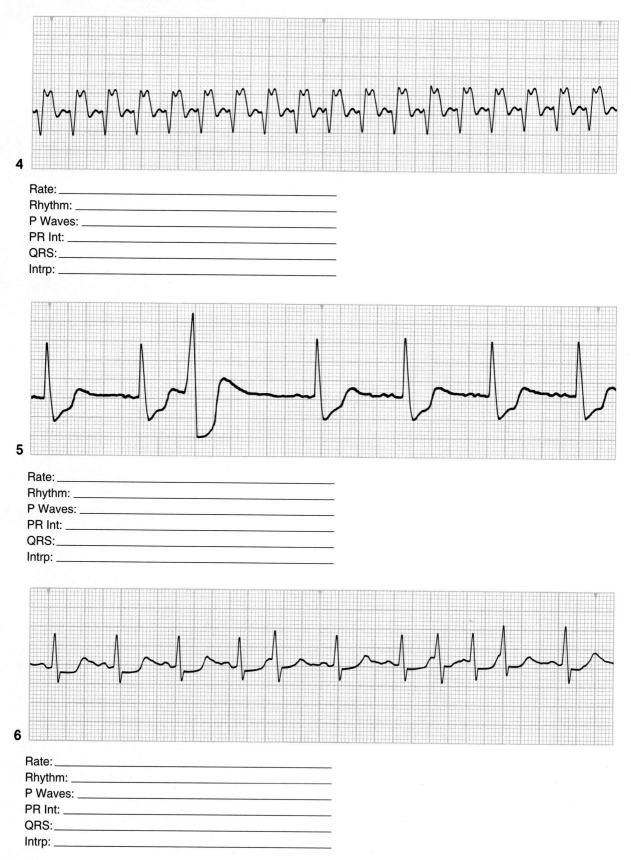

4

Rate: _____

Rhythm: _____

P Waves: _____

PR Int: _____

QRS: _____

Intrp: _____

5

Rate: _____

Rhythm: _____

P Waves: _____

PR Int: _____

QRS: _____

Intrp: _____

6

Rate: _____

Rhythm: _____

P Waves: _____

PR Int: _____

QRS: _____

Intrp: _____

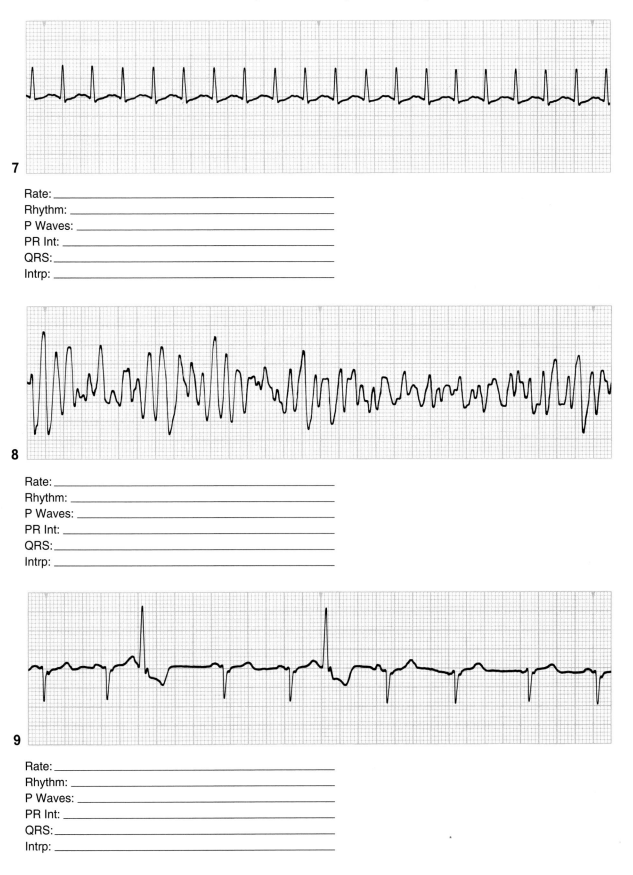

7

Rate: _____

Rhythm: _____

P Waves: _____

PR Int: _____

QRS: _____

Intrp: _____

8

Rate: _____

Rhythm: _____

P Waves: _____

PR Int: _____

QRS: _____

Intrp: _____

9

Rate: _____

Rhythm: _____

P Waves: _____

PR Int: _____

QRS: _____

Intrp: _____

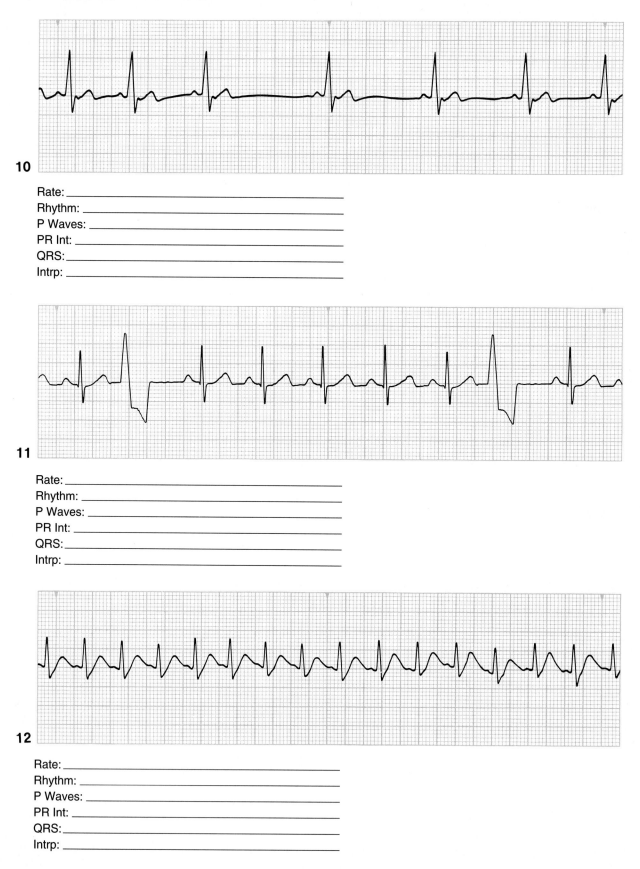

10

Rate: _____

Rhythm: _____

P Waves: _____

PR Int: _____

QRS: _____

Intrp: _____

11

Rate: _____

Rhythm: _____

P Waves: _____

PR Int: _____

QRS: _____

Intrp: _____

12

Rate: _____

Rhythm: _____

P Waves: _____

PR Int: _____

QRS: _____

Intrp: _____

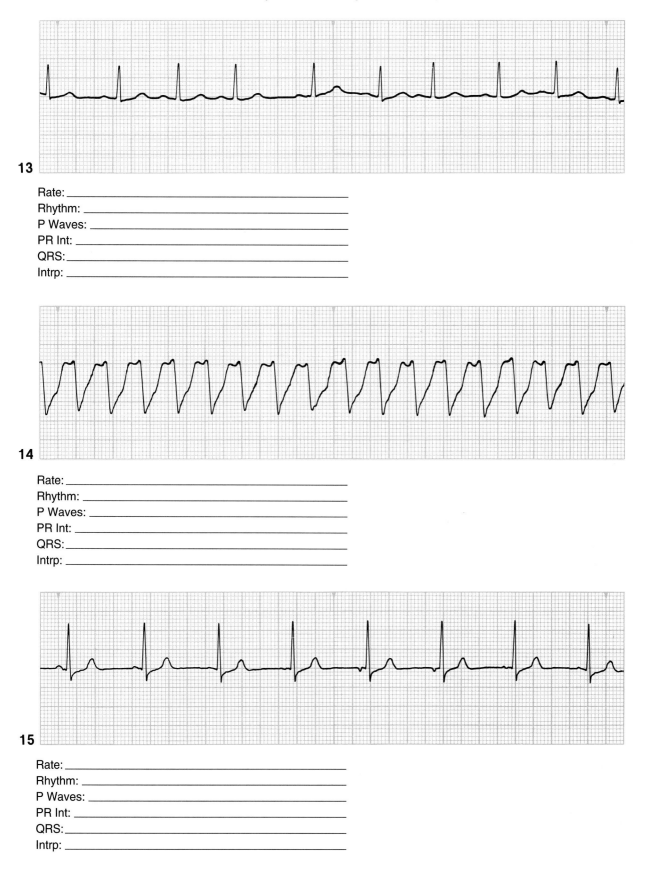

13

Rate: _____

Rhythm: _____

P Waves: _____

PR Int: _____

QRS: _____

Intrp: _____

14

Rate: _____

Rhythm: _____

P Waves: _____

PR Int: _____

QRS: _____

Intrp: _____

15

Rate: _____

Rhythm: _____

P Waves: _____

PR Int: _____

QRS: _____

Intrp: _____

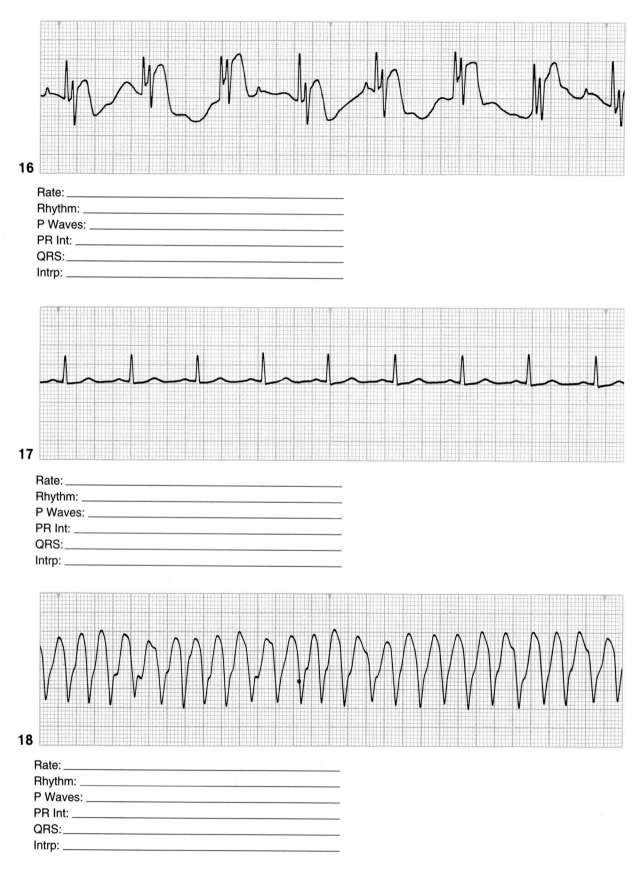

16

Rate: _____

Rhythm: _____

P Waves: _____

PR Int: _____

QRS: _____

Intrp: _____

17

Rate: _____

Rhythm: _____

P Waves: _____

PR Int: _____

QRS: _____

Intrp: _____

18

Rate: _____

Rhythm: _____

P Waves: _____

PR Int: _____

QRS: _____

Intrp: _____

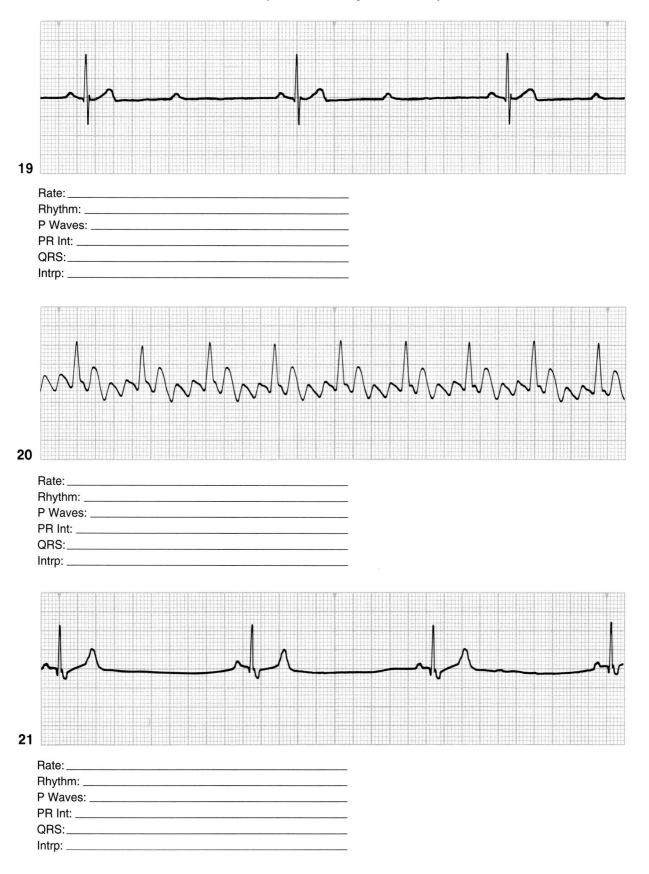

19

Rate: _____

Rhythm: _____

P Waves: _____

PR Int: _____

QRS: _____

Intrp: _____

20

Rate: _____

Rhythm: _____

P Waves: _____

PR Int: _____

QRS: _____

Intrp: _____

21

Rate: _____

Rhythm: _____

P Waves: _____

PR Int: _____

QRS: _____

Intrp: _____

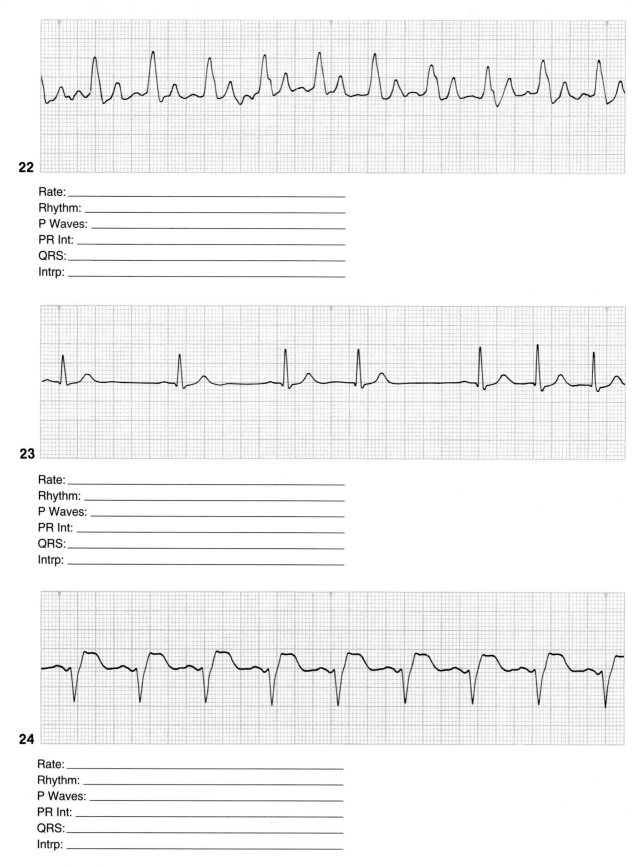

22

Rate: _____

Rhythm: _____

P Waves: _____

PR Int: _____

QRS: _____

Intrp: _____

23

Rate: _____

Rhythm: _____

P Waves: _____

PR Int: _____

QRS: _____

Intrp: _____

24

Rate: _____

Rhythm: _____

P Waves: _____

PR Int: _____

QRS: _____

Intrp: _____

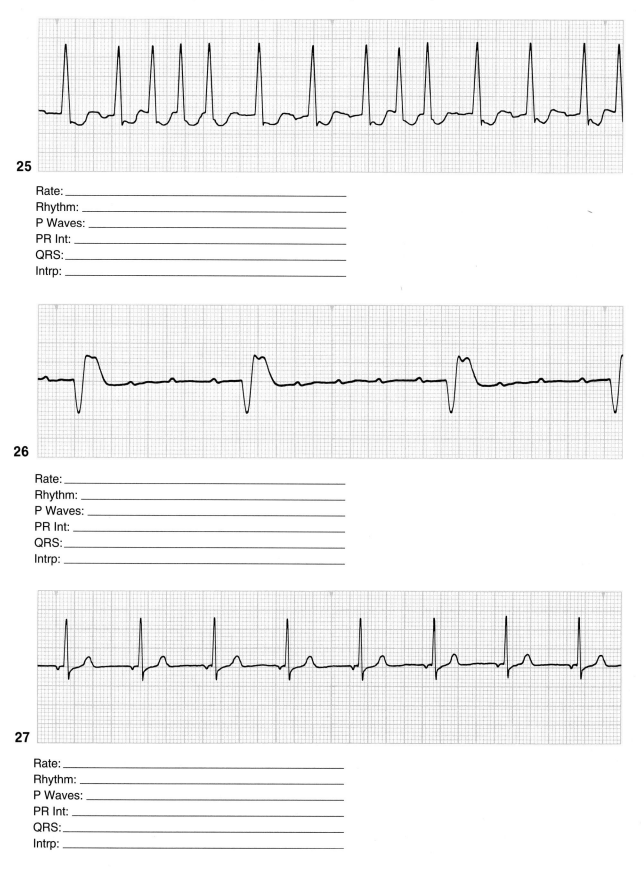

25

Rate: _____

Rhythm: _____

P Waves: _____

PR Int: _____

QRS: _____

Intrp: _____

26

Rate: _____

Rhythm: _____

P Waves: _____

PR Int: _____

QRS: _____

Intrp: _____

27

Rate: _____

Rhythm: _____

P Waves: _____

PR Int: _____

QRS: _____

Intrp: _____

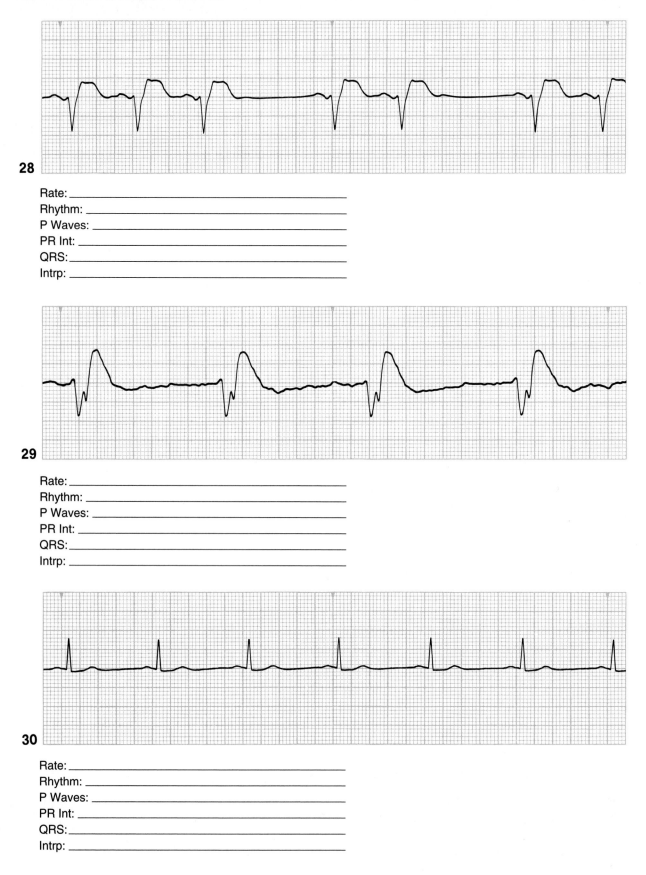

28

Rate: _____

Rhythm: _____

P Waves: _____

PR Int: _____

QRS: _____

Intrp: _____

29

Rate: _____

Rhythm: _____

P Waves: _____

PR Int: _____

QRS: _____

Intrp: _____

30

Rate: _____

Rhythm: _____

P Waves: _____

PR Int: _____

QRS: _____

Intrp: _____

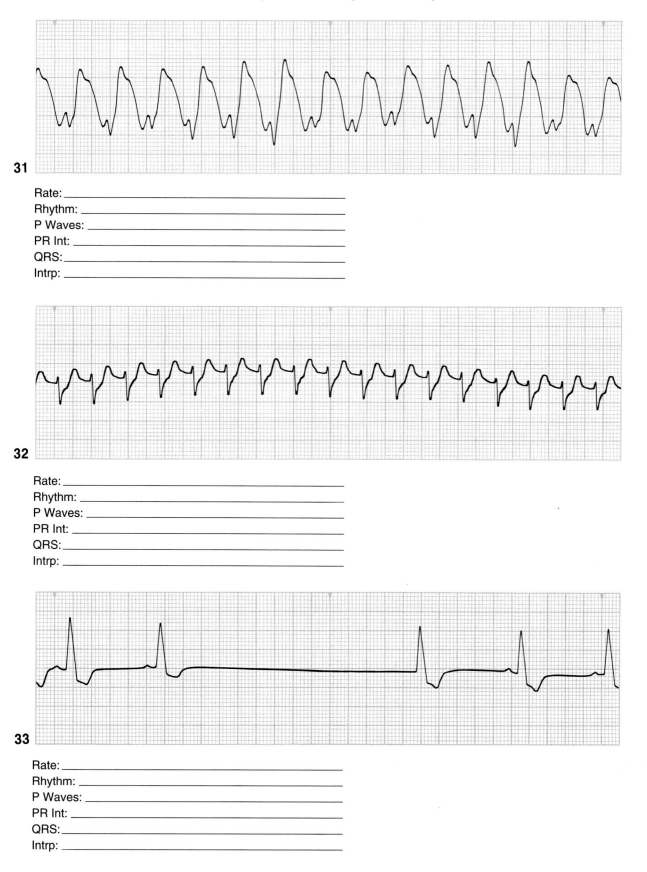

31

Rate: _____

Rhythm: _____

P Waves: _____

PR Int: _____

QRS: _____

Intrp: _____

32

Rate: _____

Rhythm: _____

P Waves: _____

PR Int: _____

QRS: _____

Intrp: _____

33

Rate: _____

Rhythm: _____

P Waves: _____

PR Int: _____

QRS: _____

Intrp: _____

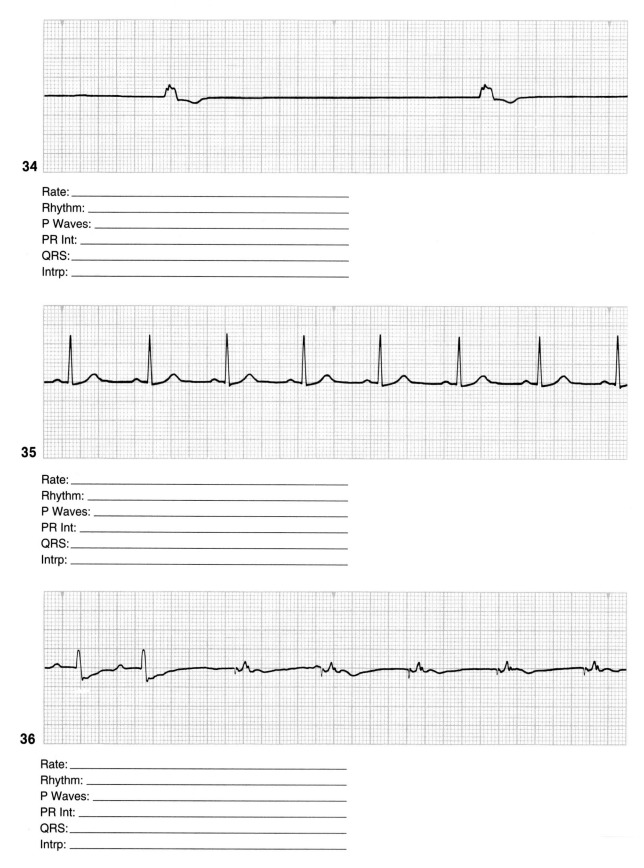

34

Rate: _____

Rhythm: _____

P Waves: _____

PR Int: _____

QRS: _____

Intrp: _____

35

Rate: _____

Rhythm: _____

P Waves: _____

PR Int: _____

QRS: _____

Intrp: _____

36

Rate: _____

Rhythm: _____

P Waves: _____

PR Int: _____

QRS: _____

Intrp: _____

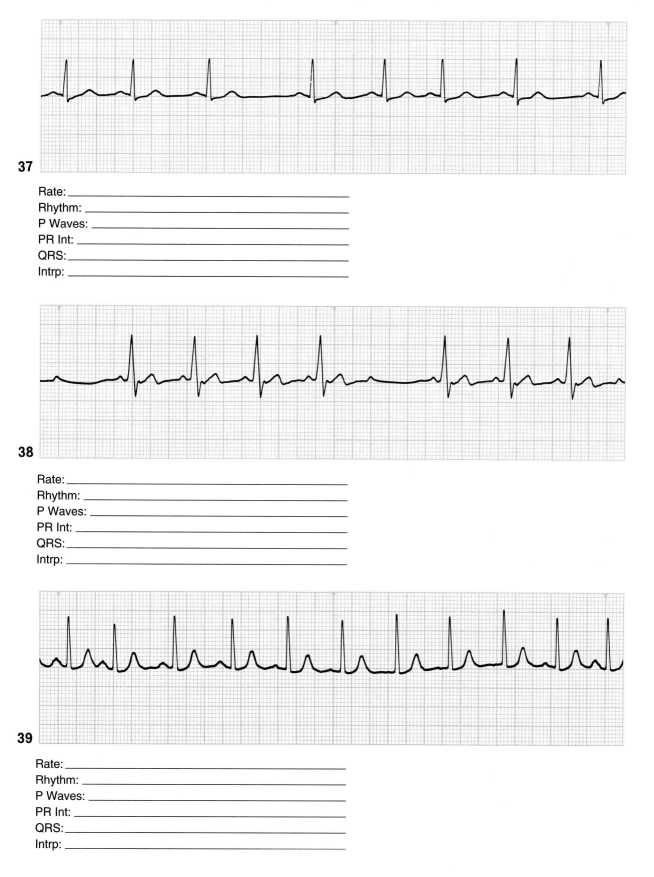

37

Rate: _____

Rhythm: _____

P Waves: _____

PR Int: _____

QRS: _____

Intrp: _____

38

Rate: _____

Rhythm: _____

P Waves: _____

PR Int: _____

QRS: _____

Intrp: _____

39

Rate: _____

Rhythm: _____

P Waves: _____

PR Int: _____

QRS: _____

Intrp: _____

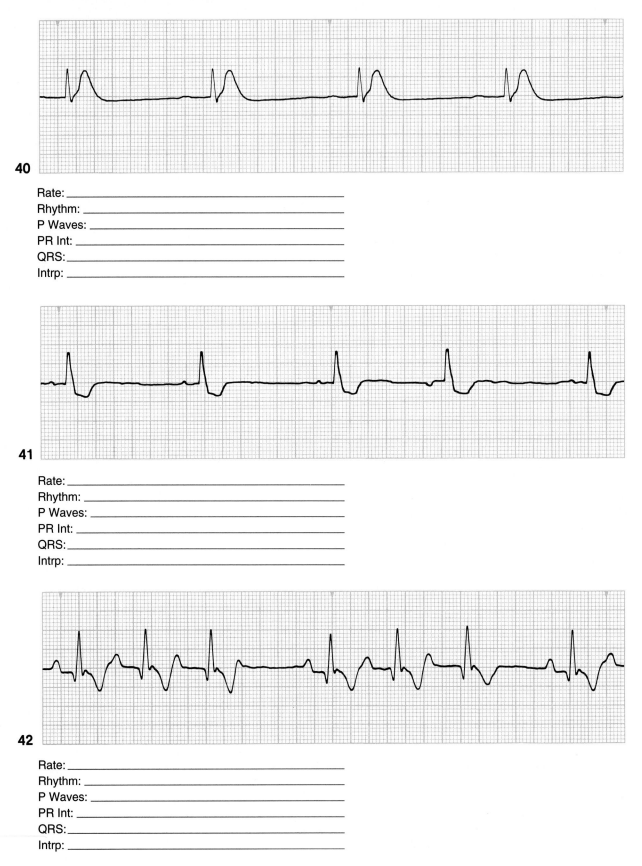

40

Rate: _____

Rhythm: _____

P Waves: _____

PR Int: _____

QRS: _____

Intrp: _____

41

Rate: _____

Rhythm: _____

P Waves: _____

PR Int: _____

QRS: _____

Intrp: _____

42

Rate: _____

Rhythm: _____

P Waves: _____

PR Int: _____

QRS: _____

Intrp: _____

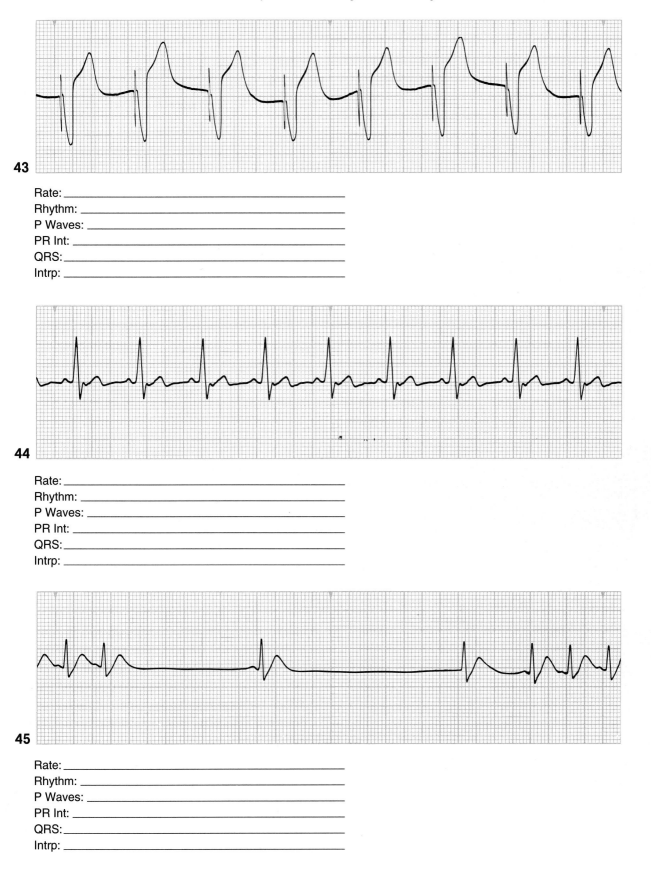

43

Rate: _____

Rhythm: _____

P Waves: _____

PR Int: _____

QRS: _____

Intrp: _____

44

Rate: _____

Rhythm: _____

P Waves: _____

PR Int: _____

QRS: _____

Intrp: _____

45

Rate: _____

Rhythm: _____

P Waves: _____

PR Int: _____

QRS: _____

Intrp: _____

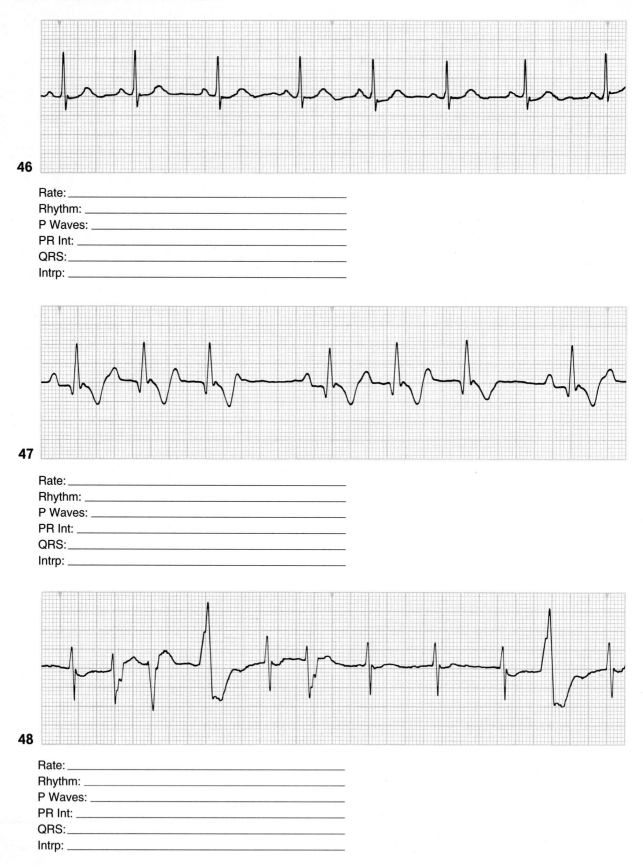

46

Rate: _____

Rhythm: _____

P Waves: _____

PR Int: _____

QRS: _____

Intrp: _____

47

Rate: _____

Rhythm: _____

P Waves: _____

PR Int: _____

QRS: _____

Intrp: _____

48

Rate: _____

Rhythm: _____

P Waves: _____

PR Int: _____

QRS: _____

Intrp: _____

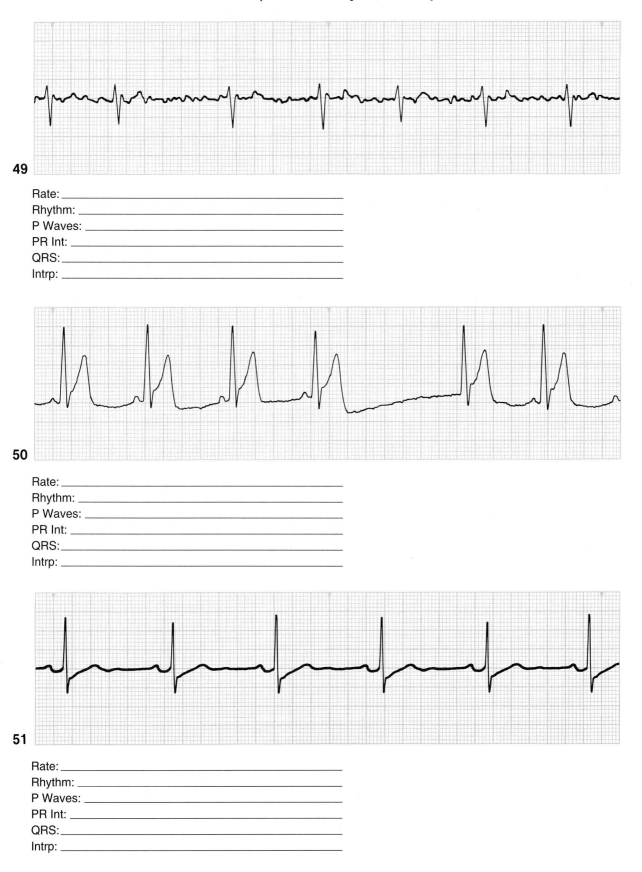

49

Rate: _____

Rhythm: _____

P Waves: _____

PR Int: _____

QRS: _____

Intrp: _____

50

Rate: _____

Rhythm: _____

P Waves: _____

PR Int: _____

QRS: _____

Intrp: _____

51

Rate: _____

Rhythm: _____

P Waves: _____

PR Int: _____

QRS: _____

Intrp: _____

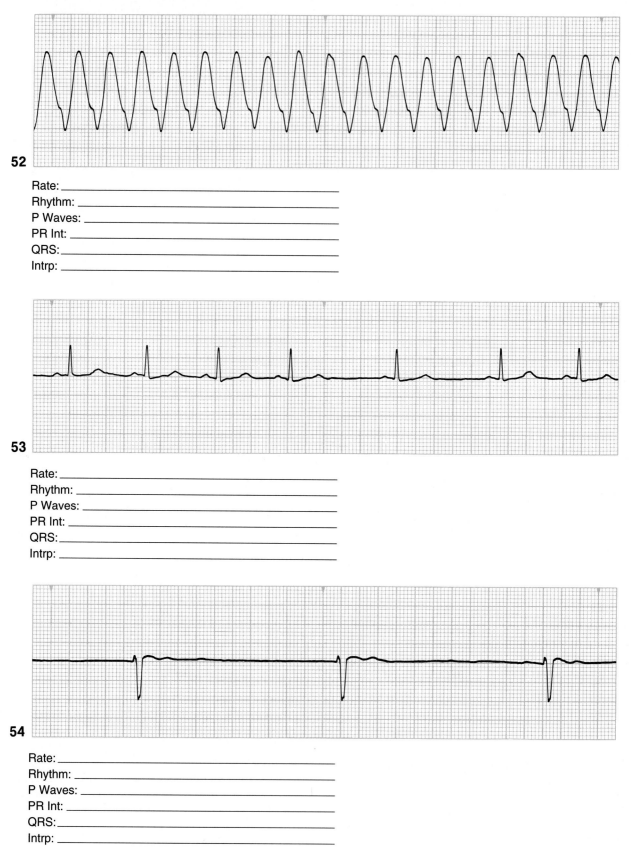

52

Rate: _____

Rhythm: _____

P Waves: _____

PR Int: _____

QRS: _____

Intrp: _____

53

Rate: _____

Rhythm: _____

P Waves: _____

PR Int: _____

QRS: _____

Intrp: _____

54

Rate: _____

Rhythm: _____

P Waves: _____

PR Int: _____

QRS: _____

Intrp: _____

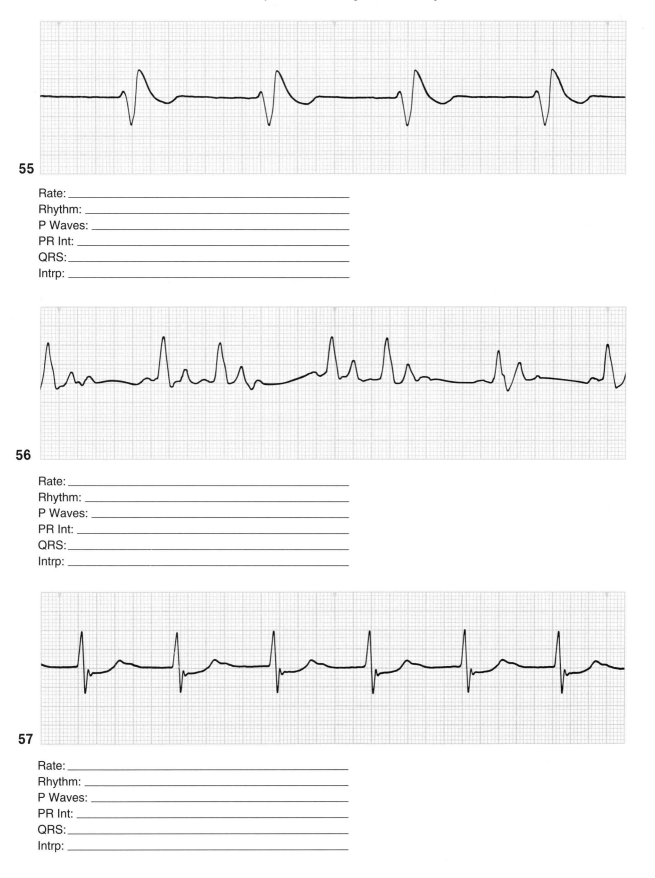

55

Rate: _____

Rhythm: _____

P Waves: _____

PR Int: _____

QRS: _____

Intrp: _____

56

Rate: _____

Rhythm: _____

P Waves: _____

PR Int: _____

QRS: _____

Intrp: _____

57

Rate: _____

Rhythm: _____

P Waves: _____

PR Int: _____

QRS: _____

Intrp: _____

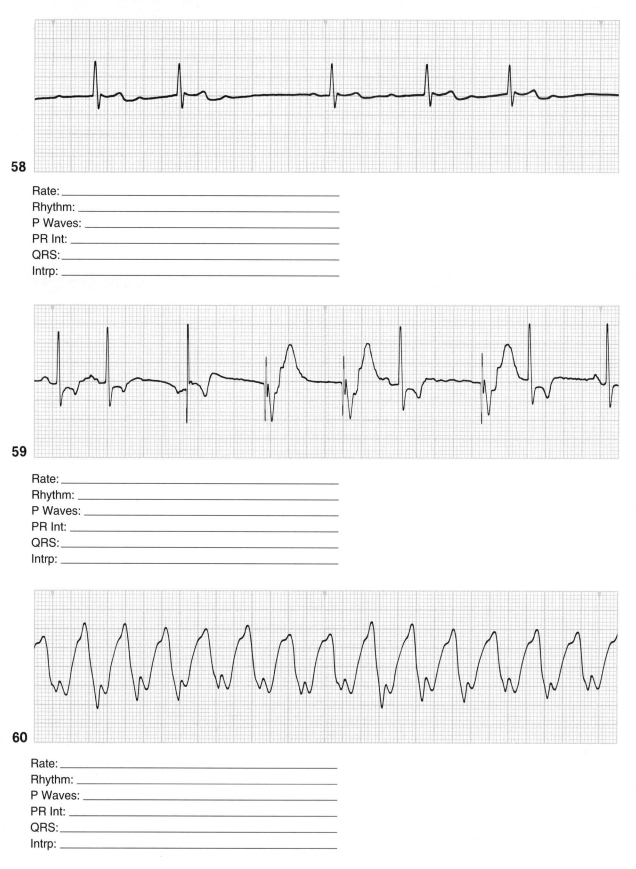

58

Rate: _____

Rhythm: _____

P Waves: _____

PR Int: _____

QRS: _____

Intrp: _____

59

Rate: _____

Rhythm: _____

P Waves: _____

PR Int: _____

QRS: _____

Intrp: _____

60

Rate: _____

Rhythm: _____

P Waves: _____

PR Int: _____

QRS: _____

Intrp: _____

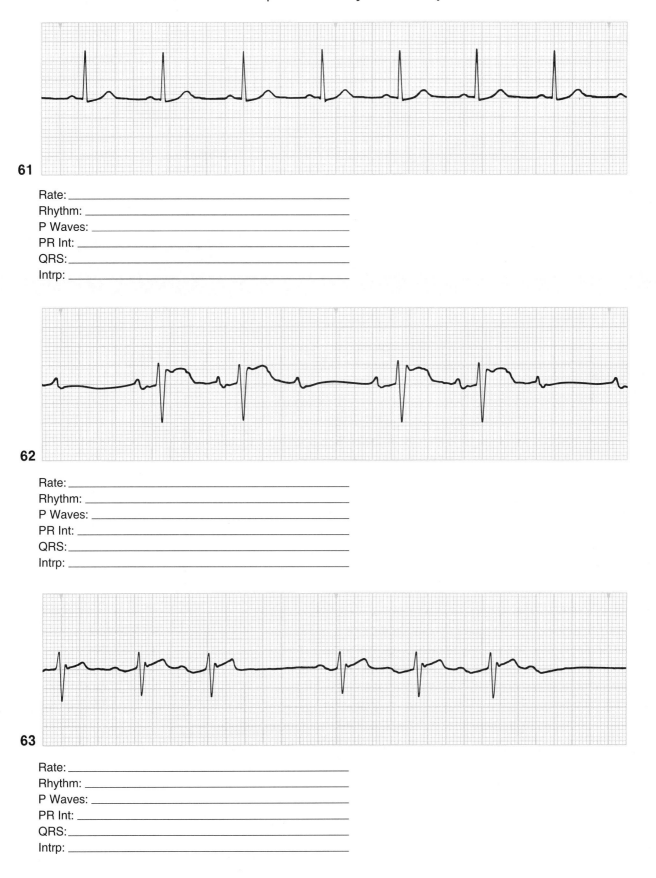

61

Rate: _____

Rhythm: _____

P Waves: _____

PR Int: _____

QRS: _____

Intrp: _____

62

Rate: _____

Rhythm: _____

P Waves: _____

PR Int: _____

QRS: _____

Intrp: _____

63

Rate: _____

Rhythm: _____

P Waves: _____

PR Int: _____

QRS: _____

Intrp: _____

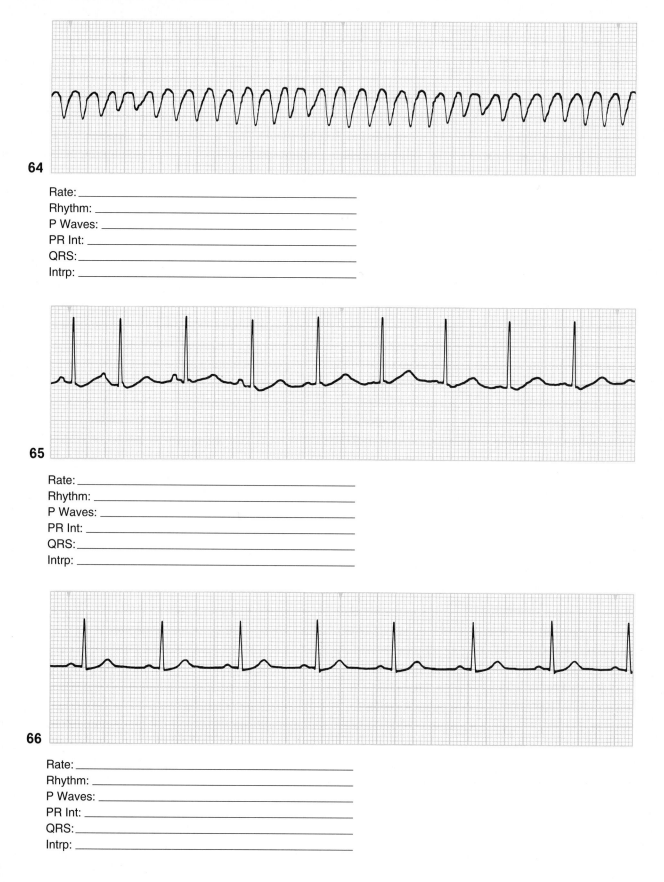

64

Rate: _____

Rhythm: _____

P Waves: _____

PR Int: _____

QRS: _____

Intrp: _____

65

Rate: _____

Rhythm: _____

P Waves: _____

PR Int: _____

QRS: _____

Intrp: _____

66

Rate: _____

Rhythm: _____

P Waves: _____

PR Int: _____

QRS: _____

Intrp: _____

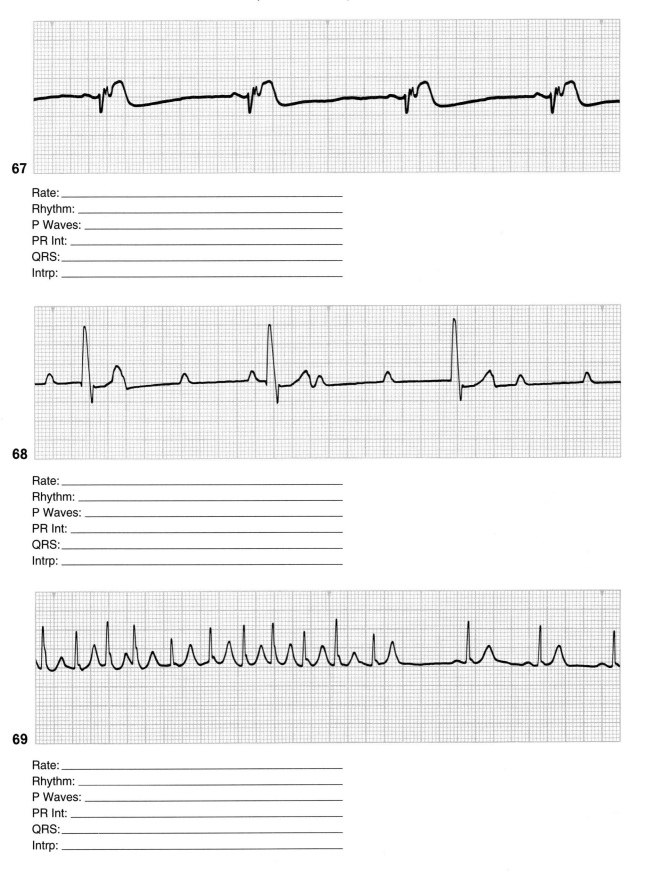

67

Rate: _____

Rhythm: _____

P Waves: _____

PR Int: _____

QRS: _____

Intrp: _____

68

Rate: _____

Rhythm: _____

P Waves: _____

PR Int: _____

QRS: _____

Intrp: _____

69

Rate: _____

Rhythm: _____

P Waves: _____

PR Int: _____

QRS: _____

Intrp: _____

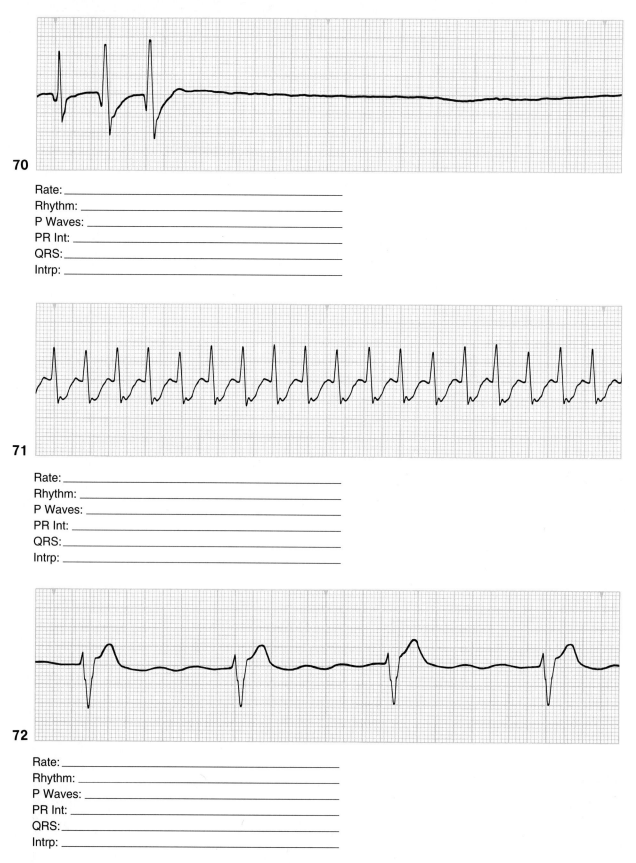

70

Rate: _____

Rhythm: _____

P Waves: _____

PR Int: _____

QRS: _____

Intrp: _____

71

Rate: _____

Rhythm: _____

P Waves: _____

PR Int: _____

QRS: _____

Intrp: _____

72

Rate: _____

Rhythm: _____

P Waves: _____

PR Int: _____

QRS: _____

Intrp: _____

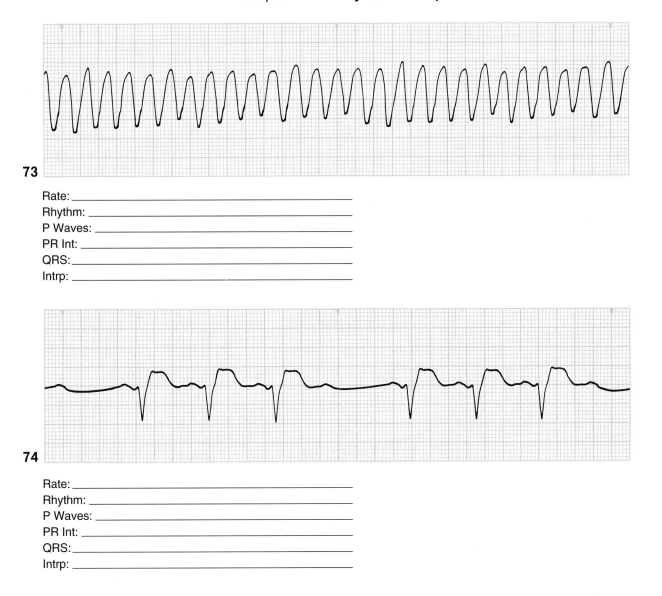

73

Rate: _____

Rhythm: _____

P Waves: _____

PR Int: _____

QRS: _____

Intrp: _____

74

Rate: _____

Rhythm: _____

P Waves: _____

PR Int: _____

QRS: _____

Intrp: _____

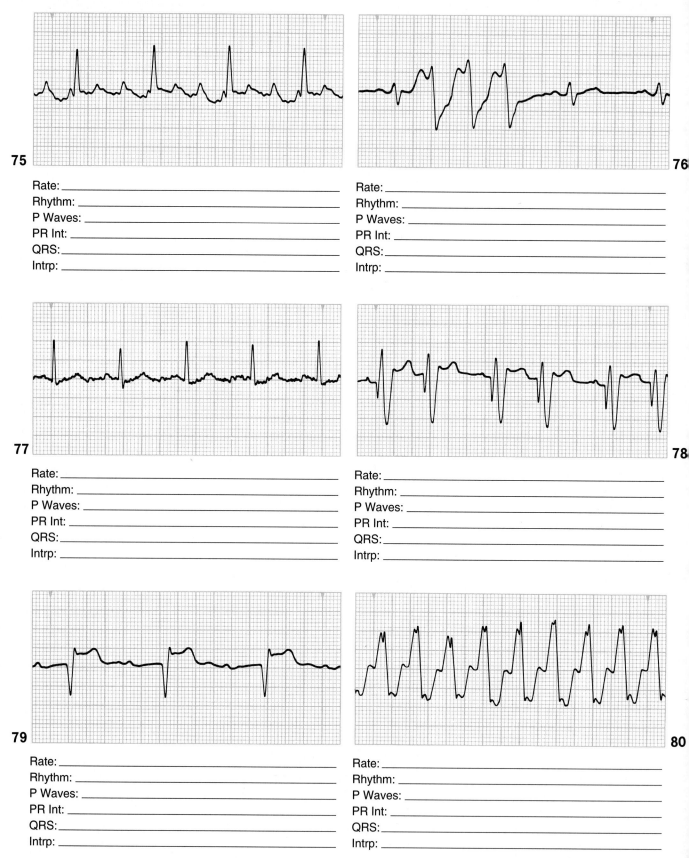

75

Rate: _____

Rhythm: _____

P Waves: _____

PR Int: _____

QRS: _____

Intrp: _____

76

Rate: _____

Rhythm: _____

P Waves: _____

PR Int: _____

QRS: _____

Intrp: _____

77

Rate: _____

Rhythm: _____

P Waves: _____

PR Int: _____

QRS: _____

Intrp: _____

78

Rate: _____

Rhythm: _____

P Waves: _____

PR Int: _____

QRS: _____

Intrp: _____

79

Rate: _____

Rhythm: _____

P Waves: _____

PR Int: _____

QRS: _____

Intrp: _____

80

Rate: _____

Rhythm: _____

P Waves: _____

PR Int: _____

QRS: _____

Intrp: _____

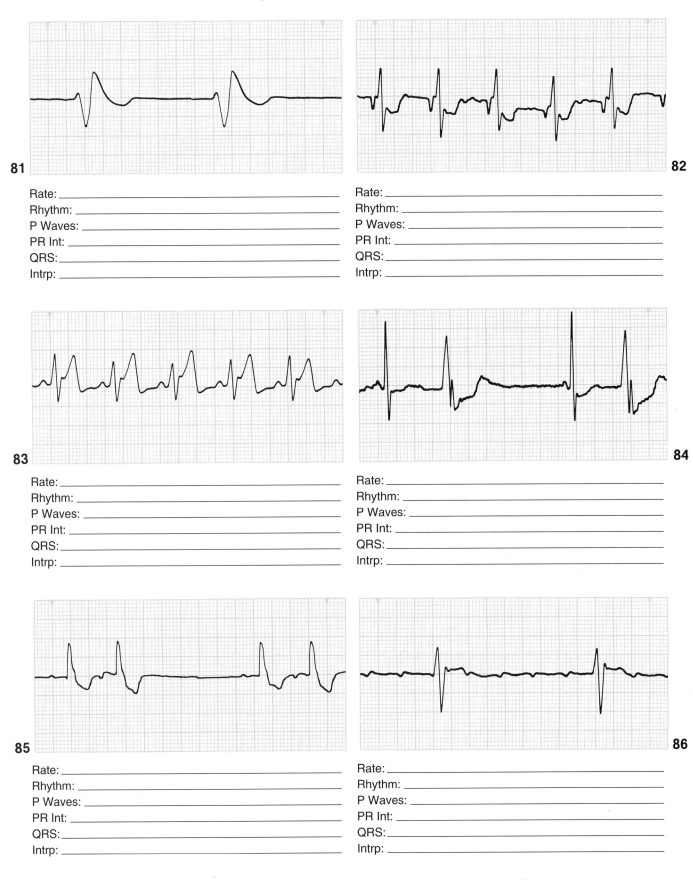

81

Rate: _____
Rhythm: _____
P Waves: _____
PR Int: _____
QRS: _____
Intrp: _____

82

Rate: _____
Rhythm: _____
P Waves: _____
PR Int: _____
QRS: _____
Intrp: _____

83

Rate: _____
Rhythm: _____
P Waves: _____
PR Int: _____
QRS: _____
Intrp: _____

84

Rate: _____
Rhythm: _____
P Waves: _____
PR Int: _____
QRS: _____
Intrp: _____

85

Rate: _____
Rhythm: _____
P Waves: _____
PR Int: _____
QRS: _____
Intrp: _____

86

Rate: _____
Rhythm: _____
P Waves: _____
PR Int: _____
QRS: _____
Intrp: _____

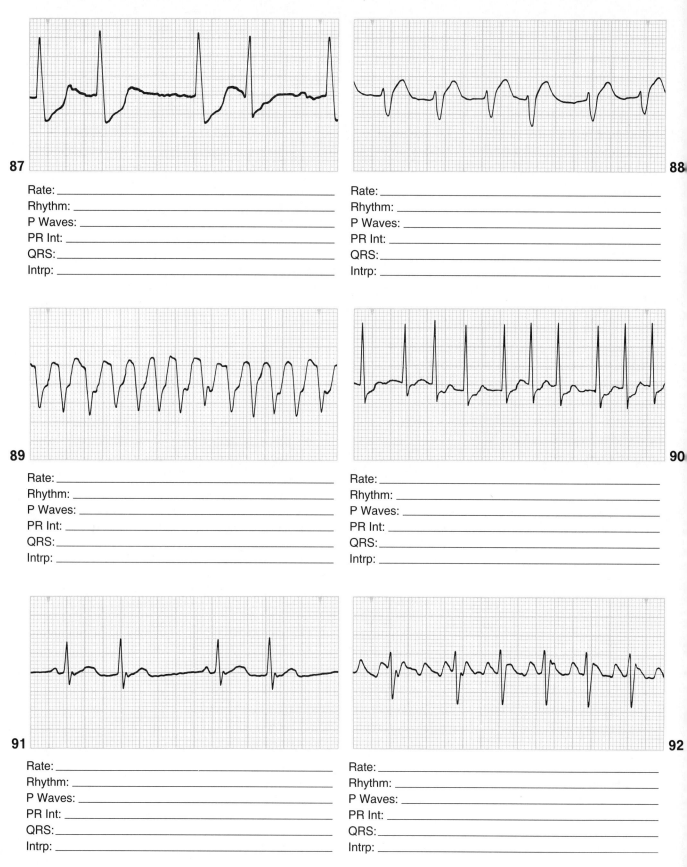

87

Rate: _____
Rhythm: _____
P Waves: _____
PR Int: _____
QRS: _____
Intrp: _____

88

Rate: _____
Rhythm: _____
P Waves: _____
PR Int: _____
QRS: _____
Intrp: _____

89

Rate: _____
Rhythm: _____
P Waves: _____
PR Int: _____
QRS: _____
Intrp: _____

90

Rate: _____
Rhythm: _____
P Waves: _____
PR Int: _____
QRS: _____
Intrp: _____

91

Rate: _____
Rhythm: _____
P Waves: _____
PR Int: _____
QRS: _____
Intrp: _____

92

Rate: _____
Rhythm: _____
P Waves: _____
PR Int: _____
QRS: _____
Intrp: _____

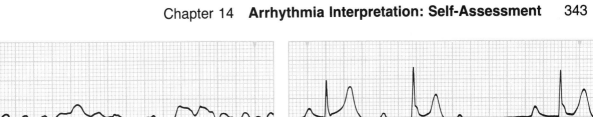

93

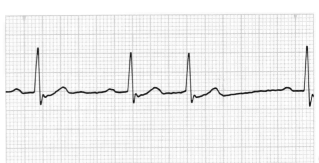

94

Rate: _____
Rhythm: _____
P Waves: _____
PR Int: _____
QRS: _____
Intrp: _____

Rate: _____
Rhythm: _____
P Waves: _____
PR Int: _____
QRS: _____
Intrp: _____

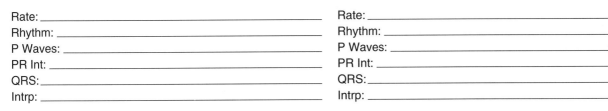

95

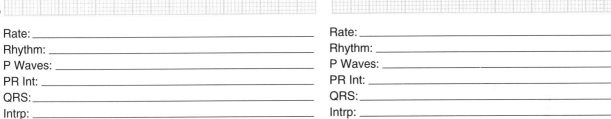

96

Rate: _____
Rhythm: _____
P Waves: _____
PR Int: _____
QRS: _____
Intrp: _____

Rate: _____
Rhythm: _____
P Waves: _____
PR Int: _____
QRS: _____
Intrp: _____

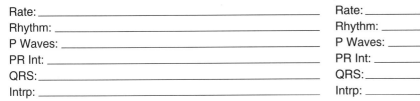

97

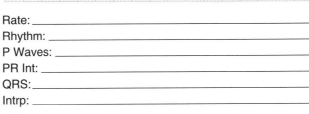
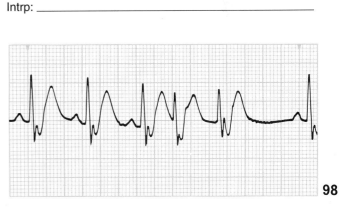

98

Rate: _____
Rhythm: _____
P Waves: _____
PR Int: _____
QRS: _____
Intrp: _____

Rate: _____
Rhythm: _____
P Waves: _____
PR Int: _____
QRS: _____
Intrp: _____

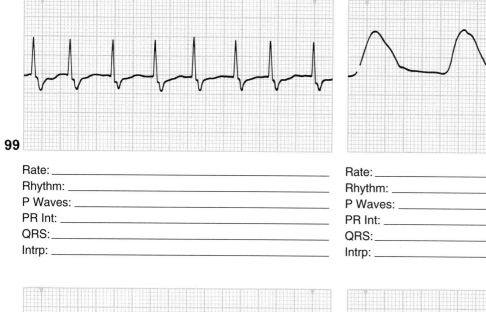

99

Rate: _____

Rhythm: _____

P Waves: _____

PR Int: _____

QRS: _____

Intrp: _____

10

Rate: _____

Rhythm: _____

P Waves: _____

PR Int: _____

QRS: _____

Intrp: _____

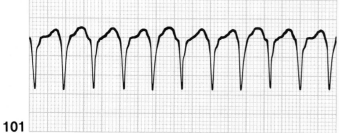

101

Rate: _____

Rhythm: _____

P Waves: _____

PR Int: _____

QRS: _____

Intrp: _____

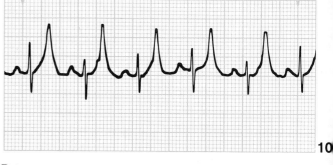

10

Rate: _____

Rhythm: _____

P Waves: _____

PR Int: _____

QRS: _____

Intrp: _____

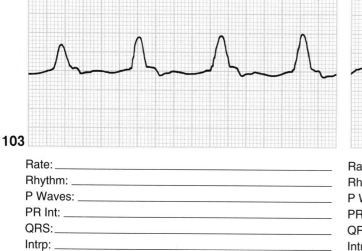

103

Rate: _____

Rhythm: _____

P Waves: _____

PR Int: _____

QRS: _____

Intrp: _____

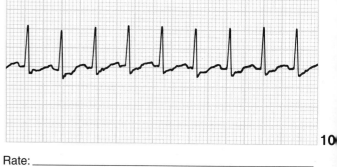

10

Rate: _____

Rhythm: _____

P Waves: _____

PR Int: _____

QRS: _____

Intrp: _____

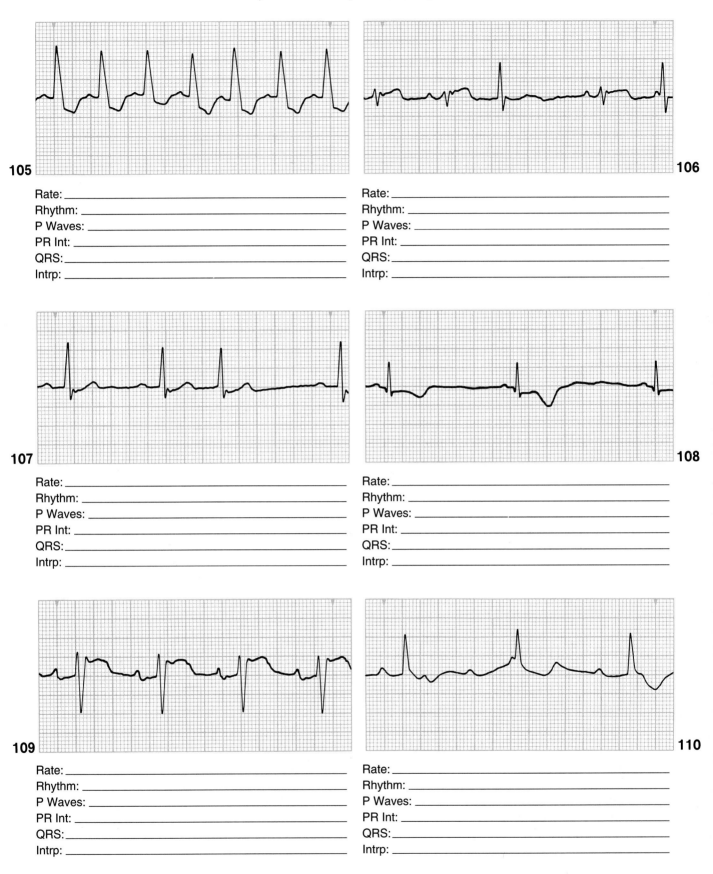

105

Rate: _____
Rhythm: _____
P Waves: _____
PR Int: _____
QRS: _____
Intrp: _____

106

Rate: _____
Rhythm: _____
P Waves: _____
PR Int: _____
QRS: _____
Intrp: _____

107

Rate: _____
Rhythm: _____
P Waves: _____
PR Int: _____
QRS: _____
Intrp: _____

108

Rate: _____
Rhythm: _____
P Waves: _____
PR Int: _____
QRS: _____
Intrp: _____

109

Rate: _____
Rhythm: _____
P Waves: _____
PR Int: _____
QRS: _____
Intrp: _____

110

Rate: _____
Rhythm: _____
P Waves: _____
PR Int: _____
QRS: _____
Intrp: _____

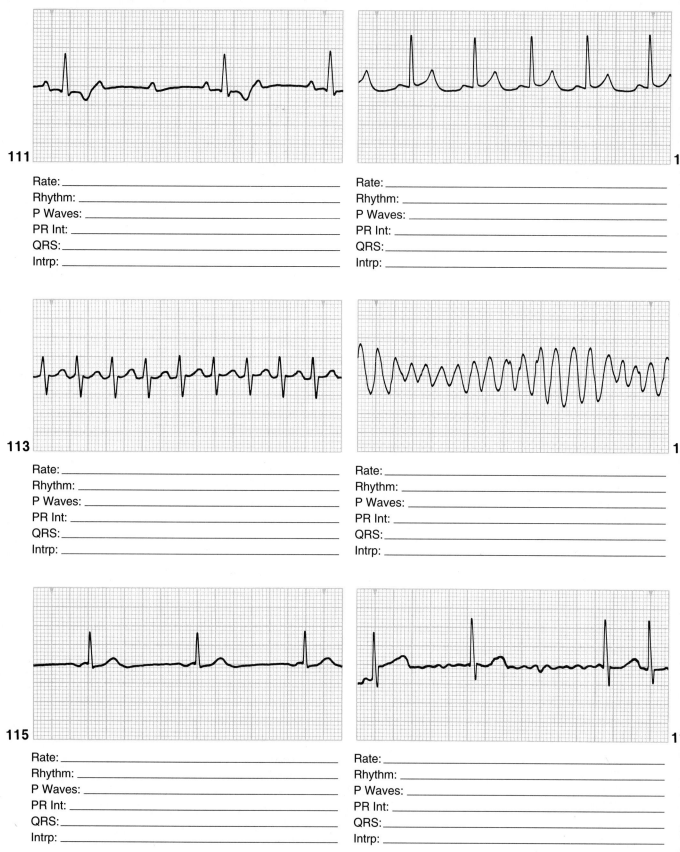

111

Rate: _____
Rhythm: _____
P Waves: _____
PR Int: _____
QRS: _____
Intrp: _____

1

Rate: _____
Rhythm: _____
P Waves: _____
PR Int: _____
QRS: _____
Intrp: _____

113

Rate: _____
Rhythm: _____
P Waves: _____
PR Int: _____
QRS: _____
Intrp: _____

11

Rate: _____
Rhythm: _____
P Waves: _____
PR Int: _____
QRS: _____
Intrp: _____

115

Rate: _____
Rhythm: _____
P Waves: _____
PR Int: _____
QRS: _____
Intrp: _____

11

Rate: _____
Rhythm: _____
P Waves: _____
PR Int: _____
QRS: _____
Intrp: _____

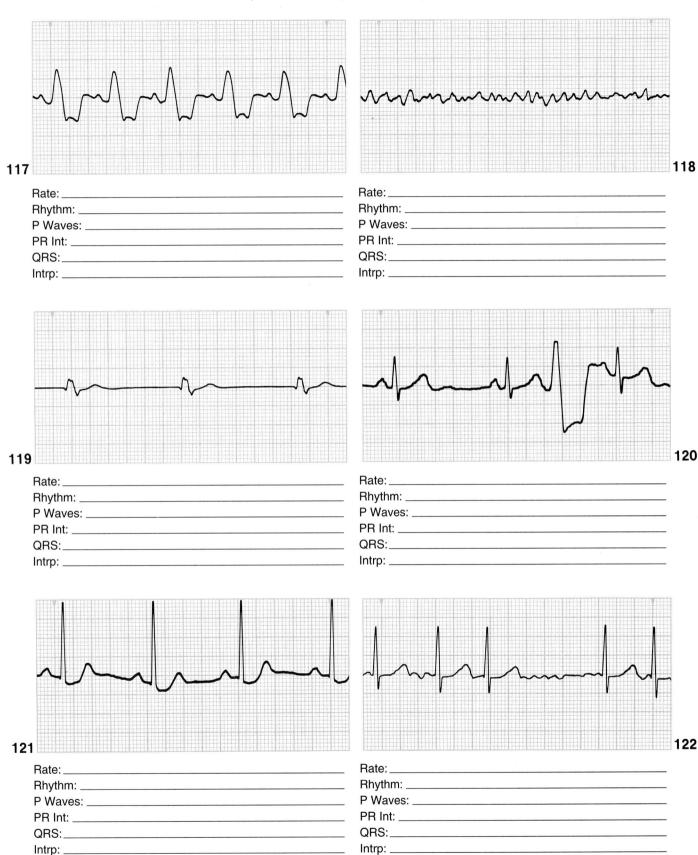

117

Rate: _____

Rhythm: _____

P Waves: _____

PR Int: _____

QRS: _____

Intrp: _____

118

Rate: _____

Rhythm: _____

P Waves: _____

PR Int: _____

QRS: _____

Intrp: _____

119

Rate: _____

Rhythm: _____

P Waves: _____

PR Int: _____

QRS: _____

Intrp: _____

120

Rate: _____

Rhythm: _____

P Waves: _____

PR Int: _____

QRS: _____

Intrp: _____

121

Rate: _____

Rhythm: _____

P Waves: _____

PR Int: _____

QRS: _____

Intrp: _____

122

Rate: _____

Rhythm: _____

P Waves: _____

PR Int: _____

QRS: _____

Intrp: _____

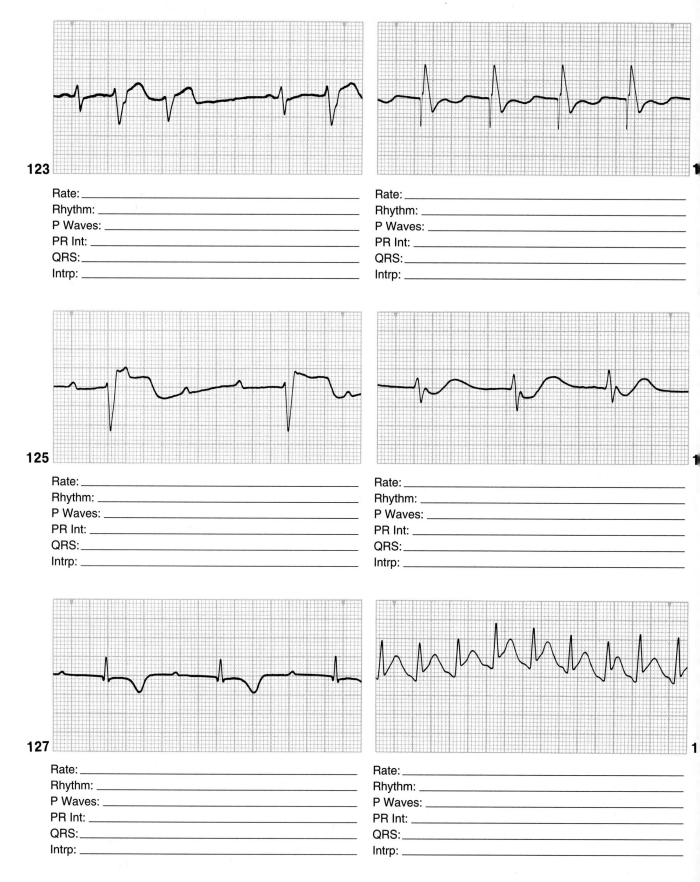

123

Rate: _____

Rhythm: _____

P Waves: _____

PR Int: _____

QRS: _____

Intrp: _____

Rate: _____

Rhythm: _____

P Waves: _____

PR Int: _____

QRS: _____

Intrp: _____

125

Rate: _____

Rhythm: _____

P Waves: _____

PR Int: _____

QRS: _____

Intrp: _____

Rate: _____

Rhythm: _____

P Waves: _____

PR Int: _____

QRS: _____

Intrp: _____

127

Rate: _____

Rhythm: _____

P Waves: _____

PR Int: _____

QRS: _____

Intrp: _____

Rate: _____

Rhythm: _____

P Waves: _____

PR Int: _____

QRS: _____

Intrp: _____

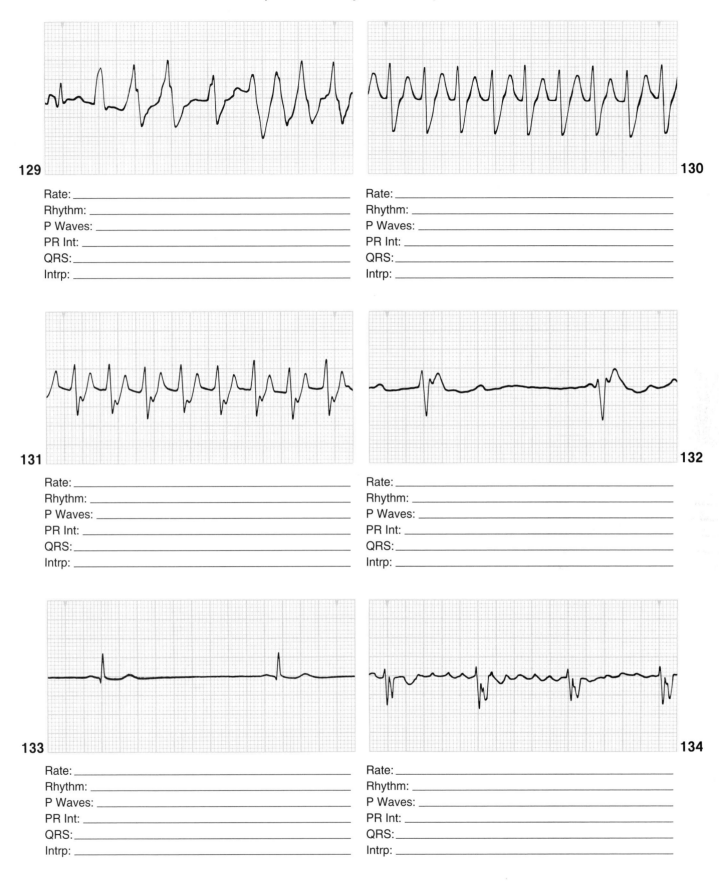

129

Rate: _____
Rhythm: _____
P Waves: _____
PR Int: _____
QRS: _____
Intrp: _____

130

Rate: _____
Rhythm: _____
P Waves: _____
PR Int: _____
QRS: _____
Intrp: _____

131

Rate: _____
Rhythm: _____
P Waves: _____
PR Int: _____
QRS: _____
Intrp: _____

132

Rate: _____
Rhythm: _____
P Waves: _____
PR Int: _____
QRS: _____
Intrp: _____

133

Rate: _____
Rhythm: _____
P Waves: _____
PR Int: _____
QRS: _____
Intrp: _____

134

Rate: _____
Rhythm: _____
P Waves: _____
PR Int: _____
QRS: _____
Intrp: _____

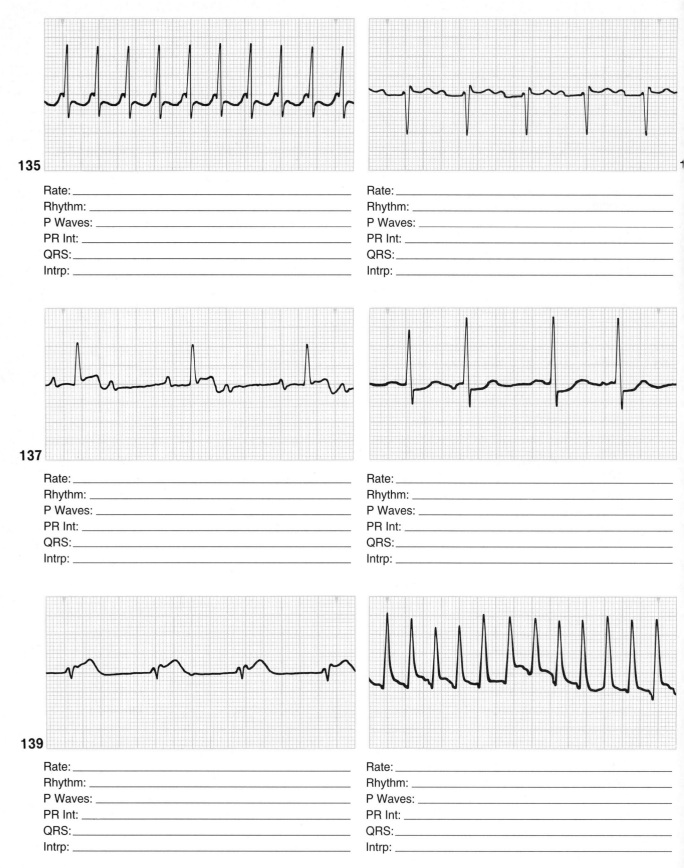

135

Rate: _____

Rhythm: _____

P Waves: _____

PR Int: _____

QRS: _____

Intrp: _____

Rate: _____

Rhythm: _____

P Waves: _____

PR Int: _____

QRS: _____

Intrp: _____

137

Rate: _____

Rhythm: _____

P Waves: _____

PR Int: _____

QRS: _____

Intrp: _____

Rate: _____

Rhythm: _____

P Waves: _____

PR Int: _____

QRS: _____

Intrp: _____

139

Rate: _____

Rhythm: _____

P Waves: _____

PR Int: _____

QRS: _____

Intrp: _____

Rate: _____

Rhythm: _____

P Waves: _____

PR Int: _____

QRS: _____

Intrp: _____

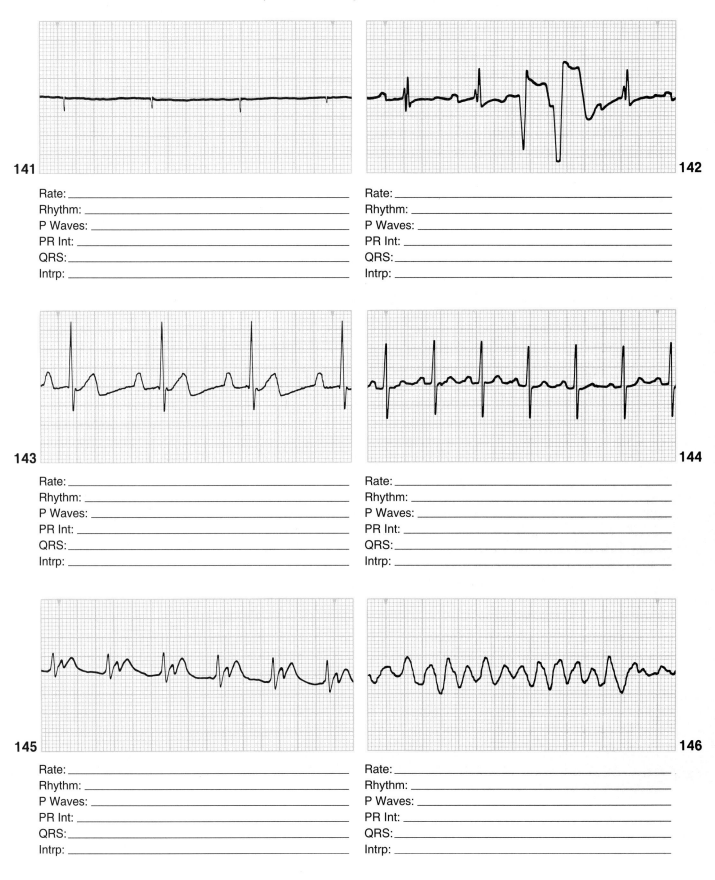

141

Rate: _____

Rhythm: _____

P Waves: _____

PR Int: _____

QRS: _____

Intrp: _____

142

Rate: _____

Rhythm: _____

P Waves: _____

PR Int: _____

QRS: _____

Intrp: _____

143

Rate: _____

Rhythm: _____

P Waves: _____

PR Int: _____

QRS: _____

Intrp: _____

144

Rate: _____

Rhythm: _____

P Waves: _____

PR Int: _____

QRS: _____

Intrp: _____

145

Rate: _____

Rhythm: _____

P Waves: _____

PR Int: _____

QRS: _____

Intrp: _____

146

Rate: _____

Rhythm: _____

P Waves: _____

PR Int: _____

QRS: _____

Intrp: _____

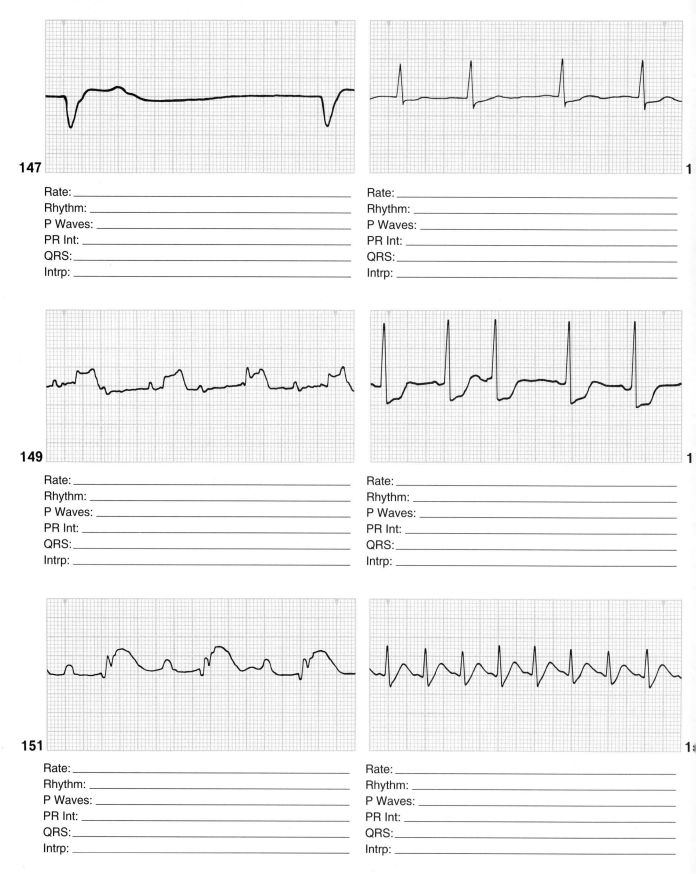

147

Rate: _____

Rhythm: _____

P Waves: _____

PR Int: _____

QRS: _____

Intrp: _____

1

Rate: _____

Rhythm: _____

P Waves: _____

PR Int: _____

QRS: _____

Intrp: _____

149

Rate: _____

Rhythm: _____

P Waves: _____

PR Int: _____

QRS: _____

Intrp: _____

1

Rate: _____

Rhythm: _____

P Waves: _____

PR Int: _____

QRS: _____

Intrp: _____

151

Rate: _____

Rhythm: _____

P Waves: _____

PR Int: _____

QRS: _____

Intrp: _____

1

Rate: _____

Rhythm: _____

P Waves: _____

PR Int: _____

QRS: _____

Intrp: _____

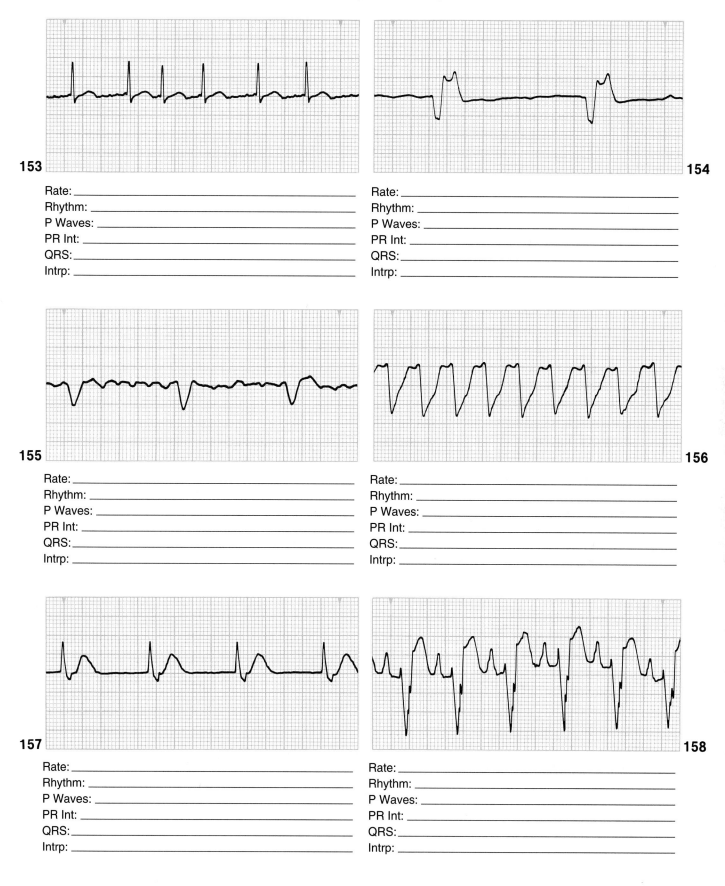

153

Rate: _____

Rhythm: _____

P Waves: _____

PR Int: _____

QRS: _____

Intrp: _____

154

Rate: _____

Rhythm: _____

P Waves: _____

PR Int: _____

QRS: _____

Intrp: _____

155

Rate: _____

Rhythm: _____

P Waves: _____

PR Int: _____

QRS: _____

Intrp: _____

156

Rate: _____

Rhythm: _____

P Waves: _____

PR Int: _____

QRS: _____

Intrp: _____

157

Rate: _____

Rhythm: _____

P Waves: _____

PR Int: _____

QRS: _____

Intrp: _____

158

Rate: _____

Rhythm: _____

P Waves: _____

PR Int: _____

QRS: _____

Intrp: _____

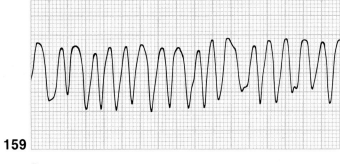

159

Rate: _____
Rhythm: _____
P Waves: _____
PR Int: _____
QRS: _____
Intrp: _____

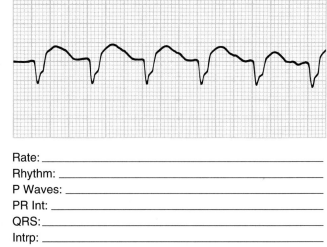

1

Rate: _____
Rhythm: _____
P Waves: _____
PR Int: _____
QRS: _____
Intrp: _____

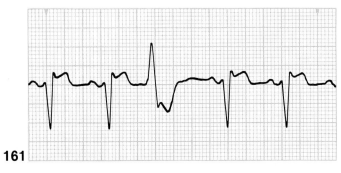

161

Rate: _____
Rhythm: _____
P Waves: _____
PR Int: _____
QRS: _____
Intrp: _____

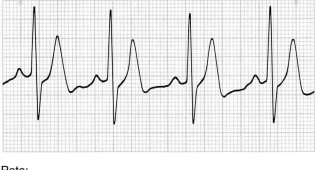

1

Rate: _____
Rhythm: _____
P Waves: _____
PR Int: _____
QRS: _____
Intrp: _____

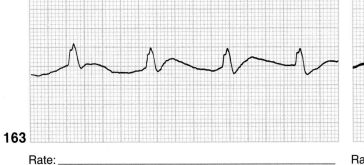

163

Rate: _____
Rhythm: _____
P Waves: _____
PR Int: _____
QRS: _____
Intrp: _____

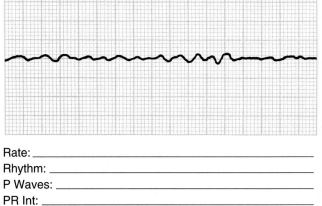

1

Rate: _____
Rhythm: _____
P Waves: _____
PR Int: _____
QRS: _____
Intrp: _____

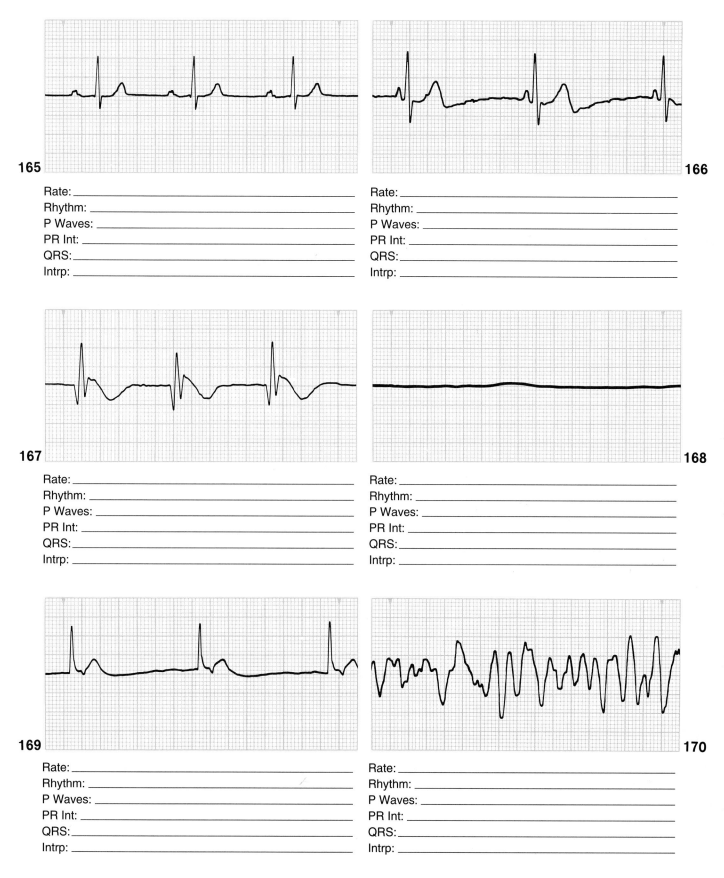

165

Rate: _____
Rhythm: _____
P Waves: _____
PR Int: _____
QRS: _____
Intrp: _____

166

Rate: _____
Rhythm: _____
P Waves: _____
PR Int: _____
QRS: _____
Intrp: _____

167

Rate: _____
Rhythm: _____
P Waves: _____
PR Int: _____
QRS: _____
Intrp: _____

168

Rate: _____
Rhythm: _____
P Waves: _____
PR Int: _____
QRS: _____
Intrp: _____

169

Rate: _____
Rhythm: _____
P Waves: _____
PR Int: _____
QRS: _____
Intrp: _____

170

Rate: _____
Rhythm: _____
P Waves: _____
PR Int: _____
QRS: _____
Intrp: _____

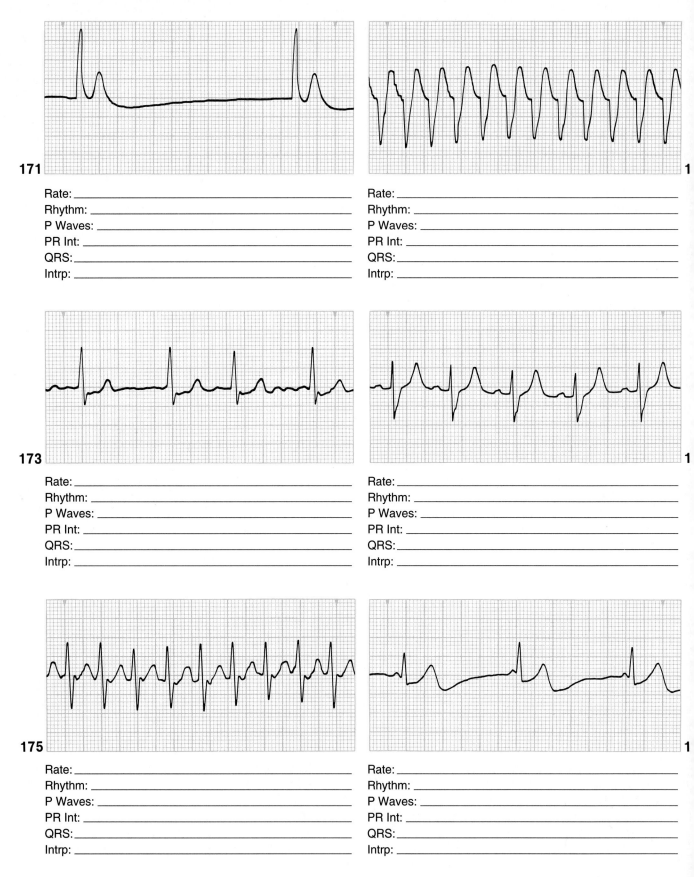

171

Rate: _____

Rhythm: _____

P Waves: _____

PR Int: _____

QRS: _____

Intrp: _____

1

Rate: _____

Rhythm: _____

P Waves: _____

PR Int: _____

QRS: _____

Intrp: _____

173

Rate: _____

Rhythm: _____

P Waves: _____

PR Int: _____

QRS: _____

Intrp: _____

1

Rate: _____

Rhythm: _____

P Waves: _____

PR Int: _____

QRS: _____

Intrp: _____

175

Rate: _____

Rhythm: _____

P Waves: _____

PR Int: _____

QRS: _____

Intrp: _____

1

Rate: _____

Rhythm: _____

P Waves: _____

PR Int: _____

QRS: _____

Intrp: _____

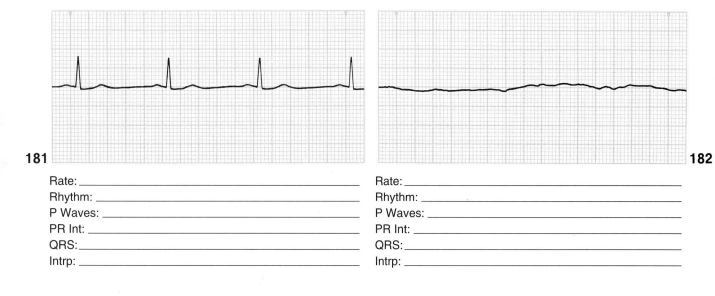
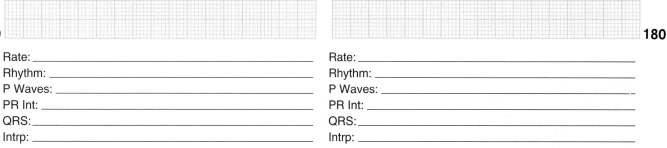

177

Rate: _____

Rhythm: _____

P Waves: _____

PR Int: _____

QRS: _____

Intrp: _____

178

Rate: _____

Rhythm: _____

P Waves: _____

PR Int: _____

QRS: _____

Intrp: _____

179

Rate: _____

Rhythm: _____

P Waves: _____

PR Int: _____

QRS: _____

Intrp: _____

180

Rate: _____

Rhythm: _____

P Waves: _____

PR Int: _____

QRS: _____

Intrp: _____

181

Rate: _____

Rhythm: _____

P Waves: _____

PR Int: _____

QRS: _____

Intrp: _____

182

Rate: _____

Rhythm: _____

P Waves: _____

PR Int: _____

QRS: _____

Intrp: _____

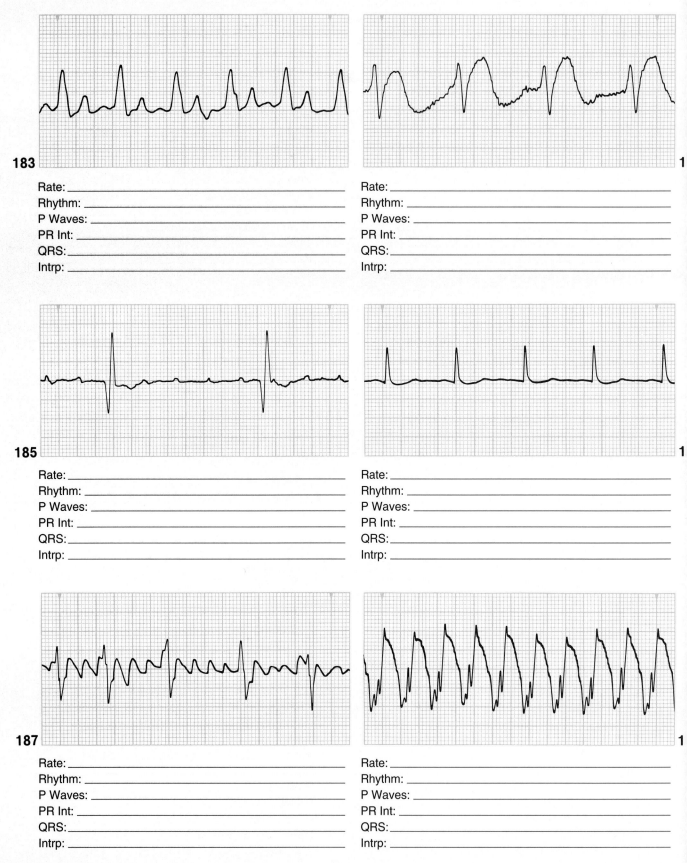

183

Rate: _____

Rhythm: _____

P Waves: _____

PR Int: _____

QRS: _____

Intrp: _____

1

Rate: _____

Rhythm: _____

P Waves: _____

PR Int: _____

QRS: _____

Intrp: _____

185

Rate: _____

Rhythm: _____

P Waves: _____

PR Int: _____

QRS: _____

Intrp: _____

1

Rate: _____

Rhythm: _____

P Waves: _____

PR Int: _____

QRS: _____

Intrp: _____

187

Rate: _____

Rhythm: _____

P Waves: _____

PR Int: _____

QRS: _____

Intrp: _____

1

Rate: _____

Rhythm: _____

P Waves: _____

PR Int: _____

QRS: _____

Intrp: _____

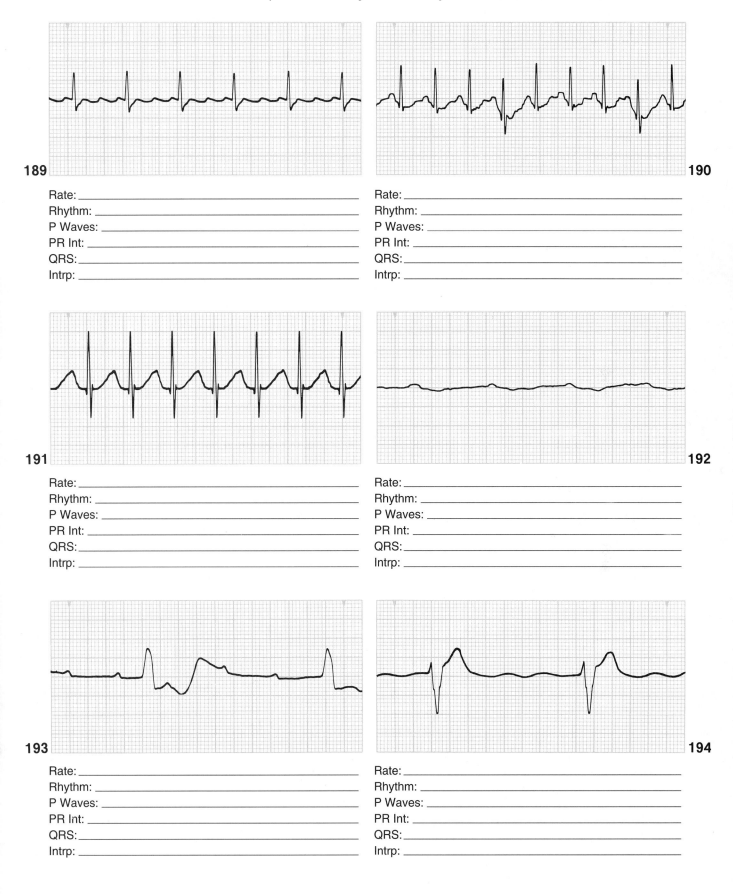

189

Rate: _____
Rhythm: _____
P Waves: _____
PR Int: _____
QRS: _____
Intrp: _____

190

Rate: _____
Rhythm: _____
P Waves: _____
PR Int: _____
QRS: _____
Intrp: _____

191

Rate: _____
Rhythm: _____
P Waves: _____
PR Int: _____
QRS: _____
Intrp: _____

192

Rate: _____
Rhythm: _____
P Waves: _____
PR Int: _____
QRS: _____
Intrp: _____

193

Rate: _____
Rhythm: _____
P Waves: _____
PR Int: _____
QRS: _____
Intrp: _____

194

Rate: _____
Rhythm: _____
P Waves: _____
PR Int: _____
QRS: _____
Intrp: _____

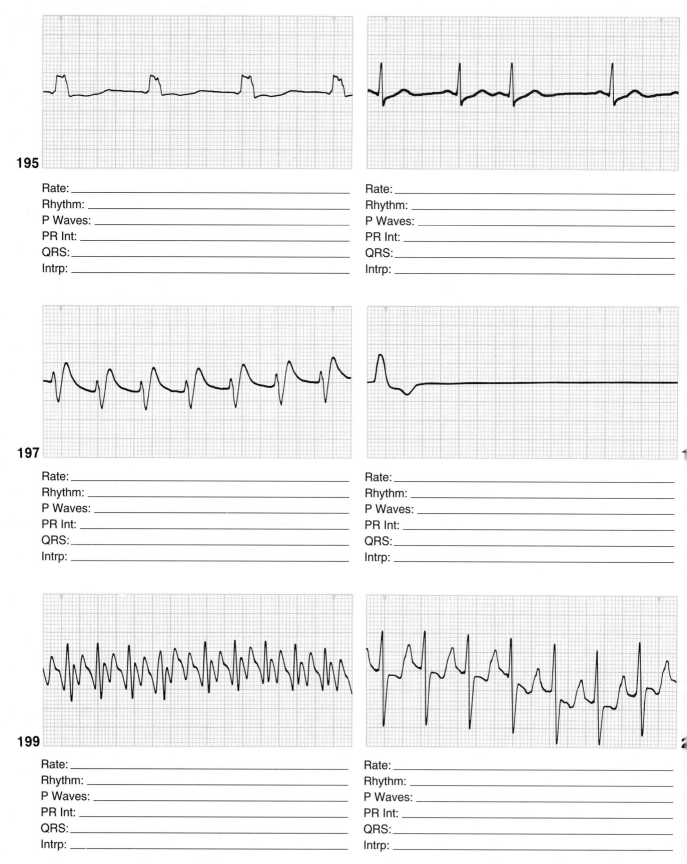

195

Rate: _____

Rhythm: _____

P Waves: _____

PR Int: _____

QRS: _____

Intrp: _____

Rate: _____

Rhythm: _____

P Waves: _____

PR Int: _____

QRS: _____

Intrp: _____

197

Rate: _____

Rhythm: _____

P Waves: _____

PR Int: _____

QRS: _____

Intrp: _____

Rate: _____

Rhythm: _____

P Waves: _____

PR Int: _____

QRS: _____

Intrp: _____

199

Rate: _____

Rhythm: _____

P Waves: _____

PR Int: _____

QRS: _____

Intrp: ___ _____

Rate: _____

Rhythm: _____

P Waves: _____

PR Int: _____

QRS: _____

Intrp: _____

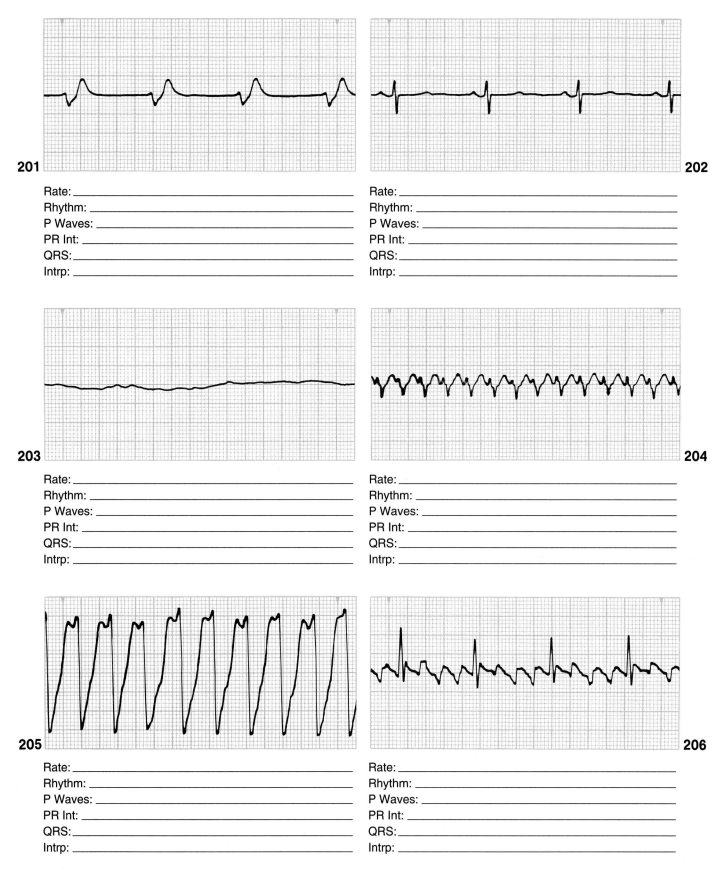

201

Rate: _____
Rhythm: _____
P Waves: _____
PR Int: _____
QRS: _____
Intrp: _____

202

Rate: _____
Rhythm: _____
P Waves: _____
PR Int: _____
QRS: _____
Intrp: _____

203

Rate: _____
Rhythm: _____
P Waves: _____
PR Int: _____
QRS: _____
Intrp: _____

204

Rate: _____
Rhythm: _____
P Waves: _____
PR Int: _____
QRS: _____
Intrp: _____

205

Rate: _____
Rhythm: _____
P Waves: _____
PR Int: _____
QRS: _____
Intrp: _____

206

Rate: _____
Rhythm: _____
P Waves: _____
PR Int: _____
QRS: _____
Intrp: _____

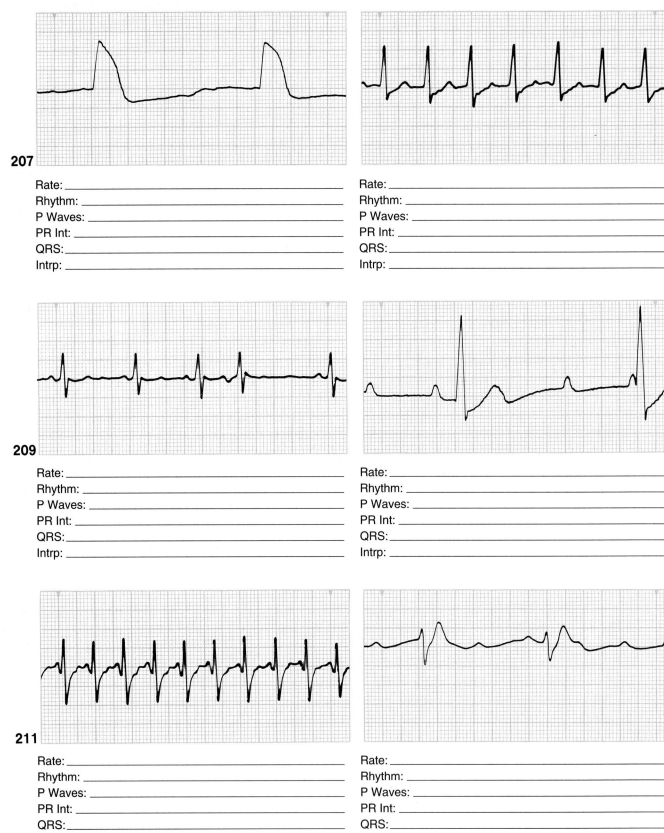

207

Rate: _____

Rhythm: _____

P Waves: _____

PR Int: _____

QRS: _____

Intrp: _____

Rate: _____

Rhythm: _____

P Waves: _____

PR Int: _____

QRS: _____

Intrp: _____

209

Rate: _____

Rhythm: _____

P Waves: _____

PR Int: _____

QRS: _____

Intrp: _____

Rate: _____

Rhythm: _____

P Waves: _____

PR Int: _____

QRS: _____

Intrp: _____

211

Rate: _____

Rhythm: _____

P Waves: _____

PR Int: _____

QRS: _____

Intrp: _____

Rate: _____

Rhythm: _____

P Waves: _____

PR Int: _____

QRS: _____

Intrp: _____

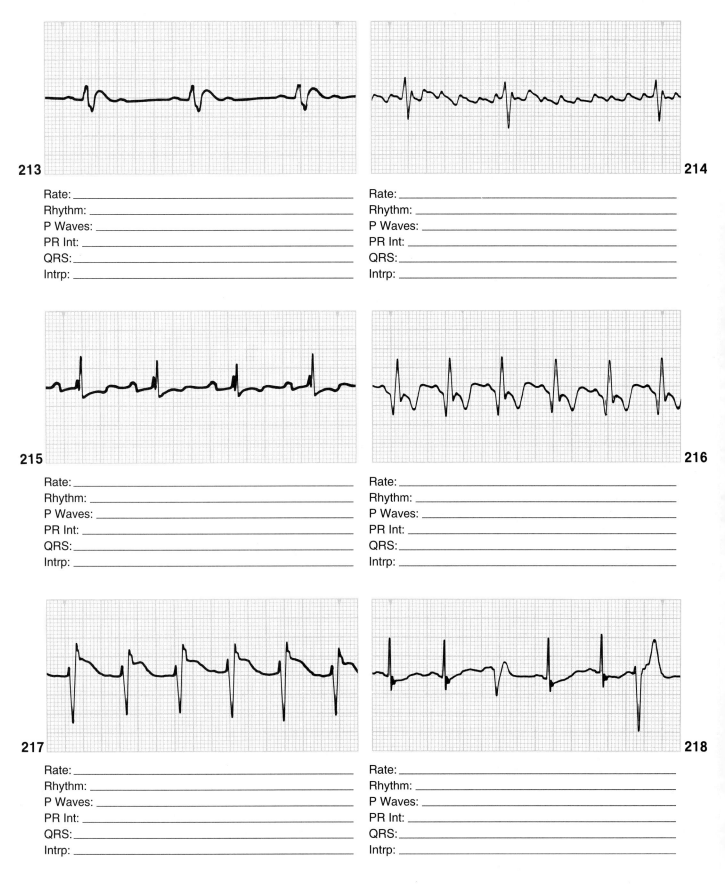

213

Rate: _____
Rhythm: _____
P Waves: _____
PR Int: _____
QRS: _____
Intrp: _____

214

Rate: _____
Rhythm: _____
P Waves: _____
PR Int: _____
QRS: _____
Intrp: _____

215

Rate: _____
Rhythm: _____
P Waves: _____
PR Int: _____
QRS: _____
Intrp: _____

216

Rate: _____
Rhythm: _____
P Waves: _____
PR Int: _____
QRS: _____
Intrp: _____

217

Rate: _____
Rhythm: _____
P Waves: _____
PR Int: _____
QRS: _____
Intrp: _____

218

Rate: _____
Rhythm: _____
P Waves: _____
PR Int: _____
QRS: _____
Intrp: _____

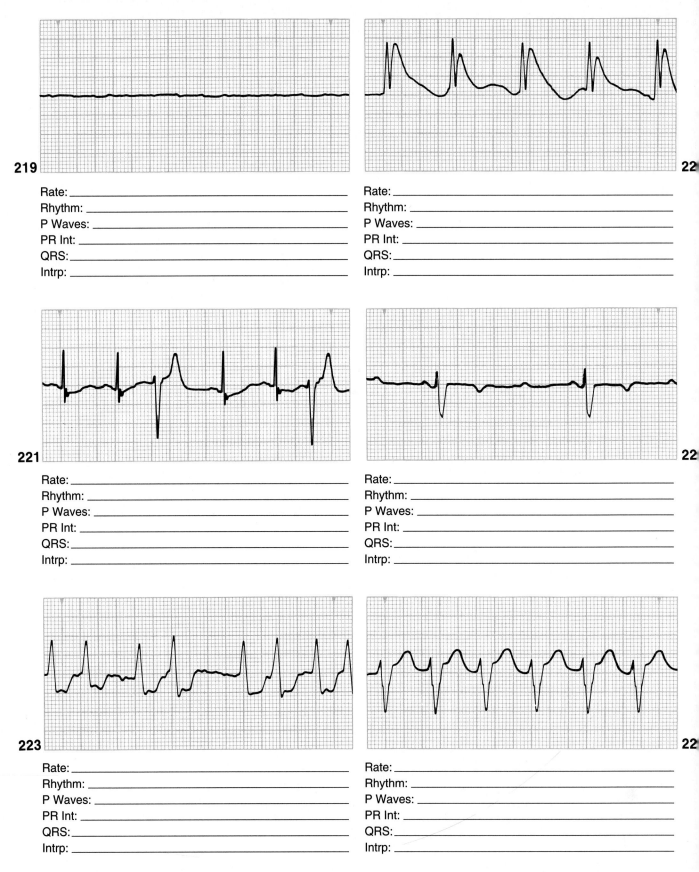

219

Rate: _____
Rhythm: _____
P Waves: _____
PR Int: _____
QRS: _____
Intrp: _____

22

Rate: _____
Rhythm: _____
P Waves: _____
PR Int: _____
QRS: _____
Intrp: _____

221

Rate: _____
Rhythm: _____
P Waves: _____
PR Int: _____
QRS: _____
Intrp: _____

22

Rate: _____
Rhythm: _____
P Waves: _____
PR Int: _____
QRS: _____
Intrp: _____

223

Rate: _____
Rhythm: _____
P Waves: _____
PR Int: _____
QRS: _____
Intrp: _____

22

Rate: _____
Rhythm: _____
P Waves: _____
PR Int: _____
QRS: _____
Intrp: _____

II. Bundle Branch and Fascicular Blocks

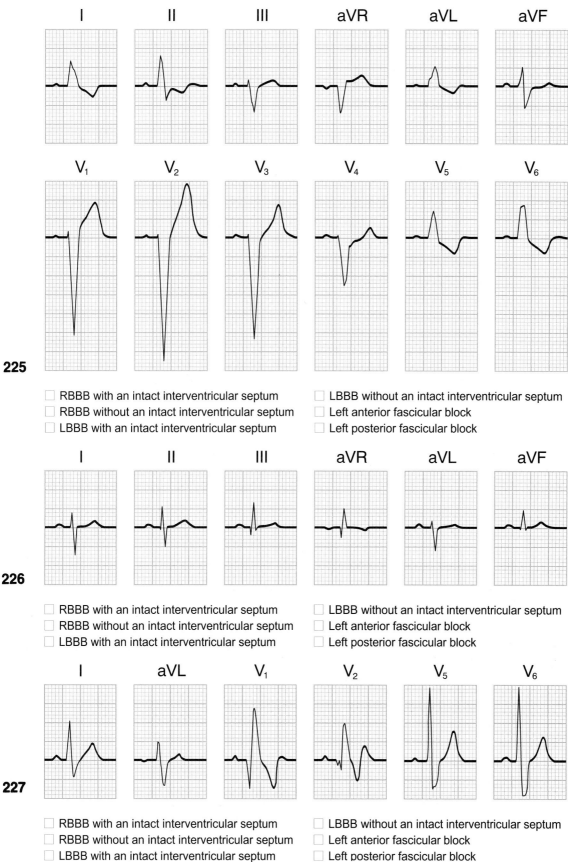

225

☐ RBBB with an intact interventricular septum
☐ RBBB without an intact interventricular septum
☐ LBBB with an intact interventricular septum

☐ LBBB without an intact interventricular septum
☐ Left anterior fascicular block
☐ Left posterior fascicular block

226

☐ RBBB with an intact interventricular septum
☐ RBBB without an intact interventricular septum
☐ LBBB with an intact interventricular septum

☐ LBBB without an intact interventricular septum
☐ Left anterior fascicular block
☐ Left posterior fascicular block

227

☐ RBBB with an intact interventricular septum
☐ RBBB without an intact interventricular septum
☐ LBBB with an intact interventricular septum

☐ LBBB without an intact interventricular septum
☐ Left anterior fascicular block
☐ Left posterior fascicular block

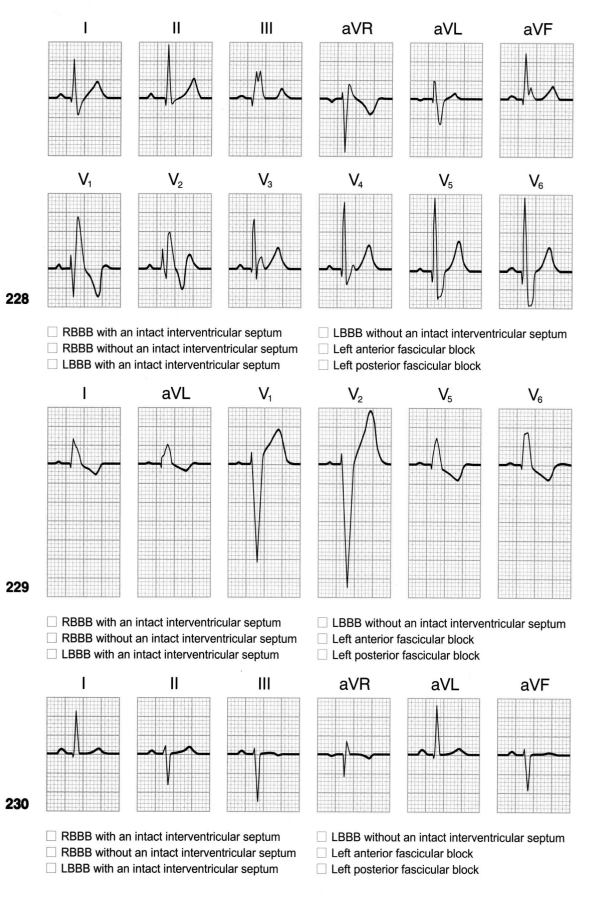

228

- ☐ RBBB with an intact interventricular septum
- ☐ RBBB without an intact interventricular septum
- ☐ LBBB with an intact interventricular septum
- ☐ LBBB without an intact interventricular septum
- ☐ Left anterior fascicular block
- ☐ Left posterior fascicular block

229

- ☐ RBBB with an intact interventricular septum
- ☐ RBBB without an intact interventricular septum
- ☐ LBBB with an intact interventricular septum
- ☐ LBBB without an intact interventricular septum
- ☐ Left anterior fascicular block
- ☐ Left posterior fascicular block

230

- ☐ RBBB with an intact interventricular septum
- ☐ RBBB without an intact interventricular septum
- ☐ LBBB with an intact interventricular septum
- ☐ LBBB without an intact interventricular septum
- ☐ Left anterior fascicular block
- ☐ Left posterior fascicular block

III. Myocardial Infarctions

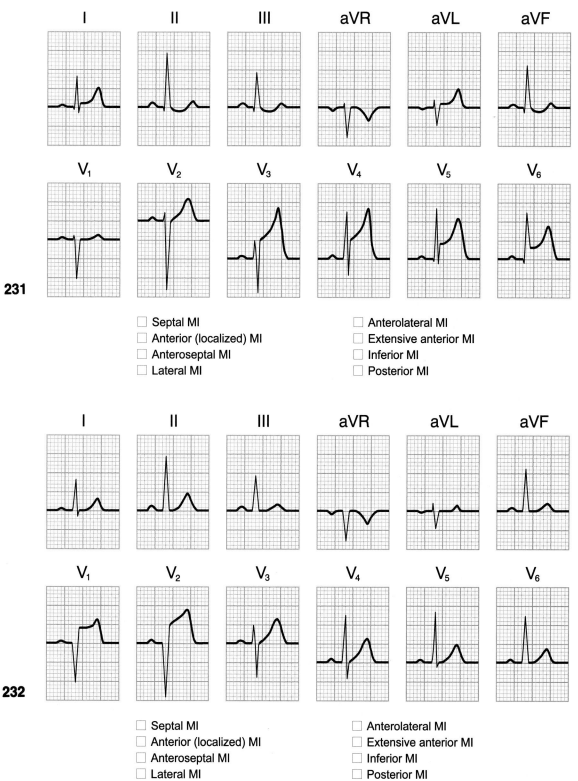

231

☐ Septal MI
☐ Anterior (localized) MI
☐ Anteroseptal MI
☐ Lateral MI

☐ Anterolateral MI
☐ Extensive anterior MI
☐ Inferior MI
☐ Posterior MI

232

☐ Septal MI
☐ Anterior (localized) MI
☐ Anteroseptal MI
☐ Lateral MI

☐ Anterolateral MI
☐ Extensive anterior MI
☐ Inferior MI
☐ Posterior MI

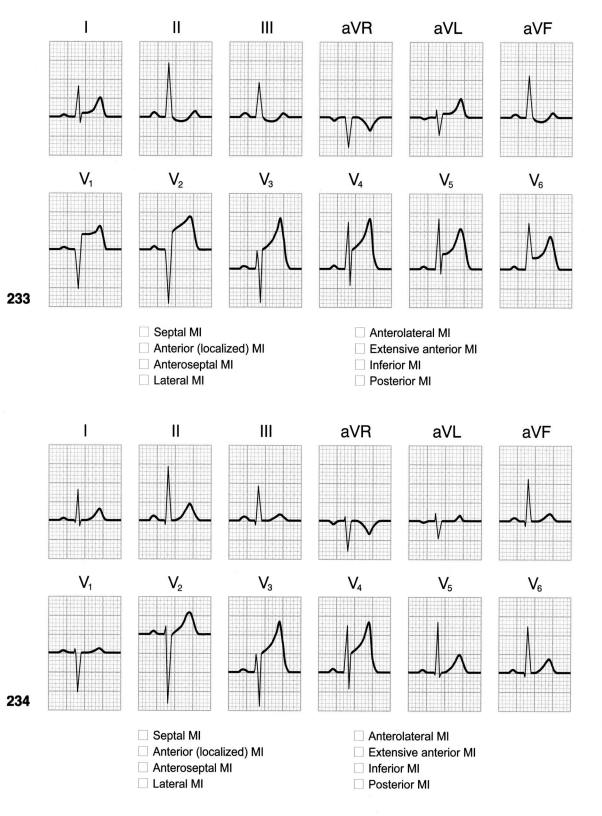

233

☐ Septal MI   ☐ Anterolateral MI
☐ Anterior (localized) MI   ☐ Extensive anterior MI
☐ Anteroseptal MI   ☐ Inferior MI
☐ Lateral MI   ☐ Posterior MI

234

☐ Septal MI   ☐ Anterolateral MI
☐ Anterior (localized) MI   ☐ Extensive anterior MI
☐ Anteroseptal MI   ☐ Inferior MI
☐ Lateral MI   ☐ Posterior MI

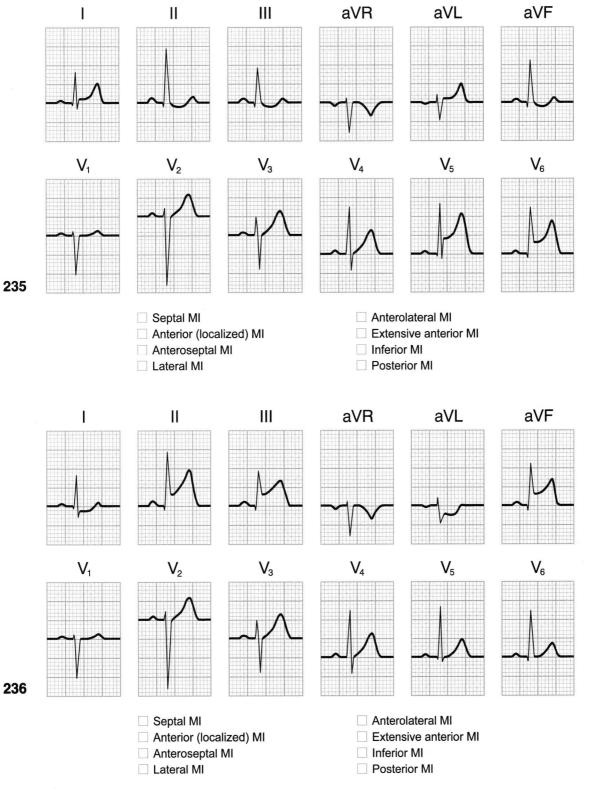

235

☐ Septal MI ☐ Anterolateral MI
☐ Anterior (localized) MI ☐ Extensive anterior MI
☐ Anteroseptal MI ☐ Inferior MI
☐ Lateral MI ☐ Posterior MI

236

☐ Septal MI ☐ Anterolateral MI
☐ Anterior (localized) MI ☐ Extensive anterior MI
☐ Anteroseptal MI ☐ Inferior MI
☐ Lateral MI ☐ Posterior MI

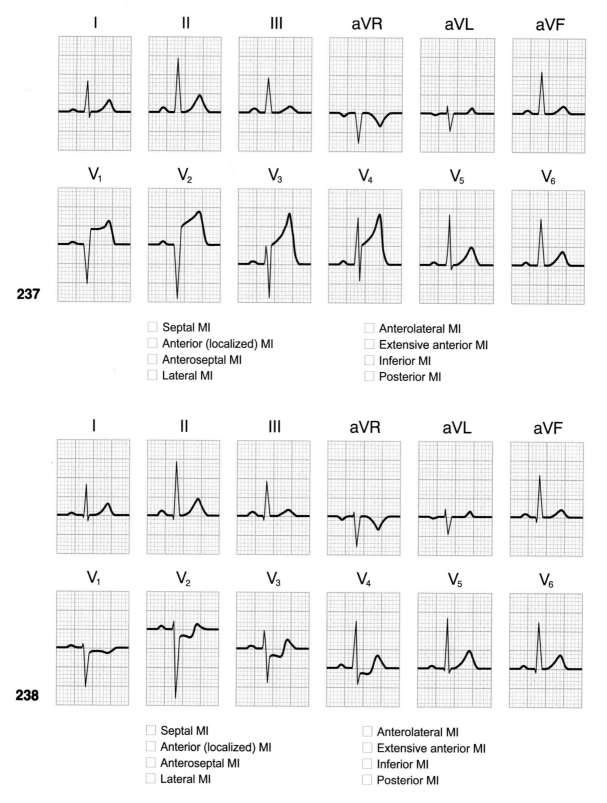

237

- ☐ Septal MI
- ☐ Anterior (localized) MI
- ☐ Anteroseptal MI
- ☐ Lateral MI
- ☐ Anterolateral MI
- ☐ Extensive anterior MI
- ☐ Inferior MI
- ☐ Posterior MI

238

- ☐ Septal MI
- ☐ Anterior (localized) MI
- ☐ Anteroseptal MI
- ☐ Lateral MI
- ☐ Anterolateral MI
- ☐ Extensive anterior MI
- ☐ Inferior MI
- ☐ Posterior MI

IV. QRS Axes

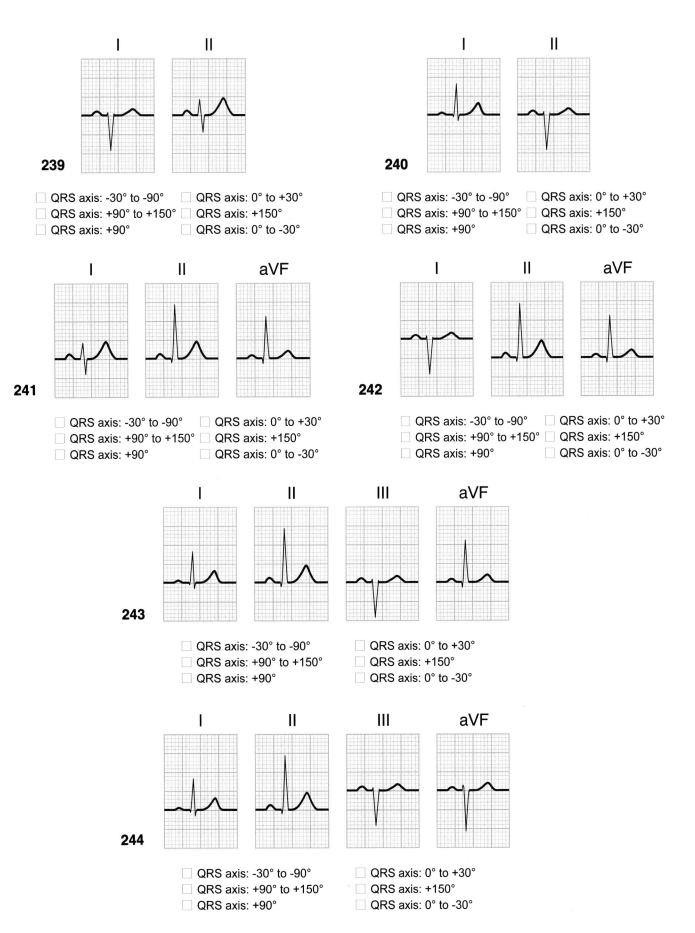

239
- ☐ QRS axis: -30° to -90°   ☐ QRS axis: 0° to +30°
- ☐ QRS axis: +90° to +150°   ☐ QRS axis: +150°
- ☐ QRS axis: +90°   ☐ QRS axis: 0° to -30°

240
- ☐ QRS axis: -30° to -90°   ☐ QRS axis: 0° to +30°
- ☐ QRS axis: +90° to +150°   ☐ QRS axis: +150°
- ☐ QRS axis: +90°   ☐ QRS axis: 0° to -30°

241
- ☐ QRS axis: -30° to -90°   ☐ QRS axis: 0° to +30°
- ☐ QRS axis: +90° to +150°   ☐ QRS axis: +150°
- ☐ QRS axis: +90°   ☐ QRS axis: 0° to -30°

242
- ☐ QRS axis: -30° to -90°   ☐ QRS axis: 0° to +30°
- ☐ QRS axis: +90° to +150°   ☐ QRS axis: +150°
- ☐ QRS axis: +90°   ☐ QRS axis: 0° to -30°

243
- ☐ QRS axis: -30° to -90°   ☐ QRS axis: 0° to +30°
- ☐ QRS axis: +90° to +150°   ☐ QRS axis: +150°
- ☐ QRS axis: +90°   ☐ QRS axis: 0° to -30°

244
- ☐ QRS axis: -30° to -90°   ☐ QRS axis: 0° to +30°
- ☐ QRS axis: +90° to +150°   ☐ QRS axis: +150°
- ☐ QRS axis: +90°   ☐ QRS axis: 0° to -30°

V. ECG Changes: Drug and Electrolyte

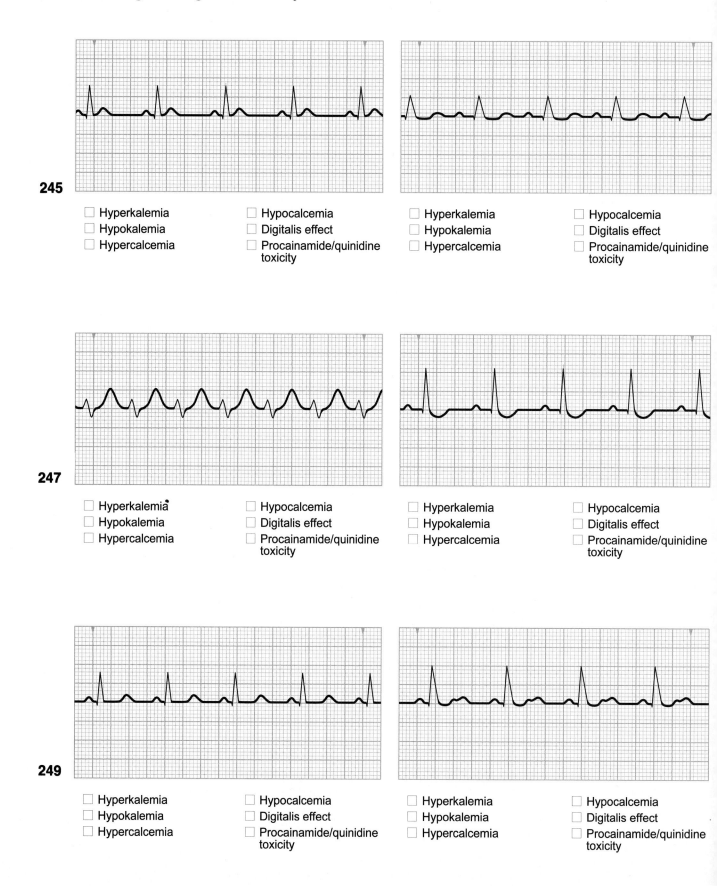

245

☐ Hyperkalemia   ☐ Hypocalcemia
☐ Hypokalemia   ☐ Digitalis effect
☐ Hypercalcemia   ☐ Procainamide/quinidine
                                  toxicity

☐ Hyperkalemia   ☐ Hypocalcemia
☐ Hypokalemia   ☐ Digitalis effect
☐ Hypercalcemia   ☐ Procainamide/quinidine
                                  toxicity

247

☐ Hyperkalemia   ☐ Hypocalcemia
☐ Hypokalemia   ☐ Digitalis effect
☐ Hypercalcemia   ☐ Procainamide/quinidine
                                  toxicity

☐ Hyperkalemia   ☐ Hypocalcemia
☐ Hypokalemia   ☐ Digitalis effect
☐ Hypercalcemia   ☐ Procainamide/quinidine
                                  toxicity

249

☐ Hyperkalemia   ☐ Hypocalcemia
☐ Hypokalemia   ☐ Digitalis effect
☐ Hypercalcemia   ☐ Procainamide/quinidine
                                  toxicity

☐ Hyperkalemia   ☐ Hypocalcemia
☐ Hypokalemia   ☐ Digitalis effect
☐ Hypercalcemia   ☐ Procainamide/quinidine
                                  toxicity

VI. ECG Changes: Miscellaneous

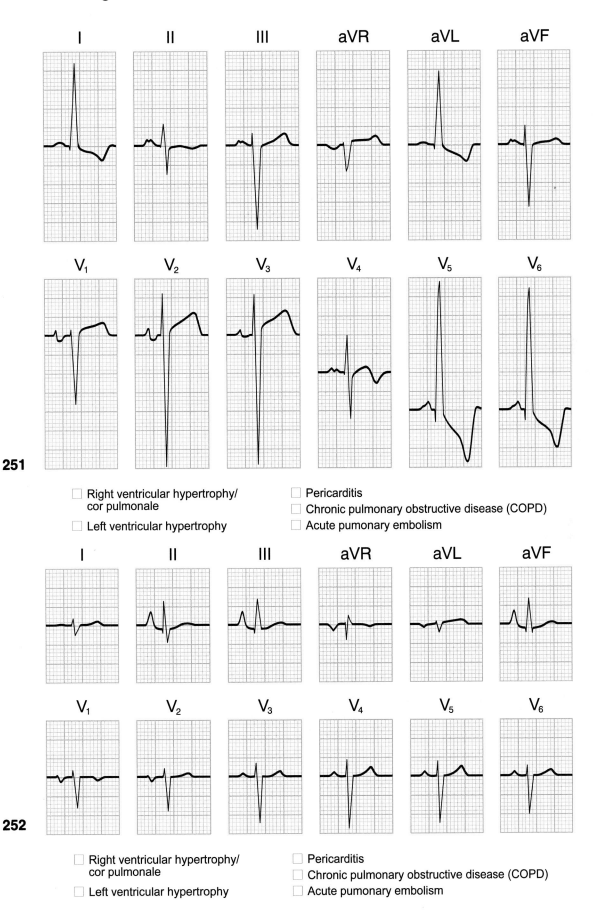

251

☐ Right ventricular hypertrophy/
    cor pulmonale
☐ Left ventricular hypertrophy

☐ Pericarditis
☐ Chronic pulmonary obstructive disease (COPD)
☐ Acute pumonary embolism

252

☐ Right ventricular hypertrophy/
    cor pulmonale
☐ Left ventricular hypertrophy

☐ Pericarditis
☐ Chronic pulmonary obstructive disease (COPD)
☐ Acute pumonary embolism

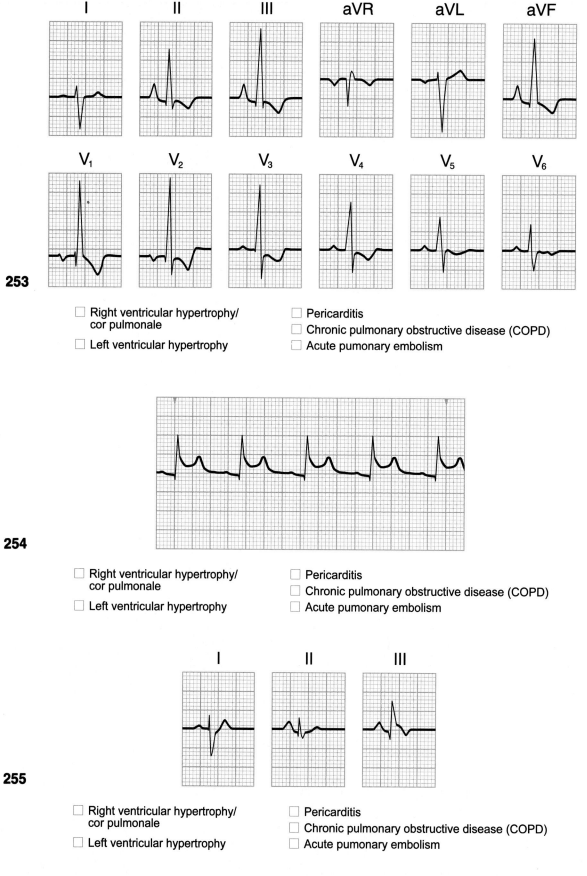

253

- ☐ Right ventricular hypertrophy/ cor pulmonale
- ☐ Left ventricular hypertrophy
- ☐ Pericarditis
- ☐ Chronic pulmonary obstructive disease (COPD)
- ☐ Acute pumonary embolism

254

- ☐ Right ventricular hypertrophy/ cor pulmonale
- ☐ Left ventricular hypertrophy
- ☐ Pericarditis
- ☐ Chronic pulmonary obstructive disease (COPD)
- ☐ Acute pumonary embolism

255

- ☐ Right ventricular hypertrophy/ cor pulmonale
- ☐ Left ventricular hypertrophy
- ☐ Pericarditis
- ☐ Chronic pulmonary obstructive disease (COPD)
- ☐ Acute pumonary embolism

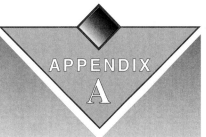

Methods of Determining the QRS Axis

Methods of Determining the QRS Axis

Method A: The Two-lead Method

Method B: The Three-lead Method

Method C: The Four-lead Method

Method D: The Six-lead Method

Method E: The "Perpendicular" Method

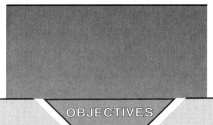

OBJECTIVES

Upon completion of all or part of this chapter you should be able to complete the following objectives indicated by your instructor:

☐ **1.** Describe in detail the steps in determining the QRS axis using one or more of the following methods:

☐ The Two-lead Method (Leads I and II)

☐ The Three-lead Method (Leads I, II, and aVF)

☐ The Four-lead Method (Leads I, II, III, and aVF)

☐ The Six-lead Method (Leads I, II, III, aVR, aVL, and aVF)

☐ The "Perpendicular" Method

Methods of Determining the QRS Axis

Various methods of determining the approximate position of the QRS axis in the frontal plane are available using the hexaxial reference figure. The methods presented in the following section are listed below.

Method A: The Two-lead Method. This method uses **leads I** and **II** to make a rapid determination of whether the QRS axis is normal or abnormally deviated to the left of right. This is one of the fastest methods in determining the QRS axis. It is especially useful in the emergency situation to spot left axis deviation since the perpendicular of lead II lies on the $-30°$ axis.

Method B: The Three-lead Method. This method uses **leads I, II,** and **aVF** to make a rapid approximation of whether the QRS axis is normal or abnormally deviated to the left or right. The positivity or negativity of **leads I** and **aVF** are determined first to determine in which of the four quadrants the QRS axis lies. Then, determining the positivity or negativity of **lead II** helps to place the QRS axis in quadrant I or III within a 30° to 60° arc.

Method C: The Four-lead Method. This method uses **leads I, II, III,** and **aVF,** and, sometimes, **aVR** in certain circumstances, to make a rapid determination of the QRS axis within a 30° arc.

Method D: The Six-lead Method. This method uses **leads I** and **aVF** to determine in which quadrant the QRS axis lies. Then, depending on which quadrant the QRS axis lies in, **leads II** and **aVR** or **leads III** and **aVL** are used to determine the position of the QRS axis in the quadrant, within a 30° arc. This method is probably too slow for use in an emergency situation.

Method E: The "Perpendicular" Method. This method is a rapid determination of the QRS axis based on the perpendicular of a bipolar or unipolar limb lead with an equiphasic QRS complex, if one is present.

Method A: The Two-lead Method.

The **Two-lead Method** uses **leads I** and **II** to determine the general position of the QRS axis and to identify left axis deviation quickly.

Determine the net **positivity** or **negativity** of the QRS complexes in **leads I** and **II.**

If **lead I** is **positive,** and:

    A. **Lead II** is **predominantly positive,** the QRS axis is between $-30°$ and $+90°$.

    B. **Lead II** is **equiphasic,** the QRS axis is exactly $-30°$.

    C. **Lead II** is **predominantly negative,** the QRS axis is between $-30°$ and $-90°$.

If **lead I** is **negative** and:

    D. **Lead II** is **predominantly positive,** the QRS axis is between $+90°$ and $+150°$.

    E. **Lead II** is **equiphasic,** the QRS axis is exactly $+150°$.

    F. **Lead II** is **predominantly negative,** the QRS axis is greater than $+150°$.

Leads		Location of
I	**II**	**QRS Axis**
+	+	$-30°$ to $+90°$
+	±	$-30°$
+	−	$-30°$ to $-90°$
−	+	$+90°$ to $+150°$
−	±	$+150°$
−	−	$>+150°$

+ = Predominantly positive   ± = Equiphasic
− = Predominantly negative

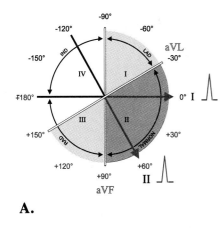

A.

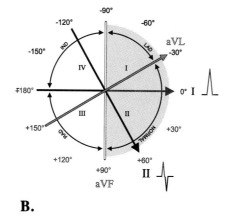

B.

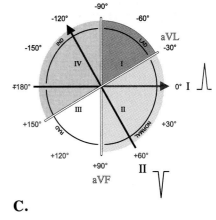

C.

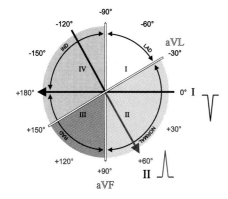

D.

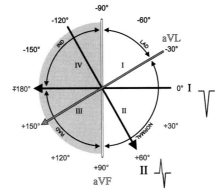

E.

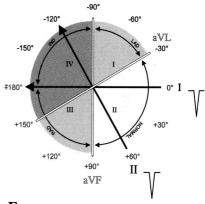

F.

Method B: The Three-lead Method

The **Three-lead Method** uses **leads I, II,** and **aVF,** and, sometimes, **aVR** in certain circumstances, to determine the general position of the QRS axis and to identify left and right axis deviation quickly.

Leads				Location of
I	aVF	II	aVR	QRS Axis
+	+	+		0° to +90°
+	−	+		0° to −30°
+	−	±		−30°
+	−	−		−30° to −90°
±	−	−		−90°
±	+	+		+90°
−	+	+		+90° to +150°
−	+	+	+	+120° to +150°
−	+	±		+150°
−	−	−		−90° to −180°

+ = Predominantly positive   ± = Equiphasic
− = Predominantly negative

Determine the net **positivity** or **negativity** of the QRS complexes in **leads I, aVF,** and **II,** in that order, and also **aVR** if lead I is negative.

If **lead I** is **positive,** and:

A. **Leads aVF** and **II** are **predominantly positive,** the QRS axis is between **0°** and **+90°.**

B. **Lead aVF** is **predominantly negative,** and **lead II, predominantly positive,** the QRS axis is between **0°** and **−30°.**

C. **Lead aVF** is **predominantly negative,** and **lead II, equiphasic,** the QRS axis is exactly **−30°.**

D. **Leads aVF** and **II** are **predominantly negative,** the QRS axis is between **−30°** and **−90°.**

If **Lead I** is **equiphasic** and:

E. **Leads aVF** and **II** are **predominantly negative,** the QRS axis is exactly **−90°.**

F. **Leads aVF** and **II** are **predominantly positive,** the QRS axis is exactly **+90°.**

If **Lead I** is **negative** and:

G.a. **Leads aVF** and **II** are **predominantly positive,** the QRS axis is between **+90°** and **+150°.**

b. If, in addition, **aVR** is also **predominantly positive,** the QRS axis is between **+120°** and **+150°.**

H. **Lead aVF** is **predominantly positive,** and **lead II, equiphasic,** the QRS axis is exactly **+150°.**

I. **Leads aVF** and **II** are **predominantly negative,** the QRS axis is between **−90°** and **−180°.**

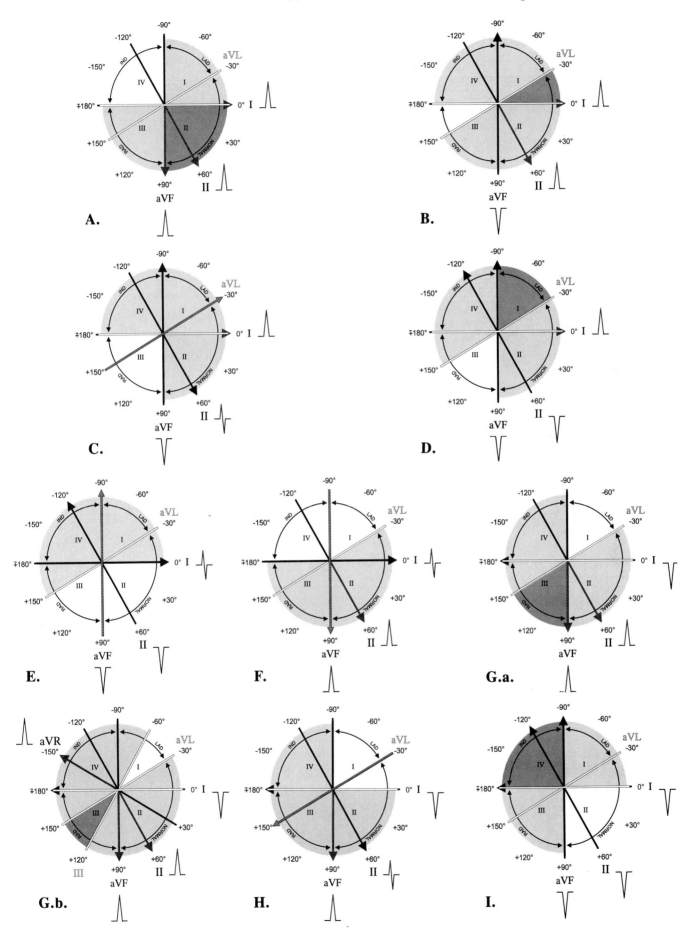

Method C: The Four-lead Method

The **Four-lead Method** uses **leads I, II, III,** and **aVF,** and, sometimes, **aVR** in certain circumstances, to determine the QRS axis within 30°.

		Leads			Location of
I	III	aVF	II	aVR	QRS Axis
+	+	+	+		+30° to +90°
+	−	+	+		0° to +30°
+	−	−	+		0° to −30°
+	−	−	±		−30°
+	−	−	−		−30° to −90°
±	−	−	−		−90°
±	+	+	+		+90°
−	+	+	+		+90° to +150°
−	+	+	+	+	+120° to +150°
−	+	+	±		+150°
−	−	−	−		−90° to −150°

+ = Predominantly positive   ± = Equiphasic
− = Predominantly negative

Determine the net **positivity** or **negativity** of the QRS complexes in **leads I, III, aVF,** and **II,** in that order, and also **aVR** if lead I is negative.

If **lead I** is **positive,** and:

A. **Leads III, aVF,** and **II** are **predominantly positive,** the QRS axis is between **+30°** and **+90°.**

B. **Lead III** is **predominantly negative,** and leads **aVF** and **II,** predominantly positive, the QRS axis is between **0°** and **+30°.**

C. **Leads III** and **aVF** are **predominantly negative,** and **lead II,** predominantly positive, the QRS axis is between **0°** and **−30°.**

D. **Leads III** and **aVF** are **predominantly negative,** and **lead II, equiphasic,** the QRS axis is exactly **−30°.**

E. **Leads III, aVF,** and **II** are **predominantly negative,** the QRS axis is between **−30°** and **−90°.**

If **lead I** is **equiphasic** and:

F. **Leads III, aVF,** and **II** are **predominantly negative,** the QRS axis is exactly **−90°.**

G. **Leads III, aVF,** and **II** are **predominantly positive,** the QRS axis is exactly **+90°.**

If **lead I** is **negative** and:

H.a. **Leads III, aVF,** and **II** are **predominantly positive,** the QRS axis is between **+90°** and **+150°.**

  b. If, in addition, **aVR** is also **predominantly positive,** the QRS axis is between **+120°** and **+150°.**

I. **Leads III** and **aVF** are **predominantly positive,** and **lead II, equiphasic,** the QRS axis is exactly **+150°.**

J. **Leads III, aVF,** and **II** are **predominantly negative,** the QRS axis is between **−90°** and **−150°.**

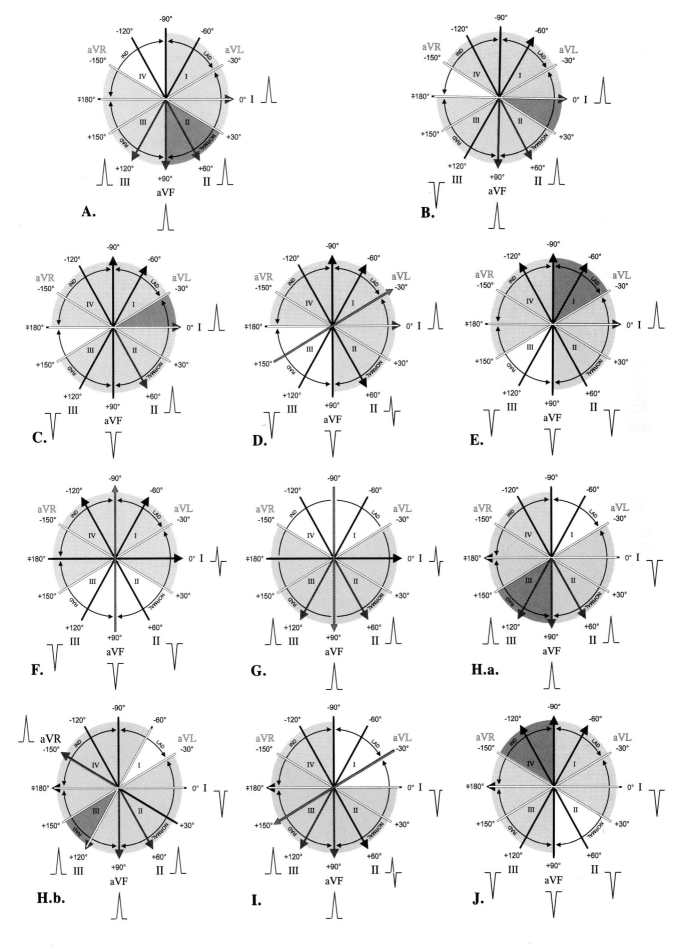

Method D: The Six-lead Method

The two-step **Six-lead Method** uses **leads I** and **aVF** in **Step 1** to determine in which quadrant the QRS axis lies. Then, in **Step 2,** depending on the quadrant initially determined, **leads II** and **aVR** or **leads III** and **aVL** are used to determine the 30° arc in which the QRS axis lies.

Step 1. Determine the quadrant in which the QRS axis lies.

Determine the net **positivity** or **negativity** of the QRS complexes in **leads I** and **aVF.**

If **lead I** is **positive,** and:

A. **Lead aVF** is **predominantly positive,** the QRS axis is in **quadrant II (0° to +90°).**

B. **Lead aVF** is **equiphasic,** the QRS axis is exactly **0°.**

C. **Lead aVF** is **predominantly negative,** the QRS axis is in **quadrant I (0° to −90°).**

If **lead I** is **equiphasic** and:

D. **Lead aVF** is **predominantly positive,** the QRS axis is exactly **+90°.**

E. **Lead aVF** is **predominantly negative,** the QRS axis is exactly **−90°.**

If **lead I** is **negative** and:

F. **Lead aVF** is **predominantly positive,** the QRS axis is in **quadrant III (+90° to +180°).**

G. **Lead aVF** is **equiphasic,** the QRS axis is exactly **±180°.**

H. **Lead aVF** is **predominantly negative,** the QRS axis is in **quadrant IV (−90° to −180°).**

| Leads | | Location of |
I	aVF	QRS Axis
+	−	I (0° to −90°)
+	±	0°
+	+	II (0° to +90°)
±	−	−90°
±	+	+90°
−	+	III (+90° to +180°)
−	±	±180°
−	−	IV (−90° to −180°)

+ = Predominantly positive   ± = Equiphasic
− = Predominantly negative

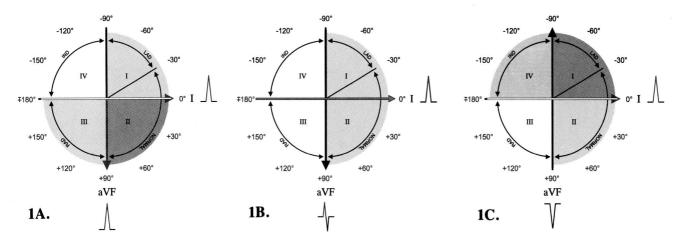

1A.

1B.

1C.

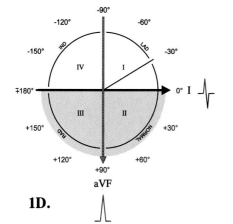

1D.

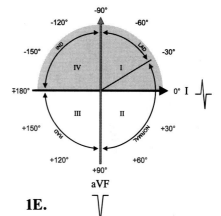

1E.

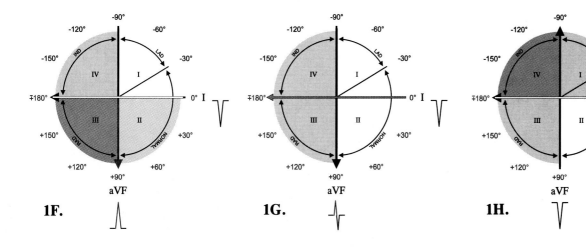

1F.

1G.

1H.

Step 2. Determine the placement of the QRS axis in the quadrant in which it lies to within a 30° arc.

If the QRS axis lies in quadrant I (0° to −90°):

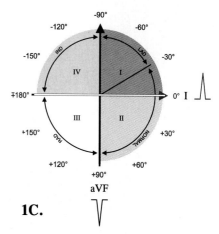

1C.

Determine the net **positivity** or **negativity** of the QRS complexes in **leads II** and **aVR**.

If **lead II** is **positive,** and:

A. **Lead aVR** is **predominantly negative,** the QRS axis is between **0°** and **−30°.**

If **lead II** is **equiphasic:**

B. The QRS axis is exactly **−30°.**

If **lead II** is **negative** and:

C. **Lead aVR** is **predominantly negative,** the QRS axis is between **−30°** and **−60°.**

D. **Lead aVR** is **equiphasic,** the QRS axis is exactly **−60°.**

E. **Lead aVR** is **predominantly positive,** the QRS axis is between **−60°** and **−90°.**

| Leads | | Location of |
II	aVR	QRS Axis
+		0° to −30°
−		−30° to −90°
	−	0° to −60°
	+	−60° to −90°
+	−	0° to −30°
±	−	**−30°**
−	−	−30° to −60°
−	±	**−60°**
−	+	−60° to −90°

+ = Predominantly positive   ± = Equiphasic
− = Predominantly negative

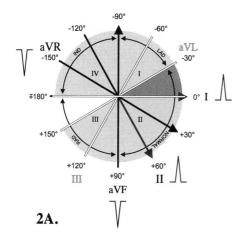

2A.

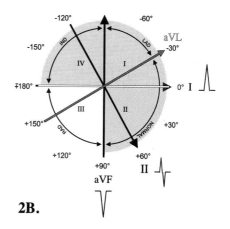

2B.

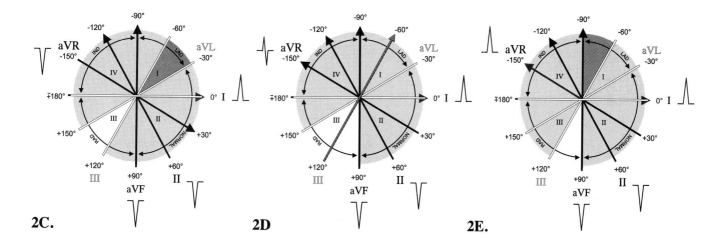

2C.

2D

2E.

Step 2. (Cont.)

If the QRS axis lies in quadrant II (0° to +90°):

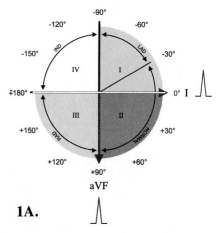

1A.

Determine the net **positivity** or **negativity** of the QRS complexes in **leads III** and **aVL.**

If **lead III** is **positive,** and:

F. **Lead aVL** is **predominantly positive,** the QRS axis is between **+30°** and **+60°.**

G. **Lead aVL** is **equiphasic,** the QRS axis is exactly **+60°.**

H. **Lead aVL** is **predominantly negative,** the QRS axis is between **+60°** and **+90°.**

If **lead III** is **equiphasic** and:

I. **Lead aVL** is **predominantly positive,** the QRS axis is exactly **+30°.**

If **Lead III** is **negative** and:

J. **Lead aVL** is **predominantly positive,** the QRS axis is between **0°** and **+30°.**

Leads		Location of
III	**aVL**	**QRS Axis**
−		0° to +30°
+		+30° to +90°
	+	0° to +60°
	−	+60° to +90°
−	+	0° to +30°
±	+	**+30°**
+	+	+30° to +60°
+	±	**+60°**
+	−	+60° to +90°

+ = Predominantly positive   ± = Equiphasic
− = Predominantly negative

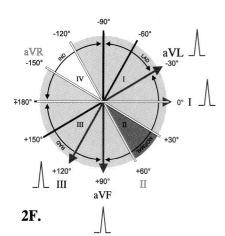

2F.

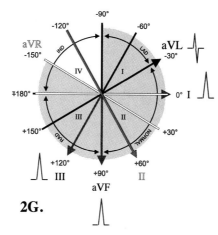

2G.

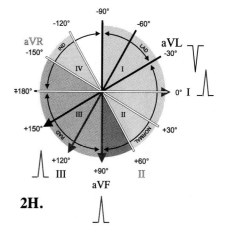

2H.

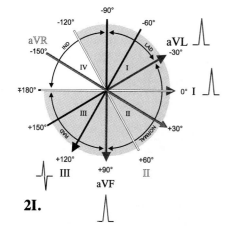

2I.

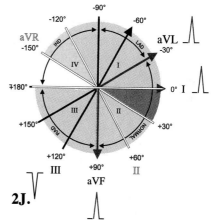

2J.

Step 2. (Cont.)

If the QRS axis lies in quadrant III (+90° to +180°):

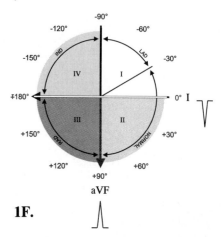

1F.

Determine the net **positivity** or **negativity** of the QRS complexes in **leads II** and **aVR.**

If **lead II** is **positive,** and:

K. **Lead aVR** is **predominantly negative,** the QRS axis is between **+90°** and **+120°.**

L. **Lead aVR** is **equiphasic,** the QRS axis is exactly **+120°.**

M. **Lead aVR** is **predominantly positive,** the QRS axis is between **+120°** and **+150°.**

If **lead II** is **equiphasic:**

N. The QRS axis is exactly **+150°.**

If **lead II** is **negative** and:

O. **Lead aVR** is **predominantly positive,** the QRS axis is between **+150°** and **+180°.**

Leads		Location of
II	**aVR**	**QRS Axis**
+		+90° to +150°
−		+150° to +180°
	−	+90° to +120°
	+	+120° to +180°
+	−	+90° to +120°
+	±	**+120°**
+	+	+120° to +150°
±	+	**+150°**
−	+	+150° to +180°

+ = Predominantly positive　± = Equiphasic
− = Predominantly negative

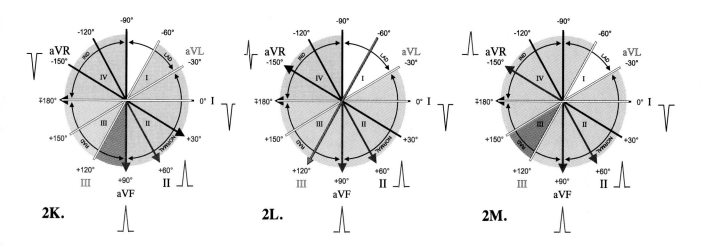

2K.

2L.

2M.

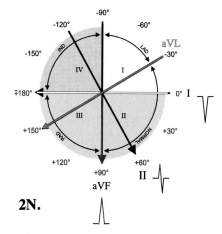

2N.

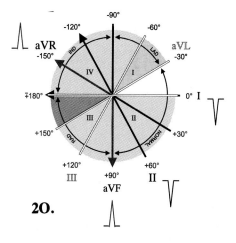

2O.

Step 2. (Cont.)

If the QRS axis lies in quadrant IV (−90° to −180°):

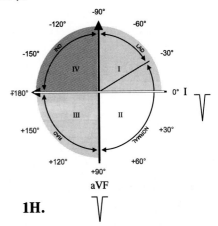

1H.

Determine the net **positivity** or **negativity** of the QRS complexes in **leads III** and **aVL.**

If **lead III** is **positive,** and:

P. Lead **aVL** is **predominantly negative,** the QRS axis is between **−150°** and **−180°.**

If **lead III** is **equiphasic:**

Q. The QRS axis is exactly **−150°.**

If **lead III** is **negative** and:

R. Lead **aVL** is **predominantly negative,** the QRS axis is between **−120°** and **−150°.**

S. Lead **aVL** is **equiphasic,** the QRS axis is exactly **−120°.**

T. Lead **aVL** is **predominantly positive,** the QRS axis is between **−90°** and **−120°.**

Leads		Location of
III	**aVL**	**QRS Axis**
+		− 150° to − 180°
−		− 90° to − 150°
	−	− 120° to − 180°
	+	− 90° to − 120°
+	−	− 150° to − 180°
±	−	**− 150°**
−	−	− 120° to − 150°
−	±	**− 120°**
−	+	− 90° to − 120°

+ = Predominantly positive   ± = Equiphasic
− = Predominantly negative

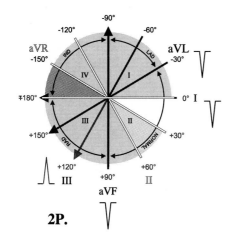

2P.

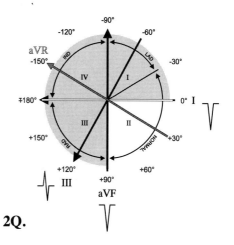

2Q.

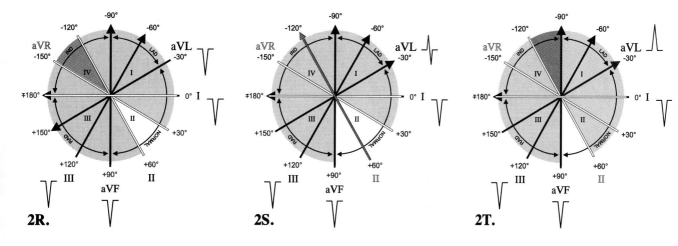

2R.

2S.

2T.

Method E: The "Perpendicular" Method

The **"Perpendicular" Method** uses the perpendicular of a lead with equiphasic or almost equiphasic QRS complexes to determine the position of the QRS axis.

Step 1. Identify the lead with **equiphasic (or almost equiphasic)** QRS complexes, and label it **"A"** on the hexaxial reference figure.

AND

Determine the **perpendicular** to this lead, and label it **"B."**

Step 2. Identify the lead axis that lies **parallel** to the **perpendicular "B,"** and label it **"C."**

AND

Determine whether the QRS complexes in the **lead represented by the lead axis "C"** are predominantly **positive** or **negative.**

Step 3. **If the QRS complexes are predominantly positive in the lead represented by lead axis "C,"** the QRS axis lies in the direction of the positive pole of **lead axis "C."**

Step 4. **If the QRS complexes are predominantly negative in the lead represented by lead axis "C,"** the QRS axis lies in the direction of the negative pole of **lead axis "C."**

Lead "A"	Lead Axis "C"*	Poles of Lead Axis "C" +	−
I	aVF	+90°	−90°
II	aVL	−30°	+150°
III	aVR	−150°	+30°
aVR	III	+120°	−60°
aVL	II	+60°	−120°
aVF	I	0°	±180°

*Lead "C" is parallel to perpendicular "B" of equiphasic lead "A."

Step 1.

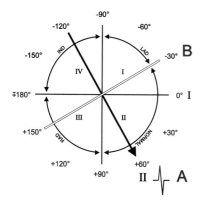

Step 2.

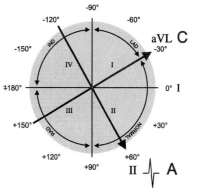

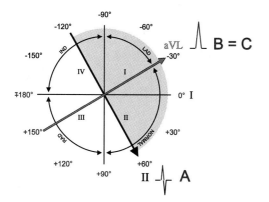

Step 3.

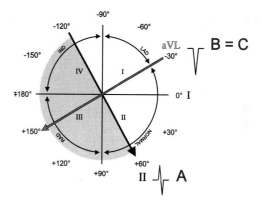

Step 4.

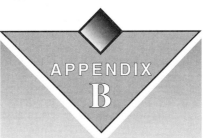

Chapter Review Questions
Answer Keys

CHAPTER 1

1.(B) The inner layer of the serous pericardium is called the visceral pericardium or **epicardium.**

2.(C) The **right** heart pumps blood into the **pulmonary** circulation (the blood vessels within the lungs and those carrying blood to and from the lungs). The **left** heart pumps blood into the **systemic** circulation (the blood vessels in the rest of the body and those carrying blood to and from the body).

3.(A) The right ventricle pumps unoxygenated blood through the **pulmonic** valve and into the lungs through the **pulmonary** artery. In the lungs, the blood picks up oxygen and releases excess carbon dioxide.

4.(C) The period of relaxation and filling of the ventricles with blood is called **ventricular diastole.**

5.(B) The electrical conduction system of the heart is composed of the following structures: the SA node, internodal atrial conduction tract, AV junction, bundle branches, and the Purkinje network. The **coronary sinus** is not a component of the electrical conduction system.

6.(A) **Conductivity** is the ability of cardiac cells to conduct electrical impulses.

7.(D) When a myocardial cell is in the resting state a high concentration of **positively** charged **sodium** ions (Na +) (cations) is present outside the cell.

8.(B) Cardiac cells cannot be stimulated to depolarize during the **absolute refractory period** because they have not sufficiently repolarized.

9.(C) The **SA node** is normally the dominant and primary pacemaker of the heart because it possesses the highest level of automaticity.

10.(B) **Reentry** is a condition in which the progression of an electrical impulse is delayed or blocked in one or more segments of the electrical conduction system while being conducted normally through the rest of the electrical conduction system.

CHAPTER 2

1.(D) When electrical activity of the heart is not being detected, the ECG is a **straight flat line,** referred to as the **baseline** or **isoelectric line.**

2.(B) The sensitivity of the ECG machine is calibrated so that a **1 millivolt** electrical signal produces a **10 mm** deflection on the ECG, equivalent to two large squares on the ECG paper.

3.(A) An ECG lead composed of a single positive electrode and a zero reference point (the central terminal) is called a **unipolar lead.**

4.(C) If the positive ECG electrode is attached to the left leg or lower left anterior chest, all the electric currents generated in the heart which flow toward the positive electrode will be recorded as **positive (upright)** deflections. The electric currents flowing away from the positive electrode will be recorded as negative (inverted) deflections.

5.(C) A lead obtained using a positive electrode and a central terminal is called a unipolar lead. Unipolar leads include the three augmented leads (aVR, aVL, aVF) and the six precordial leads (V_1, V_2, V_3, V_4, V_5, V_6).

6.(B) & 7.(D) The placement of the positive chest electrode is as follows:

V_1 - right side of the sternum in the fourth intercostal space

V_2 - **left side of the sternum in the fourth intercostal space**

V_3 - midway between V_2 and V_4

V_4 - **midclavicular line in the fifth intercostal space**

V_5 - anterior axillary line at the same level as V_4

V_6 - midaxillary line at the same level as V_4

8.(C) Leads II, III, and aVF face the **inferior** or diaphragmatic surface of the heart.

9.(D) Left axis deviation with a QRS axis greater than $-30°$ occurs in adults in the following cardiac disorders:
- left ventricular enlargement and hypertrophy
- **hypertension**
- **aortic stenosis**
- **ischemic heart disease**
- left bundle branch block and left anterior fascicular block

10.(A) A QRS axis **greater than $+90°$** (right axis deviation) occurs in adults with the following cardiac and pulmonary disorders:
- COPD
- pulmonary embolism
- congenital heart disease
- cor pulmonale
- severe pulmonary hypertension

CHAPTER 3

1.(D) Increased left atrial pressure and left atrial dilatation and hypertrophy as found in **hypertension, mitral and aortic valvular disease, acute MI,** and pulmonary edema secondary to left heart failure may cause wide, notched P waves.

2.(C) The normal PR interval is between **0.12 and 0.20 second.**

3.(C) An ectopic P wave represents atrial depolarization occurring in an **abnormal direction** or **sequence** or both.

4.(B) A normal QRS complex represents normal **depolarization of the ventricles.**

5.(A) The time from the onset of the QRS complex to the peak of the R wave is the **ventricular activation time** (VAT). The VAT represents the time taken for depolarization of the interventricular septum plus depolarization of the ventricle from the endocardium to the epicardium under the facing lead.

6.(B) Aberrant ventricular conduction may occur in the following supraventricular arrhythmias:
- **PACs**
- PJCs
- Nonparoxysmal atrial tachycardia
- **Paroxysmal atrial tachycardia**
- Atrial flutter
- Atrial fibrillation
- Nonparoxysmal junctional tachycardia
- Paroxysmal junctional tachycardia

7.(C) Abnormal ventricular repolarization (the **T** wave) may result from myocardial ischemia, acute MI, myocarditis, pericarditis, ventricular enlargement (hypertrophy), electrolyte imbalance (e.g., excess serum potassium), or administration of certain cardiac drugs (e.g., quinidine, procainamide).

8.(B) An abnormally tall U wave may be present in **hypokalemia, cardiomyopathy,** left ventricular hypertrophy, and diabetes and may follow administration of digitalis, quinidine, and procainamide.

9.(D) A **prolonged PR interval** (one that is greater in duration than 0.20 second) indicates that a delay of progression of the electrical impulse through the AV node, bundle of His, or, rarely, the bundle branches is present.

10.(A) An abnormal ST segment indicates **abnormal ventricular repolarization,** a common consequence of myocardial ischemia and acute MI. It is also present in ventricular fibrosis or aneurysm, pericarditis, left ventricular enlargement (hypertrophy), and administration of digitalis.

CHAPTER 4

1.(D) The heart rate can be determined by the **six-second count method,** a **heart rate calculator ruler,** the **R-R interval method,** or the triplicate method.

2.(C) In adults, a heart rate less than **60** beats per minute indicates a **bradycardia;** a heart rate greater than **100** beats per minute, a **tachycardia.**

3.(C) When using both the **triplicate** method and the **R-R interval** method of determining the heart rate, the rhythm must be regular or else the calculated rate could be inaccurate.

4.(B) The heart rate is **75** beats per minute. Provided the ECG has a regular rate, one method to determine the rate is to count the large squares (0.20 second squares) between the peaks of two consecutive **R** waves and divide this number into 300.

5.(D) The rate of the P waves is usually **the same as that of the QRS complexes,** but it may be **sometimes less:** if an AV block is present, it may be **greater.**

6.(A) If QRS complexes are present but do not regularly precede or follow the P waves, **a complete AV block (third-degree AV block) is present.** Another term used to describe the condition when QRS complexes occur totally unrelated to the P, P' or F waves is atrioventricular (AV) dissociation.

7.(B) If atrial flutter or fibrillation waves are present, the electrical impulses responsible for them have originated in the **atria.**

8.(D) If the P waves are inverted in lead II, the electrical impulses responsible for the P waves most likely have originated in the **lower atria,** the **AV junction,** or the **ventricles.**

9.(A) If the QRS complexes are 0.10 second or less in duration, the electrical impulses responsible for the QRS complexes most likely have originated in the **SA node,** atria, or AV junction.

10.(D) Bizarre appearing QRS complexes with a duration greater than 0.12 second most likely have a pacemaker site in the distal part of a bundle branch, the **Purkinje network,** or the **ventricular myocardium.** The pacemaker site of such abnormal QRS complexes may also be in the SA node, atria, **AV junction,** or the upper part of a bundle branch **in the presence of a bundle branch block or aberrant ventricular conduction.**

CHAPTER 5

1.(B) Typically, the heart rate **increases** during inspiration and **decreases** during expiration.

2.(C) The most common type of sinus arrhythmia, the one related to respiration, is a normal **phenomenon commonly seen in** children, **young adults,** and elderly individuals. It is caused by the inhibitory vagal effect of respiration on the SA node.

3.(D) Another less common type of sinus arrhythmia is not related to respiration. It may occur in healthy individuals but is more commonly found in adult patients **with heart disease** or **acute MI** and in those **on digitalis** or morphine.

4.(A) An arrhythmia originating in the SA node with a regular rate of less than 60 beats per minute is called **sinus bradycardia.**

5.(D) Sinus bradycardia may be caused by **excessive inhibitory vagal tone on the SA node, decrease in sympathetic tone on the SA node,** and **hypothermia,** among other things.

6.(C) An asymptomatic bradycardia has a heart beat of **50 to 59** beats per minute.

7.(B) A patient with marked sinus bradycardia who is symptomatic will likely have **hypotension and decreased cerebral perfusion.**

8.(B) Symptomatic sinus bradycardia must be promptly treated with **atropine and transcutaneous pacing.**

9.(C) **Sinus arrest** is an arrhythmia caused by episodes of failure in the automaticity of the SA node resulting in bradycardia or asystole.

10.(D) Sinoatrial (SA) exit block may result from toxicity of such medication as **quinidine, digitalis,** and **propranolol.**

CHAPTER 6

1.(B) An arrhythmia originating in pacemakers that shift back and forth between the SA node and an ectopic pacemaker in the atria or AV junction is called a **wandering atrial pacemaker.** It is characterized by P waves of varying size, shape and direction in any given lead.

2.(D) The arrhythmia described in question number 1 may normally be seen in **the very young, the elderly,** and **athletes.**

3.(C) An extra atrial contraction consisting of an abnormal P wave followed by a normal or abnormal QRS complex, occurring earlier than the next beat of the underlying rhythm, is called **a premature atrial contraction.** It is usually followed by a noncompensatory pause.

4.(B) A nonconducted or blocked PAC is **a P' wave that is not followed by a QRS complex.**

5.(A) The QRS complex of the PAC usually resembles that of **the underlying rhythm.**

6.(B) Two PACs in a row are called **a couplet.**

7.(C) The electrophysiologic mechanism responsible for PACs is **enhanced automaticity** and **reentry.**

8.(D) An arrhythmia originating in an ectopic pacemaker in the atria or the site of a rapid reentry circuit in the AV node with a rate between 160 and 240 beats per minute is called **atrial tachycardia.**

9.(D) The reduction in cardiac output accompanying atrial tachycardia can cause **syncope, lightheadedness,** and **dizziness.** In patients with coronary artery disease, it can also cause angina, congestive heart failure, or an acute MI.

10.(B) Atrial flutter is characterized by **flutter waves with a sawtooth appearance.**

CHAPTER 7

1.(C) Absent P′ waves in junctional arrhythmias indicate that either **retrograde atrial depolarizations occurred during the QRS complexes** or **atrial depolarizations have not occurred because of a retrograde AV block** between the ectopic pacemaker site in the AV junction and the atria.

2.(C) If the ectopic pacemaker in the AV junction discharges too soon after the preceding QRS complex, **the premature P′ wave may not be followed by a QRS complex.**

3.(B) An extra contraction that originates in an ectopic pacemaker in the AV junction, occurring before the next expected beat of the underlying rhythm, is called **a premature junctional contraction** or PJC.

4.(D) The QRS complex of a PJC **usually resembles that of the underlying rhythm,** being 0.10 second or less in duration. The QRS complex, however, may be 0.12 second or greater in duration and **resemble that of a premature ventricular contraction if aberrant ventricular conduction is present.** The QRS complex may **precede or follow the P′ wave with which it is associated.**

5.(B) Two PJCs in a row are called a **couplet.**

6.(D) PJCs are caused by **increased parasympathetic tone on the SA node,** congestive heart failure, damage to the AV junction, **sympathomimetic drugs, digitalis toxicity,** and an excessive dose of certain cardiac drugs like quinidine or procainamide.

7.(D) More than four to six PJCs per minute may indicate an **enhanced automaticity or a reentry mechanism in the AV junction** and **that more serious junctional arrhythmias may occur.**

8.(C) An arrhythmia originating in an escape pacemaker in the AV junction with a rate of 40 to 60 beats per minute is called a **junctional escape rhythm.**

9.(D) An arrhythmia consisting of narrow QRS complexes occurring at a rate of 55 beats per minute and P waves occurring independently at a slower rate is a **junctional escape rhythm— a supraventricular arrhythmia.** The presence of P waves occurring independently of the QRS complexes indicates the presence of **atrioventricular (AV) dissociation.**

10.(B) The usual treatment for a symptomatic junctional escape rhythm is **transcutaneous pacing.**

CHAPTER 8

1.(C) An extra contraction consisting of an abnormally wide and bizarre QRS complex originating in an ectopic pacemaker in the ventricles is called a **PVC.**

2.(B) Premature ventricular contractions that originate from a single ectopic pacemaker site are called **unifocal.**

3.(C) A PVC may **trigger ventricular fibrillation if it occurs on the T wave** or **depolarize the SA node, momentarily suppressing it, so that the next P wave of the underlying rhythm appears later than expected.**

4.(A) A PVC which appears relatively normal usually originates **near the bifurcation of the bundle of His.**

5.(C) A QRS that has characteristics of both the PVC and a QRS complex of the underlying rhythm is called a **ventricular fusion beat.**

6.(D) Groups of two or more PVCs are called **ventricular group beats, bursts,** and **salvos.**

7.(D) A reentry mechanism may precipitate **repetitive ventricular contractions, ventricular tachycardia,** or **ventricular fibrillation.**

8.(A) PVCs may occur in healthy persons with apparently healthy hearts and without apparent cause. PVCs, especially if they are frequent, may be caused by an increase in catecholamines and sympathetic tone (as in emotional stress), an increase in vagal (parasympathetic) tone, **stimulants** (e.g., alcohol, caffeine and tobacco), excessive administration of digitalis or sympathomimetic drugs (e.g., epinephrine, isoproterenol, and norepinephrine), hypoxia, acidosis, hypokalemia, congestive heart failure, or acute MI.

9.(B) A form of ventricular tachycardia characterized by QRS complexes that gradually change back and forth from one shape and direction to another over a series of beats is called **torsade de pointes.**

10.(C) When the ventricles contract between 300 and 500 times a minute in an unsynchronized, uncoordinated manner the immediate treatment is **defibrillation.**

CHAPTER 9

1.(C) An arrhythmia that occurs commonly in acute inferior myocardial infarction because of the effect of an increase in vagal tone and ischemia on the AV node is called a **first-degree AV block.**

2.(B) An arrhythmia in which there is a progressive delay following each P wave in the conduction of electrical impulses through the AV node until the conduction of the electrical impulses is completley blocked is called a **second-degree, type I AV block** or Wenckebach block.

3.(A) Second-degree, type I AV block is usually transient and reversible and asymptomatic, yet the patient should be monitored and observed because **it can progress to a higher degree AV block.**

4.(C) An arrhythmia in which a complete block of conduction of electrical impulses occurs in one bundle branch and an intermittent block in the other is called a **second-degree, type II AV block.**

5.(A) If a second-degree, type II AV block presents in the setting of an acute anteroseptal MI, the immediate treatment is **a transcutaneous pacemaker.**

6.(D) A high-degree or advanced AV block has an AV conduction ratio of **3 : 1 or greater,** i.e., 3 : 1, 4 : 1, 6 : 1, 8 : 1, or greater.

7.(C) The absence of conduction of electrical impulses through the AV node, bundle of His, or bundle branches, characterized by independent beating of the atria and ventricles, is called a **third-degree AV block.**

8.(D) An escape pacemaker in the AV junction has an inherent firing rate of **40 to 60** beats per minute.

9.(B) If an AV junctional or ventricular escape pacemaker does not take over after a sudden onset of third-degree AV block, ventricular asystole will occur. This is called an **Adams-Stokes syndrome.**

10.(A) A pacemaker that senses spontaneous occurring P waves and QRS complexes, and paces the atria when P waves fail to appear and paces the ventricles when QRS complexes fail to appear after spontaneously occurring or paced P waves, is called an **optimal sequential pacemaker.**

CHAPTER 10

1.(C) The time from the onset of the QRS complex to the peak of the R wave in the QRS complex is called **the ventricular activation time** (VAT) or **the preintrinsicoid deflection.**

2.(C) The anterior portion of the septum is supplied with blood from the **left anterior descending coronary artery.**

3.(B) The main blood supply of the AV node and proximal part of the bundle of His is the AV node artery which arises from the **right coronary artery** in 85 to 90 percent of the hearts. In the rest of the hearts, the AV node artery arises from the left circumflex coronary artery.

4.(D) Common causes of bundle branch and fascicular blocks are cardiomyopathy, **ischemic heart disease, idiopathic degenerative disease of the electrical conduction system,** and severe left ventricular hypertrophy.

5.(A) In the setting of an acute MI, an acute right bundle branch block occurs primarily in an **anteroseptal MI,** and rarely in an inferior MI.

6.(A) In patients with an acute MI complicated by a bundle branch block, **the incidence of pump failure and ventricular arrhythmias is much higher** than in those not so complicated.

7.(C) Common causes of chronic right bundle branch blocks are **myocarditis, cardiomyopathy, and cardiac surgery.**

8.(B) In a right bundle branch block with an intact interventricular septum, the QRS complex in lead V_1 is **wide with a classic triphasic rSR' pattern.**

9.(A) When the electrical impulses are prevented from directly entering the anterior and lateral walls of the left ventricle, the condition is called a **left anterior fascicular block.**

10.(C) The electrial impulses are prevented from entering the interventricular septum and posterior wall of the left ventricle directly when the patient has a **left posterior fascicular block.**

CHAPTER 11

1.(B) The artery which arises from the left main coronary artery at an obtuse angle and runs posteriorly along the left atrioventricular groove to end in back of the left ventricle is called the **left circumflex coronary artery.** This is the case in 85 to 90 percent of hearts. In the remaining percentage of hearts, the left circumflex coronary artery continues along the atrioventricular groove to become the posterior descending coronary artery while giving rise to the posterior left ventricular arteries and the AV node artery.

2.(C) The SA node is supplied with blood by the sinoatrial node artery which arises from either **the left circumflex coronary artery** (in 40 to 50 percent of hearts) or **the right coronary artery** (in 50 to 60 percent of hearts).

3.(D) Myocardial ischemia or infarction may be caused by an **occlusion of an atherosclerotic coronary artery, coronary artery spasm, increased myocardial workload,** toxic exposure to cocaine or ethanol, decreased level of oxygen in the blood delivered to the myocardium, and decreased coronary artery blood flow from whatever cause.

4.(A) The most common cause of acute MI (occurring in about 90 percent of acute MIs) is a **coronary thrombosis.**

5.(B) Upon revascularization or reoxygenation, necrotic cells **do not return to normal function.**

6.(C) A myocardial infarction in which the zone of infarction involves the entire full thickness of the ventricular wall, from the endocardium to the epicardial surface, is called a **transmural infarction.**

7.(A) By 6 hours following an acute transmural MI, **only a small percentage of cells remain viable** in the involved myocardium.

8.(C) Inverted or tall peaked T waves in the facing leads during the early phase of an acute MI are an indication of **ischemia.**

9.(D) The most likely cause of an inferior MI is an occlusion of the **posterior left ventricular arteries.**

10.(C) ST segment elevation in **leads V_1-V_4** is diagnostic of an acute anteroseptal MI during the early phase.

CHAPTER 12

1.(C) A chronic condition of the heart characterized by an increase in the thickness of a chamber's myocardial wall secondary to the increase in the size of the muscle fibers is called **hypertrophy.**

2.(B) A patient with mitral valve insufficiency or left heart failure may develop **left atrial and ventricular enlargement.**

3.(D) Left ventricular hypertrophy, a condition usually caused by increased pressure or volume in the left ventricle, is often found in **systemic hypertension, acute MI, mitral insufficiency, hypertrophic cardiomyopathy, and aortic stenosis or insufficiency.**

4.(A) The diagnosis of left ventricular hypertrophy is based upon the ECG characteristics of increased amplitude or depth of the R and S waves in specific limb and precordial leads, **a QRS axis greater than $-15°$,** and ST segment depression (not ST segment elevation).

5.(A) **Pericarditis** is an inflammatory disease directly involving the epicardium with deposition of inflammatory cells and a variable amount of serous, fibrous, purulent, or hemorrhagic exudate within the sac surrounding the heart.

6.(D) Signs and symptoms of pericarditis include **chest pain, dyspnea, weakness, malaise, chills and fever.**

7.(C) In a diffuse pericarditis the ST segment is elevated in **all leads except aVR and V_1.**

8.(D) **Hyperkalemia** is an excess of serum potassium above normal levels of 3.5 to 5.0 milliequivalents per liter (mEq/L).

9.(D) The ECG changes that occur at various levels of excess serum potassium are: **the QRS complexes widen and the T waves become tall; the ST segments disappear and the T waves become peaked; and the PR intervals become prolonged and a "sine wave" QRS-ST-T pattern appears.**

10.(B) A medication normally prescribed to heart patients which when taken in excess causes depression of myocardial contractility, AV block, ventricular asystole, and PVCs is **procainamide.**

CHAPTER 13

1.(C) In a patient with symptomatic bradycardia and an ECG showing a second-degree, type II AV block, you should administer oxygen, start an IV line, and begin **transcutaneous pacing.**

2.(D) Patients with symptomatic sinus tachycardia should be treated with the **appropriate treatment for the underlying cause of the tachycardia** (i.e., anxiety, exercise, pain, fever, congestive heart failure, hypoxemia, hypovolemia, hypotension, or shock).

3.(A) If a patient is stable with an ECG showing PSVT after administering oxygen and starting an IV line, you should **attempt vagal maneuvers.** Make sure to verify the absence of known carotid artery disease or carotid bruits before attempting carotid sinus massage.

4.(C) Your patient presents with chest pain and signs and symptoms of an acute MI. His ECG shows PAT. After administering oxygen and starting an IV line, you should immediately consider delivering **a synchronized countershock of 50 joules.**

5.(B) Your patient is conscious and hemodynamically stable with an ECG indicative of ventricular tachycardia. After administering oxygen and starting an IV, you should **administer a 1 to 1.5 mg/kg bolus of lidocaine.**

6.(A) If your patient in question number 5 begins to complain of chest pain as his blood pressure drops to 70/50 mm Hg, you should immediately deliver **an unsynchronized shock of 100 joules.**

7.(D) Pulseless electrical activity (PEA) is the absence of a detectable pulse and blood pressure in the presence of electrical activity of the heart on the ECG. It may result from a complete absence of ventricular contractions **(electromechanical dissociation [EMD])** or marked decrease in cardiac output because of a variety of causes, such as **hypovolemia, cardiac rupture,** pericardial tamponade, hypothermia, and so forth.

8.(D) PVCs should be treated if they occur in a patient with chest pain or if they **are frequent (six or more per minute), occur in groups of two or more (group beats), have different QRS configurations (multiform),** arise from different ventricular ectopic pacemakers (multifocal), are close coupled, or fall on the T wave (R-on-T phenomenon).

9.(C) In a cardiac arrest when you are having difficulty starting a peripheral IV and your patient has just been defibrillated three times, you should **administer epinephrine at 2 to 2.5 times the normal dose down the ET tube.**

10.(D) If you suspect asystole, you should **confirm the arrhythmia in two ECG leads, consider delivering three defibrillation shocks if asystole cannot be definitely confirmed, consider transcutaneous pacing after confirming the presence of asystole,** and continue CPR as necessary, all in this order.

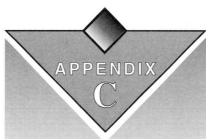

Self-Assessment Answer Keys

I. Arrhythmias

1. **Rate:** 126 beats/minute.*
   Rhythm: Irregular.
   P Waves: None; fine atrial fibrillation waves are present.
   PR Int: None.
   QRS: 0.10 second.
   Intrp: Atrial fibrillation (fine).

2. **Rate:** 33 beats/minute.
   Rhythm: Irregular.
   P Waves: Present; the first, second, third, and fifth P waves are followed by QRS complexes.
   PR Int: 0.22 to 0.36 second. The PR intervals progressively increase until a QRS complex fails to follow the P wave.
   QRS: 0.10 second.
   Intrp: Sinus rhythm with second-degree, Type I AV block (Wenckebach).

3. **Rate:** 41 beats/minute.
   Rhythm: Irregular.
   P Waves: Present; precede each QRS complex.
   PR Int: 0.16 second.
   QRS: 0.08 second.
   Intrp: Sinus bradycardia with sinus arrhythmia.

4. **Rate:** 170 beats/minute.
   Rhythm: Regular.
   P Waves: Present; precede each QRS complex.
   PR Int: 0.12 second.
   QRS: 0.12 second.
   Intrp: Atrial tachycardia with bundle branch block.

5. **Rate:** 62 beats/minute.
   Rhythm: Irregular.
   P Waves: Present; precede the second, fourth, fifth, sixth, and seventh QRS complexes. The P waves are abnormal (0.16 second in duration and notched).
   PR Int: 0.26 second.
   QRS: 0.12 second (all QRS complexes except the third QRS complex); 0.14 second (third QRS complex).
   Intrp: Sinus rhythm with first-degree AV block, bundle branch block, and an isolated premature ventricular contraction.

6. **Rate:** 107 beats/minute.
   Rhythm: Irregular.
   P Waves: Present; precede all QRS complexes except the fifth, eighth, ninth, and tenth QRS complexes.
   PR Int: 0.16 second.
   QRS: 0.09 to 0.10 second.
   Intrp: Normal sinus rhythm with premature junctional contractions (fifth, eighth, ninth, and tenth QRS complexes) occurring singly and in group beats; the latter may be considered a short episode of paroxysmal junctional tachycardia.

7. **Rate:** 182 beats/minute.
   Rhythm: Regular.
   P Waves: Present; precede each QRS complex.
   PR Int: 0.08 second.
   QRS: 0.09 second.
   Intrp: Atrial tachycardia.

*The heart rates were calculated using R-R interval method 3.

8. **Rate:** Unmeasurable.
   Rhythm: Irregular.
   P Waves: None; coarse ventricular fibrillation waves are present.
   PR Int: None.
   QRS: None.
   Intrp: Ventricular fibrillation (coarse).
9. **Rate:** 89 beats/minute.
   Rhythm: Irregular.
   P Waves: Present; precede all except the third and sixth QRS complexes. The shape and direction of the P waves vary from positive to negative.
   PR Int: 0.14 second.
   QRS: 0.10 second (all QRS complexes except the third and sixth QRS complexes); 0.12 second (third and sixth QRS complexes).
   Intrp: Wandering atrial pacemaker with unifocal premature ventricular contractions. Trigeminy is present in the first part of the tracing.
10. **Rate:** 61 beats/minute.
    Rhythm: Irregular.
    P Waves: Present; precede each QRS complex.
    PR Int: 0.12 second.
    QRS: 0.14 second.
    Intrp: Sinus arrhythmia with bundle branch block.
11. **Rate:** 89 beats/minute.
    Rhythm: Irregular.
    P Waves: Present; precede all QRS complexes except the second and eighth QRS complexes.
    PR Int: 0.18 second.
    QRS: 0.08 second (all QRS complexes except the second and eighth QRS complexes); 0.12 second (second and eighth QRS complexes).
    Intrp: Normal sinus rhythm with isolated unifocal premature ventricular contractions.
12. **Rate:** 145 beats/minute.
    Rhythm: Regular.
    P Waves: Present; precede each QRS complex.
    PR Int: 0.12 second.
    QRS: 0.08 second.
    Intrp: Sinus tachycardia.
13. **Rate:** 87 beats/minute.
    Rhythm: Irregular.
    P Waves: Present; precede each QRS complex.
    PR Int: 0.18 second.
    QRS: 0.05 second.
    Intrp: Sinus arrhythmia.
14. **Rate:** 164 beats/minute.
    Rhythm: Regular.
    P Waves: None.
    PR Int: None.
    QRS: 0.12 second.
    Intrp: Ventricular tachycardia.

15. **Rate:** 74 beats/minute.
    Rhythm: Regular.
    P Waves: Present; precede each QRS complex; shape and direction vary from positive to negative.
    PR Int: 0.08 to 0.12 second.
    QRS: 0.08 second.
    Intrp: Wandering atrial pacemaker.
16. **Rate:** 70 beats/minute (atrial rate: 52 beats/minute).
    Rhythm: Regular.
    P Waves: Present, but have no set relation to the QRS complexes.
    PR Int: None.
    QRS: 0.14 second.
    Intrp: Accelerated idioventricular rhythm with AV dissociation.
17. **Rate:** 83 beats/minute.
    Rhythm: Regular.
    P Waves: Present; precede each QRS complex.
    PR Int: 0.16 second.
    QRS: 0.06 second.
    Intrp: Normal sinus rhythm.
18. **Rate:** 229 beats/minute.
    Rhythm: Regular.
    P Waves: None.
    PR Int: None.
    QRS: 0.12 second.
    Intrp: Ventricular tachycardia.
19. **Rate:** 26 beats/minute.
    Rhythm: Regular.
    P Waves: Present; the first, third, and fifth P waves are followed by QRS complexes. AV conduction ratio is 2:1.
    PR Int: 0.19 second.
    QRS: 0.10 second.
    Intrp: Sinus rhythm with second-degree, 2:1 AV block.
20. **Rate:** 84 beats/minute.
    Rhythm: Regular.
    P Waves: None; atrial flutter waves are present.
    PR Int: None.
    QRS: 0.08 second.
    Intrp: Atrial flutter.
21. **Rate:** 30 beats/minute.
    Rhythm: Regular.
    P Waves: Present; precede each QRS complex.
    PR Int: 0.17 to 0.18 second.
    QRS: 0.12 second.
    Intrp: Sinus bradycardia with bundle branch block.
22. **Rate:** 98 beats/minute.
    Rhythm: Regular.
    P Waves: Present; precede each QRS complex.
    PR Int: About 0.16 second.
    QRS: About 0.19 second.
    Intrp: Normal sinus rhythm with bundle branch block.

23. Rate: 62 beats/minute.
   Rhythm: Irregular.
   P Waves: Present; precede the first, second, third, and fifth QRS complexes.
   PR Int: 0.18 second.
   QRS: 0.12 second.
   Intrp: Normal sinus rhythm with bundle branch block and premature junctional contractions.

24. Rate: 82 beats/minute.
   Rhythm: Regular.
   P Waves: Present; precede each QRS complex. The P waves are abnormally wide.
   PR Int: 0.16 second.
   QRS: 0.16 second.
   Intrp: Normal sinus rhythm with bundle branch block.

25. Rate: 129 beats/minute.
   Rhythm: Irregular.
   P Waves: None; fine atrial fibrillation waves are present.
   PR Int: None.
   QRS: 0.08 second.
   Intrp: Atrial fibrillation (fine).

26. Rate: 31 beats/minute.
   Rhythm: Irregular.
   P Waves: Present; a QRS complex follows the first, fifth, and tenth P waves. AV conduction ratios are 4:1 and 5:1.
   PR Int: 0.34 second.
   QRS: 0.16 second.
   Intrp: Sinus rhythm with second-degree, high-degree AV block and bundle branch block.

27. Rate: 75 beats/minute.
   Rhythm: Regular.
   P Waves: Present; negative P waves precede each QRS complex.
   PR Int: 0.08 second.
   QRS: 0.08 second.
   Intrp: Accelerated junctional rhythm.

28. Rate: 62 beats/minute.
   Rhythm: Irregular. The R-R intervals between the third and fourth QRS complexes and the fifth and sixth QRS complexes are twice the R-R interval of the underlying sinus rhythm.
   P Waves: Present; precede each QRS complex.
   PR Int: 0.18 second.
   QRS: 0.16 second.
   Intrp: Sinus rhythm with sinoatrial (SA) exit block and bundle branch block.

29. Rate: 37 beats/minute.
   Rhythm: Regular.
   P Waves: None; atrial fibrillation waves are present.
   PR Int: None.
   QRS: About 0.24 second.
   Intrp: Atrial fibrillation (fine) with third-degree AV block, bundle branch block, and ventricular escape rhythm. AV dissociation is present.

30. Rate: 60 beats/minute.
   Rhythm: Regular.
   P Waves: Present; precede each QRS complex.
   PR Int: 0.16 second.
   QRS: 0.16 second.
   Intrp: Normal sinus rhythm with bundle branch block.

31. Rate: 135 beats/minute.
   Rhythm: Regular.
   P Waves: None.
   PR Int: None.
   QRS: 0.26 second.
   Intrp: Ventricular tachycardia.

32. Rate: 163 beats/minute.
   Rhythm: Regular.
   P Waves: None.
   PR Int: None.
   QRS: 0.10 second.
   Intrp: Junctional tachycardia.

33. Rate: 41 beats/minute.
   Rhythm: Irregular.
   P Waves: Present; precede the first, second, fourth, and fifth QRS complexes. The R-R interval between the second and fourth QRS complexes is four times the R-R interval of the underlying sinus rhythm.
   PR Int: 0.14 second.
   QRS: 0.12 second.
   Intrp: Sinus rhythm with sinoatrial (SA) exit block, first-degree AV block, bundle branch block, and an isolated junctional escape beat (third QRS complex).

34. Rate: 17 beats/minute.
   Rhythm: Undeterminable.
   P Waves: None.
   PR Int: None.
   QRS: 0.14 second.
   Intrp: Ventricular escape rhythm.

35. Rate: 70 beats/minute.
   Rhythm: Regular.
   P Waves: Present; precede each QRS complex.
   PR Int: 0.16 second.
   QRS: 0.06 second.
   Intrp: Normal sinus rhythm.

36. Rate: 64 beats/minute.
   Rhythm: Irregular.
   P Waves: Present; precede the first and second QRS complexes. Pacemaker spikes precede the rest of the QRS complexes.
   PR Int: 0.26 second.
   QRS: 0.08 second (first and second QRS complexes); 0.16 second (third, fourth, fifth, sixth, and seventh QRS complexes).
   Intrp: Sinus rhythm with first-degree AV block followed by ventricular asystole and a ventricular demand pacemaker rhythm.

37. Rate: 72 beats/minute.
Rhythm: Irregular.
P Waves: Present; precede each QRS complex.
PR Int: 0.16 second.
QRS: 0.08 second.
Intrp: Sinus arrhythmia.

38. Rate: 75 beats/minute.
Rhythm: Irregular.
P Waves: Present; all but the first and sixth P waves are followed by QRS complexes. AV conduction ratio is 3:4.
PR Int: 0.12 to 0.13 second.
QRS: 0.14 second.
Intrp: Sinus rhythm with second-degree, type II AV block and bundle branch block.

39. Rate: 101 beats/minute.
Rhythm: Irregular.
P Waves: Present; precede each QRS complex. The shape and direction of the P waves vary from positive to negative.
PR Int: 0.12 to 0.18 second.
QRS: 0.06 second.
Intrp: Wandering atrial pacemaker.

40. Rate: 37 beats/minute.
Rhythm: Regular.
P Waves: Present; precede each QRS complex.
PR Int: 0.34 second.
QRS: 0.08 second.
Intrp: Sinus bradycardia with first-degree AV block.

41. Rate: 42 beats/minute.
Rhythm: Irregular.
P Waves: Present; precede each QRS complex. The fourth P wave is negative; the rest are positive.
PR Int: 0.18 to 0.20 second.
QRS: 0.12 second.
Intrp: Sinus bradycardia with bundle branch block and an isolated premature atrial contraction.

42. Rate: 66 beats/minute.
Rhythm: Irregular.
P Waves: Present; all the P waves except the fourth and eighth P waves are followed by QRS complexes.
PR Int: 0.22 to 0.36 second. The PR intervals progressively increase until a QRS complex fails to follow the P wave.
QRS: 0.14 second.
Intrp: Sinus rhythm with second-degree, type I AV block (Wenckebach) and bundle branch block.

43. Rate: 74 beats/minute.
Rhythm: Regular.
P Waves: None.
PR Int: None.
QRS: 0.12 second.
Intrp: Pacemaker rhythm (ventricular pacemaker).

44. Rate: 88 beats/minute.
Rhythm: Regular.
P Waves: Present; precede each QRS complex.
PR Int: 0.12 second.
QRS: 0.14 second.
Intrp: Normal sinus rhythm with bundle branch block.

45. Rate: 61 beats/minute.
Rhythm: Irregular.
P Waves: Present; precede all but the fourth QRS complex.
PR Int: 0.12 second.
QRS: 0.08 second.
Intrp: Sinus rhythm with sinus arrest.

46. Rate: 71 beats/minute.
Rhythm: Regular.
P Waves: Present; precede each QRS complex.
PR Int: 0.18 second.
QRS: 0.08 second.
Intrp: Normal sinus rhythm.

47. Rate: 66 beats/minute.
Rhythm: Irregular.
P Waves: Present; all but the fourth and eighth P waves are followed by QRS complexes.
PR Int: 0.22 to 0.40 second. The PR intervals progressively increase until a QRS complex fails to follow the P wave.
QRS: About 0.15 second.
Intrp: Sinus rhythm with second-degree, type I AV block (Wenckebach) and bundle branch block.

48. Rate: 102 beats/minute.
Rhythm: Irregular.
P Waves: None; fine atrial fibrillation waves are present.
PR Int: None.
QRS: 0.09 to 0.10 second (first, fifth, seventh, eighth, ninth, and tenth QRS complexes); 0.12 to 0.16 second (second, third, fourth, sixth, and tenth QRS complexes). The shape and direction of the second, third, and fourth QRS complexes differ from each other. The second QRS complex is similar to the sixth QRS complex; the fourth QRS complex is similar to the tenth QRS complex.
Intrp: Atrial fibrillation (fine) with third-degree AV block, accelerated junctional rhythm, multifocal (multiform) premature ventricular contractions (group beats), and a short burst of ventricular tachycardia. AV dissociation is present.

49. Rate: 63 beats/minute.
Rhythm: Irregular.
P Waves: None; coarse atrial fibrillation waves are present.
PR Int: None.
QRS: 0.13 second.
Intrp: Atrial fibrillation (coarse) with bundle branch block.

50. Rate: 57 beats/minute.
Rhythm: Irregular. The R-R interval between the fourth and fifth QRS complexes is less than twice the R-R interval of the underlying sinus rhythm.
P Waves: Present; precede all but the fifth QRS complex.
PR Int: 0.12 second.
QRS: 0.11 second.
Intrp: Sinus rhythm with sinus arrest and incomplete bundle branch block.

51. Rate: 52 beats/minute.
Rhythm: Regular.
P Waves: Present; precede each QRS complex.
PR Int: 0.20 second.
QRS: 0.06 second.
Intrp: Normal sinus rhythm.

52. Rate: 183 beats/minute.
Rhythm: Regular.
P Waves: None.
PR Int: None.
QRS: 0.12 second.
Intrp: Ventricular tachycardia.

53. Rate: 65 beats/minute.
Rhythm: Irregular.
P Waves: Present; precede each QRS complex.
PR Int: 0.16 second.
QRS: 0.08 second.
Intrp: Sinus arrhythmia.

54. Rate: 27 beats/minute.
Rhythm: Regular.
P Waves: None.
PR Int: None.
QRS: 0.12 second.
Intrp: Junctional escape rhythm with bundle branch block.

55. Rate: 40 beats/minute.
Rhythm: Regular.
P Waves: None.
PR Int: None.
QRS: 0.16 second.
Intrp: Ventricular escape rhythm.

56. Rate: 59 beats/minute.
Rhythm: Irregular.
P Waves: Present; the second, third, fifth, sixth, eighth, and tenth P waves are followed by QRS complexes. AV conduction ratios are 3:1 and 2:1.
PR Int: About 0.16 second.
QRS: About 0.16 second.
Intrp: Sinus rhythm with second-degree, 2:1 and high-degree AV block and bundle branch block.

57. Rate: 58 beats/minute.
Rhythm: Regular.
P Waves: Present; negative P waves follow each QRS complex.
PR Int: None.
QRS: 0.11 second.
Intrp: Accelerated junctional rhythm with incomplete bundle branch block.

58. Rate: 53 beats/minute.
Rhythm: Irregular.
P Waves: Present; the first, second, fourth, fifth, and sixth P waves are followed by QRS complexes.
PR Int: 0.22 to 0.46 second. The PR intervals progressively increase until a QRS complex fails to follow the P wave.
QRS: 0.08 second.
Intrp: Sinus rhythm with second-degree, type I AV block (Wenckebach).

59. Rate: 80 beats/minute.
Rhythm: Irregular.
P Waves: Present; precede the first, second, third, sixth, eighth, and ninth QRS complexes. The third P wave is negative; the fifth wave is buried in the preceding T wave. Pacemaker spikes precede the third, fourth, fifth, and seventh QRS complexes.
PR Int: 0.12 to 0.18 second.
QRS: 0.07 second (first, second, sixth, eighth, and ninth QRS complexes); 0.16 second (fourth, fifth, and seventh QRS complexes). The third QRS complex is a fusion beat—a combination of the normally conducted QRS complex and the pacemaker induced ventricular QRS complex.
Intrp: Sinus rhythm with episodes of ventricular demand pacemaker rhythm.

60. Rate: 134 beats/minute.
Rhythm: Regular.
P Waves: None.
PR Int: None.
QRS: About 0.32 to 0.36 second.
Intrp: Ventricular tachycardia.

61. Rate: 70 beats/minute.
Rhythm: Regular.
P Waves: Present; precede each QRS complex.
PR Int: 0.15 second.
QRS: 0.06 second.
Intrp: Normal sinus rhythm.

62. Rate: 52 beats/minute.
Rhythm: Irregular.
P Waves: Present; the second, third, fifth, and sixth P waves are followed by QRS complexes. The AV conduction ratio is 3:2.
PR Int: 0.24 to 0.26 second.
QRS: 0.16 second.
Intrp: Sinus rhythm with second-degree, type II AV block and bundle branch block.

63. Rate: 64 beats/minute.
Rhythm: Irregular.
P Waves: Present; the first, second, fourth, fifth, and sixth P waves are followed by QRS complexes.
PR Int: 0.24 to 0.36 second. The PR intervals progressively increase until a QRS complex fails to follow the P wave.
QRS: 0.12 second.
Intrp: Sinus rhythm with second-degree, type I AV block (Wenckebach) and bundle branch block.

64. Rate: 284 beats/minute.
Rhythm: Regular.
P Waves: None.
PR Int: None.
QRS: About 0.12 second.
Intrp: Ventricular tachycardia.

65. Rate: 87 beats/minute.
Rhythm: Irregular.
P Waves: Present; precede each QRS complex.
PR Int: 0.12 to 0.16 second.
QRS: 0.04 second.
Intrp: Wandering atrial pacemaker.

66. Rate: 70 beats/minute.
Rhythm: Regular.
P Waves: Present; precede each QRS complex.
PR Int: 0.16 second.
QRS: 0.05 second.
Intrp: Normal sinus rhythm.

67. Rate: 37 beats/minute.
Rhythm: Regular.
P Waves: Present; precede each QRS complex.
PR Int: 0.18 second.
QRS: 0.12 second.
Intrp: Sinus bradycardia with bundle branch block.

68. Rate: 30 beats/minute (atrial rate: 82 beats/minute).
Rhythm: Regular.
P Waves: Present, but have no set relation to the QRS complexes.
PR Int: None.
QRS: 0.14 second.
Intrp: Third-degree AV block with wide QRS complexes.

69. Rate: 125 beats/minute (average); 165 beats/minute (first part); 79 beats/minute (second part).
Rhythm: Irregular.
P Waves: Present; precede each QRS complex. In the first part, the P waves are superimposed on the preceding T waves.
PR Int: 0.16 second.
QRS: About 0.04 second.
Intrp: Paroxysmal atrial tachycardia with reversion to normal sinus rhythm.

70. Rate: 120 beats/minute (three beats).
Rhythm: Regular (three beats).
P Waves: None.
PR Int: None.
QRS: 0.14 second.
Intrp: Supraventricular tachycardia with wide QRS complexes or ventricular tachycardia followed by ventricular asystole.

71. Rate: 174 beats/minute.
Rhythm: Regular.
P Waves: None.
PR Int: None.
QRS: 0.10 second.
Intrp: Supraventricular tachycadia.

72. Rate: 36 beats/minute.
Rhythm: Regular.
P Waves: None.
PR Int: None.
QRS: 0.18 second.
Intrp: Junctional escape rhythm with bundle branch block or ventricular escape rhythm.

73. Rate: 263 beats/minute.
Rhythm: Regular.
P Waves: None.
PR Int: None.
QRS: About 0.12 second.
Intrp: Ventricular tachycardia.

74. Rate: 69 beats/minute.
Rhythm: Irregular.
P Waves: Present; the second, third, fourth, sixth, seventh, and eighth P waves are followed by QRS complexes. AV conduction ratio is 4:3.
PR Int: 0.30 second.
QRS: 0.12 second.
Intrp: Sinus rhythm with second-degree, type II AV block and bundle branch block.

75. Rate: 72 beats/minute.
Rhythm: Regular.
P Waves: Ectopic atrial P waves are present. A QRS complex follows every third P' wave.
PR Int: Unmeasurable.
QRS: 0.08 second.
Intrp: Atrial tachycardia with AV block.

76. Rate: 104 beats/minute.
Rhythm: Irregular.
P Waves: Present; precede the first, fifth, and sixth QRS complex.
PR Int: 0.18 second.
QRS: 0.12 second (first, fifth, and sixth complexes); About 0.16 second (second, third, and fourth QRS complex).
Intrp: Sinus rhythm with bundle branch block and unifocal premature ventricular contractions occurring in a burst of three (ventricular tachycardia); R-on-T phenomenon.

77. Rate: 82 beats/minute.
Rhythm: Regular.
P Waves: Present; precede each QRS complex.
PR Int: About 0.16 second.
QRS: 0.08 second.
Intrp: Normal sinus rhythm.

78. Rate: 100 beats/minute.
Rhythm: Irregular.
P Waves: Present; precede each QRS complex.
PR Int: 0.12 to 0.14 second.
QRS: 0.16 second.
Intrp: Sinus rhythm with bundle branch block and premature atrial contractions (atrial bigeminy).

79. Rate: 56 beats/minute.
Rhythm: Regular.
P Waves: Present; precede each QRS complex.
PR Int: 0.36 to 0.42 second. The PR intervals progressively increase.
QRS: About 0.12 second.
Intrp: Sinus rhythm with second-degree AV block (type undeterminable, probably type I AV block [Wenckebach]) and bundle branch block.

80. Rate: 181 beats/minute.
Rhythm: Regular.
P Waves: None.
PR Int: None.
QRS: About 0.18 second.
Intrp: Supraventricular tachycardia with wide QRS complexes or ventricular tachycardia.

81. Rate: 40 beats/minute.
Rhythm: Undeterminable.
P Waves: None.
PR Int: None.
QRS: 0.16 second.
Intrp: Ventricular escape rhythm.

82. Rate: 94 beats/minute.
Rhythm: Regular.
P Waves: Present; negative P waves precede each QRS complex.
PR Int: 0.08 second.
QRS: 0.10 second.
Intrp: Accelerated junctional rhythm.

83. Rate: 94 beats/minute.
Rhythm: Regular.
P Waves: Present; precede each QRS complex.
PR Int: 0.12 second.
QRS: 0.12 second.
Intrp: Normal sinus rhythm with bundle branch block.

84. Rate: 68 beats/minute.
Rhythm: Irregular.
P Waves: Present; precede the first and third QRS complexes.
PR Int: About 0.08 second.
QRS: 0.08 second (first and third QRS complex); 0.18 second (second and fourth QRS complex).
Intrp: Atrial rhythm with premature ventricular contractions (ventricular bigeminy).

85. Rate: 68 beats/minute.
Rhythm: Irregular.
P Waves: Present; precede each QRS complex. The first and third P waves are positive; the second and fourth P waves are negative.
PR Int: 0.20 second.
QRS: 0.12 second.
Intrp: Sinus rhythm with first-degree AV block, bundle branch block, and premature atrial contractions (atrial bigeminy).

86. Rate: 34 beats/minute (atrial rate: 163 beats/minute).
Rhythm: Undeterminable.
P Waves: Present, but the negative P waves have no set relation to the QRS complexes.
PR Int: None.
QRS: 0.16 second.
Intrp: Third-degree AV block with wide QRS complexes.

87. Rate: 75 beats/minute.
Rhythm: Irregular.
P Waves: None; fine atrial fibrillation waves are present.
PR Int: None.
QRS: 0.16 second.
Intrp: Atrial fibrillation (fine).

88. Rate: 107 beats/minute.
Rhythm: Irregular.
P Waves: Present; precede each QRS complex.
PR Int: 0.14 second.
QRS: 0.12 second.
Intrp: Sinus tachycardia with first-degree AV block, bundle branch block, and an isolated premature junctional contraction (fourth QRS complex).

89. Rate: 230 beats/minute.
Rhythm: Slightly irregular.
P Waves: None.
PR Int: None.
QRS: 0.12 second.
Intrp: Ventricular tachycardia.

90. Rate: 170 beats/minute.
Rhythm: Irregular.
P Waves: None; fine atrial fibrillation waves are present.
PR Int: None.
QRS: 0.08 second.
Intrp: Atrial fibrillation (fine).

91. Rate: 80 second beats/minute.
Rhythm: Irregular.
P Waves: Present; precede the first and third QRS complexes.
PR Int: 0.14 second.
QRS: 0.12 second.
Intrp: Sinus rhythm with bundle branch block and premature junctional contractions (bigeminy).

92. Rate: 115 beats/minute.
Rhythm: Irregular.
P Waves: None; atrial flutter waves are present.
PR Int: None.
QRS: 0.12 second.
Intrp: Atrial flutter.

93. Rate: Unmeasurable.
Rhythm: Irregular.
P Waves: None; coarse ventricular fibrillation waves are present.
PR Int: None.
QRS: None.
Intrp: Ventricular fibrillation (coarse).

94. Rate: 46 beats/minute.
Rhythm: Irregular.
P Waves: Present; the first, second, and fourth P waves are followed by QRS complexes.
PR Int: 0.20 to 0.32 second. The PR intervals progressively increase until a QRS complex fails to follow the P wave.
QRS: 0.10 second.
Intrp: Sinus rhythm with second-degree, type I AV block (Wenckebach).

95. Rate: 82 beats/minute.
Rhythm: Regular.
P Waves: None; atrial and ventricular pacemaker spikes are present.
PR Int: None.
QRS: 0.16 second.
Intrp: Pacemaker rhythm (AV sequential pacemaker).

96. Rate: 61 beats/minute.
Rhythm: Irregular.
P Waves: Present; precede the first, second, and fourth QRS complexes.
PR Int: 0.22 second.
QRS: 0.11 second.
Intrp: Normal sinus rhythm with incomplete bundle branch block and an isolated premature junctional contraction (third QRS complex).

97. Rate: 224 beats/minute.
Rhythm: Regular.
P Waves: None.
PR Int: None.
QRS: 0.06 second.
Intrp: Supraventricular tachycardia.

98. Rate: 98 beats/minute.
Rhythm: Irregular.
P Waves: Present; precede the first, second, third, and sixth QRS complexes.
PR Int: 0.16 second.
QRS: 0.16 to 0.18 second.
Intrp: Normal sinus rhythm with bundle branch block and premature junctional contractions (group beats).

99. Rate: 136 beats/minute.
Rhythm: Regular.
P Waves: Present; negative P waves follow each QRS complex.
PR Int: None.
QRS: 0.06 second.
Intrp: Junctional tachycardia.

100. Rate: 63 beats/minute.
Rhythm: None.
P Waves: None; positive wide artifacts are present.
PR Int: None.
QRS: None.
Intrp: Ventricular asystole with artifacts (chest compressions).

101. Rate: 184 beats/minute.
Rhythm: Regular.
P Waves: None.
PR Int: None.
QRS: 0.10 second.
Intrp: Supraventricular tachycardia.

102. Rate: 102 beats/minute.
Rhythm: Regular.
P Waves: Present; precede each QRS complex.
PR Int: 0.16 second.
QRS: 0.06 second.
Intrp: Sinus tachycardia. Abnormally tall T waves characteristic of hyperkalemia are present.

103. Rate: 68 beats/minute.
Rhythm: Regular.
P Waves: None.
PR Int: None.
QRS: 0.18 to 0.24 second.
Intrp: Accelerated idioventricular rhythm.

104. Rate: 164 beats/minute.
Rhythm: Regular.
P Waves: Present; precede each QRS complex.
PR Int: 0.12 second.
QRS: 0.08 second.
Intrp: Atrial tachycardia.

105. Rate: 123 beats/minute.
Rhythm: Regular.
P Waves: Present; precede each QRS complex.
PR Int: 0.14 second.
QRS: 0.12 second.
Intrp: Sinus tachycardia with bundle branch block.

106. **Rate:** 76 beats/minute.
Rhythm: Irregular.
P Waves: Present; precede the second and fourth QRS complex. The fifth QRS complex is superimposed on a P wave.
PR Int: 0.16 second.
QRS: 0.08 second (third and fifth QRS complexes); 0.12 second (first, second, and fourth QRS complexes).
Intrp: Normal sinus rhythm with bundle branch block and premature junctional contractions.

107. **Rate:** 61 beats/minute.
Rhythm: Irregular.
P Waves: Present; precede the first, second, and fourth QRS complexes.
PR Int: 0.24 second.
QRS: 0.10 second.
Intrp: Sinus rhythm with first-degree AV block and an isolated premature junctional contraction.

108. **Rate:** 41 beats/minute.
Rhythm: Regular.
P Waves: Present; precede each QRS complex.
PR Int: About 0.14 second.
QRS: 0.08 second.
Intrp: Sinus bradycardia.

109. **Rate:** 69 beats/minute.
Rhythm: Regular.
P Waves: Present; precede each QRS complex.
PR Int: 0.22 to 0.26 second.
QRS: 0.16 second.
Intrp: Sinus rhythm with first-degree AV block and bundle branch block.

110. **Rate:** 48 beats/minute (atrial rate: 125 beats/minute).
Rhythm: Regular.
P Waves: Present, but have no set relation to the QRS complexes.
PR Int: None.
QRS: 0.10 second.
Intrp: Third-degree AV block.

111. **Rate:** 41 beats/minute.
Rhythm: Irregular.
P Waves: Present; the first, fourth, and sixth P waves are followed by QRS complexes. AV conduction ratios are 2:1 and 3:1.
PR Int: 0.20 second.
QRS: 0.12 second.
Intrp: Sinus rhythm with second-degree, 2:1 and high-degree AV block.

112. **Rate:** 92 beats/minute.
Rhythm: Regular.
P Waves: Present; precede each QRS complex.
PR Int: 0.14 second.
QRS: About 0.06 second.
Intrp: Normal sinus rhythm.

113. **Rate:** 161 beats/minute.
Rhythm: Regular.
P Waves: None.
PR Int: None.
QRS: 0.09 second.
Intrp: Supraventricular tachycardia.

114. **Rate:** 320 beats/minute.
Rhythm: Slightly irregular.
P Waves: None.
PR Int: None.
QRS: 0.14 to 0.20 second.
Intrp: Torsade de pointes.

115. **Rate:** 50 beats/minute.
Rhythm: Regular.
P Waves: Present; precede each QRS complex.
PR Int: 0.16 second.
QRS: 0.05 second.
Intrp: Junctional escape rhythm with first-degree AV block.

116. **Rate:** 60 beats/minute.
Rhythm: Irregular.
P Waves: None; fine atrial fibrillation waves are present.
PR Int: None.
QRS: 0.07 second.
Intrp: Atrial fibrillation (fine).

117. **Rate:** 97 beats/minute.
Rhythm: Regular.
P Waves: Present; precede each QRS complex.
PR Int: 0.16 second.
QRS: 0.16 second.
Intrp: Normal sinus rhythm with bundle branch block.

118. **Rate:** Unmeasurable.
Rhythm: Irregular.
P Waves: None; coarse ventricular fibrillation waves present.
PR Int: None.
QRS: None.
Intrp: Ventricular fibrillation (coarse).

119. **Rate:** 48 beats/minute.
Rhythm: Regular.
P Waves: Present; follow each QRS complex.
PR Int: None.
QRS: 0.11 to 0.12 second.
Intrp: Junctional escape rhythm with bundle branch block.

120. **Rate:** 73 beats/minute.
Rhythm: Irregular.
P Waves: Present; precede the first, second, and fourth QRS complexes.
PR Int: 0.18 second.
QRS: 0.08 second (first, second, and fourth QRS complexes); 0.16 second (third QRS complex).
Intrp: Normal sinus rhythm with an isolated premature ventricular contraction (interpolated).

121. Rate: 62 beats/minute.
Rhythm: Regular.
P Waves: Present; precede each QRS complex.
PR Int: 0.20 second.
QRS: 0.10 second.
Intrp: Normal sinus rhythm.

122. Rate: 78 beats/minute.
Rhythm: Irregular.
P Waves: None; fine atrial fibrillation waves are present.
PR Int: None.
QRS: 0.08 second.
Intrp: Atrial fibrillation (fine).

123. Rate: 87 beats/minute.
Rhythm: Irregular.
P Waves: Present; precede the first and fourth QRS complexes.
PR Int: 0.16 second.
QRS: 0.09 second (first and fourth QRS complexes); 0.16 second (second, third, and fifth QRS complexes).
Intrp: Normal sinus rhythm with multiform premature ventricular contractions (group beats).

124. Rate: 80 beats/minute.
Rhythm: Regular.
P Waves: None; ventricular pacemaker spikes are present.
PR Int: None.
QRS: 0.12 second.
Intrp: Pacemaker rhythm (ventricular pacemaker).

125. Rate: 31 beats/minute (atrial rate: 97 beats/minute).
Rhythm: Undeterminable.
P Waves: Present, but have no set relation to the QRS complexes.
PR Int: None.
QRS: 0.12 to 0.14 second.
Intrp: Third-degree AV block with wide QRS complexes.

126. Rate: 57 beats/minute.
Rhythm: Regular.
P Waves: None.
PR Int: None.
QRS: 0.11 to 0.13 second.
Intrp: Junctional escape rhythm with bundle branch block.

127. Rate: 47 beats/minute.
Rhythm: Regular.
P Waves: Present; precede each QRS complex.
PR Int: 0.48 second.
QRS: 0.08 second.
Intrp: Sinus bradycardia with first-degree AV block.

128. Rate: 149 beats/minute.
Rhythm: Regular.
P Waves: Present; precede each QRS complex.
PR Int: Unmeasurable.
QRS: 0.08 second.
Intrp: Atrial tachycardia.

129. Rate: 160 beats/minute.
Rhythm: Irregular.
P Waves: Undeterminable.
PR Int: Undeterminable.
QRS: 0.12 second. (first QRS complex); 0.16 second (rest of the QRS complexes).
Intrp: A wide QRS complex followed by multiform ventricular tachycardia.

130. Rate: 160 beats/minute.
Rhythm: Regular.
P Waves: None.
PR Int: None.
QRS: 0.14 second.
Intrp: Supraventricular tachycardia with wide QRS complexes or ventricular tachycardia.

131. Rate: 150 beats/minute.
Rhythm: Regular.
P Waves: Present; follow each QRS complex.
PR Int: None.
QRS: 0.10 second.
Intrp: Junctional tachycardia.

132. Rate: 31 beats/minute (atrial rate: unmeasurable).
Rhythm: Undeterminable.
P Waves: Present, but have no set relation to the QRS complexes.
PR Int: None.
QRS: About 0.15 second.
Intrp: Third-degree AV block with wide QRS complexes.

133. Rate: 31 beats/minute.
Rhythm: Undeterminable.
P Waves: Present; precede each QRS complex.
PR Int: 0.14 second.
QRS: 0.08 second.
Intrp: Sinus bradycardia.

134. Rate: 59 beats/minute.
Rhythm: Regular.
P Waves: None; atrial flutter waves are present.
PR Int: None.
QRS: 0.12 to 0.14 second.
Intrp: Atrial flutter with bundle branch block.

135. Rate: 178 beats/minute.
Rhythm: Regular.
P Waves: None.
PR Int: None.
QRS: 0.08 second.
Intrp: Supraventricular tachycardia.

136. Rate: 91 beats/minute.
Rhythm: Regular.
P Waves: Present; precede each QRS complex.
PR Int: 0.28 second.
QRS: 0.12 second.
Intrp: Sinus rhythm with first-degree AV block and bundle branch block.

137. Rate: 47 beats/minute.
Rhythm: Regular.
P Waves: Present; the first, third, and fifth P waves are followed by QRS complexes.
PR Int: 0.28 second.
QRS: 0.12 second.
Intrp: Sinus rhythm with second-degree, 2:1 AV block and bundle branch block.

138. Rate: 78 beats/minute.
Rhythm: Irregular.
P Waves: Present; precede each QRS complex. The second and fourth P waves are abnormal, each in a different way.
PR Int: 0.20 second (first and third PR intervals); 0.11 to 0.12 second (second and fourth PR intervals).
QRS: 0.08 to 0.09 second.
Intrp: Sinus rhythm with multifocal premature atrial contractions.

139. Rate: 64 beats/minute.
Rhythm: Regular.
P Waves: None.
PR Int: None.
QRS: About 0.10 second.
Intrp: Accelerated junctional rhythm.

140. Rate: 222 beats/minute.
Rhythm: Regular.
P Waves: None.
PR Int: None.
QRS: 0.12 second.
Intrp: Supraventricular tachycardia with wide QRS complexes or ventricular tachycardia.

141. Rate: None (pacemaker spikes: 63 beats/minute).
Rhythm: Regular.
P Waves: None; pacemaker spikes are present.
PR Int: None.
QRS: None.
Intrp: Ventricular asystole with pacemaker spikes without capture.

142. Rate: 99 beats/minute.
Rhythm: Irregular.
P Waves: Present; precede the first, second, and fifth QRS complexes.
PR Int: 0.28 second.
QRS: 0.10 second (first, second, and fifth QRS complexes); 0.12 to 0.16 second (third and fourth QRS complexes).
Intrp: Sinus rhythm with first-degree AV block and multiform premature ventricular contractions (group beats).

143. Rate: 61 beats/minute.
Rhythm: Regular.
P Waves: Present; precede each QRS complex. P waves are abnormally tall (P pulmonale).
PR Int: 0.26 second.
QRS: 0.10 to 0.12 second.
Intrp: Sinus rhythm with first-degree AV block and bundle branch block.

144. Rate: 114 beats/minute.
Rhythm: Regular.
P Waves: Present; precede each QRS complex.
PR Int: 0.16 second.
QRS: 0.08 second.
Intrp: Sinus tachycardia.

145. Rate: 100 beats/minute.
Rhythm: Regular.
P Waves: Present; negative P waves follow each QRS complex.
PR Int: None.
QRS: 0.10 second.
Intrp: Junctional tachycardia.

146. Rate: Unmeasurable.
Rhythm: Irregular.
P Waves: None; coarse ventricular fibrillation waves are present.
PR Int: None.
QRS: None.
Intrp: Ventricular fibrillation (coarse).

147. Rate: 21 beats/minute.
Rhythm: Undeterminable.
P Waves: None.
PR Int: None.
QRS: 0.16 second.
Intrp: Ventricular escape rhythm.

148. Rate: 68 beats/minute.
Rhythm: Irregular.
P Waves: None; fine atrial fibrillation waves are present.
PR Int: None.
QRS: 0.10 second.
Intrp: Atrial fibrillation (fine).

149. Rate: 65 beats/minute (atrial rate: 113 beats/minute).
Rhythm: Regular.
P Waves: Present, but have no set relation to the QRS complexes.
PR Int: None.
QRS: About 0.10 second.
Intrp: Third-degree AV block.

150. Rate: 88 beats/minute.
Rhythm: Irregular.
P Waves: None; fine atrial fibrillation waves are present.
PR Int: None.
QRS: About 0.08 second.
Intrp: Atrial fibrillation (fine).

151. Rate: 55 beats/minute.
Rhythm: Regular.
P Waves: Present; abnormally wide, positive P waves precede each QRS complex.
PR Int: About 0.40 second.
QRS: About 0.10 second.
Intrp: Sinus rhythm with first-degree AV block.

152. Rate: 148 beats/minute.
Rhythm: Regular.
P Waves: Present; precede each QRS complex.
PR Int: Undeterminable; P waves are buried in the preceding QRS complexes.
QRS: 0.10 second.
Intrp: Atrial tachycardia.

153. Rate: 118 beats/minute.
Rhythm: Irregular.
P Waves: None; fine atrial fibrillation waves are present.
PR Int: None.
QRS: 0.10 second.
Intrp: Atrial fibrillation (fine).

154. Rate: 36 beats/minute.
Rhythm: Undeterminable.
P Waves: None.
PR Int: None.
QRS: About 0.16 second.
Intrp: Ventricular escape rhythm.

155. Rate: 50 beats/minute.
Rhythm: Regular.
P Waves: None; atrial flutter waves are present.
PR Int: None.
QRS: 0.16 second.
Intrp: Atrial flutter with bundle branch block.

156. Rate: 163 beats/minute.
Rhythm: Regular.
P Waves: None.
PR Int: None.
QRS: 0.16 second.
Intrp: Ventricular tachycardia.

157. Rate: 63 beats/minute.
Rhythm: Regular.
P Waves: Present; negative P waves follow each QRS complex.
PR Int: None.
QRS: 0.06 second.
Intrp: Accelerated junctional rhythm.

158. Rate: 103 beats/minute.
Rhythm: Regular.
P Waves: Present; P waves precede each QRS complex. The P waves are abnormally tall (P pulmonale).
PR Int: 0.19 second.
QRS: 0.14 second.
Intrp: Sinus tachycardia with bundle branch block.

159. Rate: 312 beats/minute.
Rhythm: Slightly irregular.
P Waves: None.
PR Int: None.
QRS: 0.12 to 0.14 second.
Intrp: Ventricular tachycardia (multiform).

160. Rate: 101 beats/minute.
Rhythm: Regular.
P Waves: None.
PR Int: None.
QRS: 0.14 second.
Intrp: Accelerated junctional rhythm with wide QRS complexes or accelerated idioventricular rhythm.

161. Rate: 92 beats/minute.
Rhythm: Irregular.
P Waves: Present; precede the first, second, fourth, and fifth QRS complexes.
PR Int: 0.14 second.
QRS: 0.16 second.
Intrp: Normal sinus rhythm with bundle branch block and an isolated premature ventricular contraction (interpolated).

162. Rate: 70 beats/minute.
Rhythm: Regular.
P Waves: Present; precede each QRS complex.
PR Int: 0.16 to 0.18 second.
QRS: 0.12 second.
Intrp: Normal sinus rhythm with bundle branch block.

163. Rate: 72 beats/minute.
Rhythm: Regular.
P Waves: None.
PR Int: None.
QRS: 0.12 to 0.16 second.
Intrp: Accelerated idioventricular rhythm.

164. Rate: Unmeasurable.
Rhythm: Irregular.
P Waves: None; fine ventricular waves are present.
PR Int: None.
QRS: None.
Intrp: Ventricular fibrillation (fine).

165. Rate: 57 beats/minute.
Rhythm: Regular.
P Waves: Present; precede each QRS complex.
PR Int: 0.24 second.
QRS: 0.08 second.
Intrp: Sinus bradycardia with first-degree AV block.

166. Rate: 43 beats/minute.
Rhythm: Regular.
P Waves: Present; positive P waves precede each QRS complex.
PR Int: 0.10 second.
QRS: 0.09 second.
Intrp: Bradycardia, probably atrial in origin.

167. Rate: 57 beats/minute.
Rhythm: Regular.
P Waves: None.
PR Int: None.
QRS: About 0.16 second.
Intrp: Accelerated idioventricular rhythm.

168. Rate: None.
Rhythm: None.
P Waves: None.
PR Int: None.
QRS: None.
Intrp: Ventricular asystole.

169. Rate: 43 beats/minute.
Rhythm: Regular.
P Waves: Present; negative P waves follow each QRS complex.
PR Int: None.
QRS: 0.09 second.
Intrp: Junctional escape rhythm.

170. Rate: Unmeasurable.
Rhythm: Irregular.
P Waves: None; coarse ventricular fibrillation waves are present.
PR Int: None.
QRS: None.
Intrp: Ventricular fibrillation (coarse).

171. Rate: 25 beats/minute.
Rhythm: Undeterminable.
P Waves: None.
PR Int: None.
QRS: 0.12 second.
Intrp: Junctional escape rhythm with bundle branch block.

172. Rate: 213 beats/minute.
Rhythm: Regular.
P Waves: None.
PR Int: None.
QRS: 0.12 second.
Intrp: Supraventricular tachycardia with wide QRS complexes or ventricular tachycardia.

173. Rate: 70 beats/minute.
Rhythm: Irregular.
P Waves: None; fine atrial fibrillation waves are present.
PR Int: None.
QRS: 0.10 second.
Intrp: Atrial fibrillation (fine).

174. Rate: 89 beats/minute.
Rhythm: Regular.
P Waves: Present; precede each QRS complex.
PR Int: About 0.18 second.
QRS: 0.12 second.
Intrp: Normal sinus rhythm with bundle branch block.

175. Rate: 165 beats/minute.
Rhythm: Regular.
P Waves: None.
PR Int: None.
QRS: 0.10 second.
Intrp: Supraventricular tachycardia.

176. Rate: 48 beats/minute.
Rhythm: Regular.
P Waves: Present; appear to precede each QRS complex.
PR Int: 0.08 second.
QRS: 0.08 second.
Intrp: Bradycardia, probably atrial in origin. (A third-degree AV block cannot be ruled out.)

177. Rate: 79 beats/minute.
Rhythm: Irregular.
P Waves: Present; positive P waves precede the first, second, fourth, and fifth QRS complexes. A negative P wave precedes the third QRS complex.
PR Int: 0.12 second (first, second, fourth, and fifth QRS complexes); 0.09 second (third QRS complex).
QRS: 0.10 second.
Intrp: Normal sinus rhythm with an isolated premature junctional contraction.

178. Rate: 33 beats/minute (atrial rate: 39 beats/minute).
Rhythm: Undeterminable.
P Waves: Present, but have no set relation to the QRS complexes.
PR Int: None.
QRS: 0.12 second.
Intrp: Third-degree AV block with wide QRS complexes.

179. Rate: 59 beats/minute.
Rhythm: Irregular.
P Waves: Present; the first, third, and fourth P waves are followed by QRS complexes.
PR Int: 0.20 to 0.28 second.
QRS: About 0.05 second.
Intrp: Sinus rhythm with second-degree AV block (probably Type I [Wenckebach]).

180. Rate: 96 beats/minute.
Rhythm: Irregular. An incomplete compensatory pause follows the fourth QRS complex.
P Waves: Present; precede the second, third, fifth, and sixth QRS complexes.
PR Int: 0.18 second.
QRS: 0.10 second.
Intrp: Normal sinus rhythm with an isolated premature junctional contraction.

181. Rate: 60 beats/minute.
Rhythm: Regular.
P Waves: Present; precede each QRS complex.
PR Int: 0.15 second.
QRS: 0.09 second.
Intrp: Normal sinus rhythm.

182. Rate: Unmeasurable.
Rhythm: Irregular.
P Waves: None; fine ventricular fibrillation waves are present.
PR Int: None.
QRS: None.
Intrp: Ventricular fibrillation (fine).

183. Rate: 98 beats/minute.
Rhythm: Regular.
P Waves: Present; precede each QRS complex.
PR Int: About 0.20 second.
QRS: About 0.19 second.
Intrp: Normal sinus rhythm with bundle branch block.

184. Rate: 64 beats/minute.
Rhythm: Regular.
P Waves: None.
PR Int: None.
QRS: About 0.16 second.
Intrp: Accelerated idioventricular rhythm.

185. Rate: 35 beats/minute (atrial rate: 167 beats/minute).
Rhythm: Undeterminable.
P Waves: Present, but have no set relation to the QRS complexes.
PR Int: None.
QRS: 0.12 second.
Intrp: Third-degree AV block with wide QRS complexes.

186. Rate: 79 beats/minute.
Rhythm: Regular.
P Waves: Present; precede each QRS complex.
PR Int: 0.15 second.
QRS: 0.08 second.
Intrp: Normal sinus rhythm.

187. Rate: 87 beats/minute.
Rhythm: Irregular.
P Waves: None; atrial flutter waves are present. The AV conduction ratios vary.
PR Int: None.
QRS: 0.10 second.
Intrp: Atrial flutter.

188. Rate: 181 beats/minute.
Rhythm: Regular.
P Waves: None.
PR Int: None.
QRS: About 0.22 second.
Intrp: Supraventricular tachycardia with wide QRS complexes or ventricular tachycardia.

189. Rate: 103 beats/minute.
Rhythm: Regular.
P Waves: None; atrial flutter waves are present.
PR Int: None.
QRS: 0.06 second.
Intrp: Atrial flutter.

190. Rate: 161 beats/minute.
Rhythm: Regular.
P Waves: Present; precede each QRS complex.
PR Int: 0.12 second.
QRS: 0.09 second.
Intrp: Atrial tachycardia.

191. Rate: 130 beats/minute.
Rhythm: Regular.
P Waves: None.
PR Int: None.
QRS: About 0.10 second.
Intrp: Supraventricular tachycardia.

192. Rate: Ventricular rate: none (atrial rate: 70 beats/minute).
Rhythm: Regular.
P Waves: Present.
Pr Int: None.
QRS: None.
Intrp: Ventricular asystole.

193. Rate: 31 beats/minute (atrial rate 106 beats/minute).
Rhythm: Undeterminable.
P Waves: Present, but have no set relation to the QRS complexes.
PR Int: None.
QRS: About 0.14 second.
Intrp: Third-degree AV block with wide QRS complexes.

194. Rate: 36 beats/minute.
Rhythm: Undeterminable.
P Waves: None.
PR Int: None.
QRS: 0.16 second.
Intrp: Junctional escape rhythm with wide QRS complexes or ventricular escape rhythm.

195. Rate: 59 beats/minute.
Rhythm: Regular.
P Waves: Present; negative P waves precede each QRS complex.
PR Int: 0.05 to 0.06 second.
QRS: About 0.14 second.
Intrp: Junctional escape rhythm with bundle branch block.

196. Rate: 71 beats/minute.
Rhythm: Irregular. A complete compensatory pause follows the third QRS complex.
P Waves: Present; precede each QRS complex.
PR Int: 0.16 second.
QRS: 0.08 second.
Intrp: Normal sinus rhythm with an isolated premature atrial contraction.

197. Rate: 122 beats/minute.
Rhythm: Regular.
P Waves: None.
PR Int: None.
QRS: 0.12 second.
Intrp: Junctional tachycardia with wide QRS complexes.

198. Rate: None.
Rhythm: None.
P Waves: None.
PR Int: None.
QRS: 0.16 second.
Intrp: A single wide QRS complex followed by ventricular asystole.

199. Rate: 169 beats/minute.
Rhythm: Irregular.
P Waves: None; atrial flutter waves are present. The AV conduction ratios vary.
PR Int: None.
QRS: 0.08 second.
Intrp: Atrial flutter.

200. Rate: 128 beats/minute.
Rhythm: Regular.
P Waves: Present; precede each QRS complex. The P waves are abnormally tall (P pulmonale).
PR Int: 0.20 second.
QRS: About 0.11 second.
Intrp: Sinus tachycardia with incomplete bundle branch block.

201. Rate: 63 beats/minute.
Rhythm: Regular.
P Waves: None.
PR Int: None.
QRS: About 0.12 second.
Intrp: Accelerated junctional rhythm with wide QRS complexes or accelerated idioventricular rhythm.

202. Rate: 60 beats/minute.
Rhythm: Regular.
P Waves: Present; precede each QRS complex.
PR Int: 0.16 second.
QRS: 0.07 second.
Intrp: Normal sinus rhythm.

203. Rate: Unmeasurable.
Rhythm: None.
P Waves: None; fine ventricular fibrillation waves are present.
PR Int: None.
QRS: None.
Intrp: Ventricular fibrillation (fine).

204. Rate: 238 beats/minute.
Rhythm: Regular.
P Waves: Present; precede each QRS complex.
PR Int: Unmeasurable.
QRS: 0.04 second.
Intrp: Atrial tachycardia.

205. Rate: 165 beats/minute.
Rhythm: Regular.
P Waves: None.
PR Int: None.
QRS: About 0.24 second.
Intrp: Ventricular tachycardia.

206. Rate: 72 beats/minute.
Rhythm: Regular.
P Waves: None; atrial flutter waves are present.
PR Int: None.
QRS: 0.08 second.
Intrp: Atrial flutter.

207. Rate: 33 beats/minute.
Rhythm: Undeterminable.
P Waves: None.
PR Int: None.
QRS: Unmeasurable; greater than 0.12 second.
Intrp: Ventricular escape rhythm.

208. Rate: 126 beats/minute.
Rhythm: Regular.
P Waves: None.
PR Int: None.
QRS: 0.11 second.
Intrp: Junctional tachycardia with incomplete bundle branch block.

209. Rate: 81 beats/minute.
Rhythm: Irregular.
P Waves: Present; precede each QRS complex. The shape and direction of the fourth P wave differs from the others.
PR Int: 0.13 second (first, second, third, and fifth PR intervals); 0.18 second (fourth PR interval).
QRS: 0.09 second (first, second, third, and fifth QRS complexes); 0.10 second (fourth QRS complex).
Intrp: Normal sinus rhythm with an isolated premature atrial contraction.

210. Rate: 31 beats/minute (atrial rate: 83 beats/minute).
Rhythm: Undeterminable.
P Waves: Present, but have no set relation to the QRS complexes.
PR Int: None.
QRS: 0.12 second.
Intrp: Third-degree AV block with wide QRS complexes.

211. Rate: 180 beats/minute.
Rhythm: Regular.
P Waves: Present; precede each QRS complex.
PR Int: 0.08 second.
QRS: 0.08 second.
Intrp: Atrial tachycardia.

212. Rate: 45 beats/minute (atrial rate 111 beats/minute).
Rhythm: Regular.
P Waves: Present, but have no set relation to the QRS complexes.
PR Int: None.
QRS: 0.10 second.
Intrp: Third-degree AV block.

213. Rate: 52 beats/minute.
Rhythm: Regular.
P Waves: Present; the first, third, and fifth P waves are followed by QRS complexes. The AV condution ratio is 2:1.
PR Int: 0.20 second.
QRS: 0.14 second.
Intrp: Sinus rhythm with second-degree, 2:1 AV block and bundle branch block.

214. Rate: 44 beats/minute.
Rhythm: Irregular.
P Waves: None; atrial flutter waves are present. The AV conduction ratios vary.
PR Int: None.
QRS: 0.10 second.
Intrp: Atrial flutter.

215. Rate: 71 beats/minute.
Rhythm: Regular.
P Waves: Present; precede each QRS complex.
PR Int: 0.26 second.
QRS: 0.08 second.
Intrp: Sinus rhythm with first-degree AV block.

216. Rate: 103 beats/minute.
Rhythm: Regular.
P Waves: Present; precede each QRS complex.
PR Int: 0.12 second.
QRS: 0.14 second.
Intrp: Sinus tachycardia with bundle branch block.

217. Rate: 104 beats/minute.
Rhythm: Regular.
P Waves: None.
PR Int: None.
QRS: 0.12 second.
Intrp: Junctional tachycardia with wide QRS complexes or ventricular tachycadia.

218. Rate: 109 beats/minute.
Rhythm: Irregular
P Waves: Present; precede the first, second, third, fourth, and fifth QRS complexes.
PR Int: 0.14 second.
QRS: 0.09 second (first, second, third, fourth, and fifth QRS complexes); 0.11 second (sixth QRS complex).
Intrp: Normal sinus rhythm with premature ventricular contractions and a fusion beat (third QRS complex).

219. Rate: None.
Rhythm: None.
P Waves: None.
PR Int: None.
QRS: None.
Intrp: Ventricular asystole.

220. Rate: 81 beats/minute.
Rhythm: Regular.
P Waves: None.
PR Int: None.
QRS: 0.10 second.
Intrp: Accelerated junctional rhythm.

221. Rate: 109 beats/minute.
Rhythm: Irregular.
P Waves: Present; precede the first, second, fourth, and fifth QRS complexes.
PR Int: About 0.12 second.
QRS: 0.08 second (first, second, fourth, and fifth QRS complexes); 0.12 second (third and sixth QRS complexes).
Intrp: Normal sinus rhythm with unifocal premature ventricular contractions (trigeminy).

222. Rate: 37 beats/minute.
Rhythm: Undeterminable.
P Waves: Present; the second and fifth P waves are followed by QRS complexes. The third and sixth P waves are buried in the preceding T waves. The AV conduction ratio is 3:1.
PR Int: 0.14 second.
QRS: 0.13 second.
Intrp: Sinus rhythm with second-degree, high-degree AV block and bundle branch block.

223. Rate: 128 beats/minute.
Rhythm: Irregular.
P Waves: None; fine atrial fibrillation waves are present.
PR Int: None.
QRS: 0.12 to 0.16 second.
Intrp: Atrial fibrillation (fine) with bundle branch block.

224. Rate: 108 beats/minute.
Rhythm: Regular.
P Waves: None.
PR Int: None.
QRS: 0.16 second.
Intrp: Ventricular tachycardia.

II. Bundle Branch and Fascicular Blocks
225. Left bundle branch block with an intact interventricular septum.
226. Left posterior fascicular block.
227. Right bundle branch block without an intact interventricular septum.
228. Right bundle branch block with an intact interventricular septum.
229. Left bundle branch block without an intact interventricular septum.
230. Left anterior fascicular block.

III. Myocardial Infarctions
231. Anterolateral myocardial infarction.
232. Septal myocardial infarction.
233. Extensive anterior myocardial infarction.
234. Anterior (localized) myocardial infarction.
235. Lateral myocardial infarction.
236. Inferior myocardial infarction.
237. Anteroseptal myocardial infarction.
238. Posterior myocardial infarction.

IV. QRS Axes
239. QRS axis: +150°.
240. QRS axis: −30° to −90°.
241. QRS axis: +90°.
242. QRS axis: +90° to +150°.
243. QRS axis: 0° to −30°.
244. QRS axis: 0° to +30°.

V. ECG Changes: Drug and Electrolyte
245. Hypercalcemia.
246. Procainamide/quinidine toxicity.
247. Hyperkalemia.
248. Digitalis effect.
249. Hypocalcemia.
250. Hypokalemia.

VI. ECG Changes: Miscellaneous
251. Left ventricular hypertrophy.
252. Chronic obstructive pulmonary disease (COPD).
253. Right ventricular hypertrophy/cor pulmonale.
254. Pericarditis.
255. Acute pulmonary embolism.

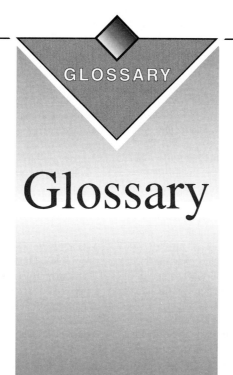

Glossary

ABCs. Airway, breathing, and circulation. The determination of unresponsiveness, breathlessness, and pulselessness and their management.

Aberrancy. See *Aberrant ventricular conduction (aberrancy).*

Aberrant ventricular conduction (aberrancy). An electrical impulse originating in the SA node, atria, or AV junction that is temporarily conducted abnormally through the bundle branches resulting in a bundle branch block. This is usually caused by the appearance of the electrical impulse at the bundle branches prematurely, before the bundle branches have been sufficiently repolarized. Aberrancy may occur with atrial fibrillation, atrial flutter, premature atrial and junctional contractions, and sinus, atrial and junctional tachycardias. Also referred to simply as **ventricular aberrancy.**

Absolute refractory period (ARP) of the ventricles. The period of ventricular depolarization and most of ventricular repolarization during which the ventricles cannot be stimulated to depolarize. It begins with the onset of the QRS complex and ends at about the peak of the T wave.

Accelerated idioventricular rhythm (AIVR). An arrhythmia originating in an ectopic pacemaker in the ventricles with a rate between 40 and 100 beats per minute. Also referred **to as accelerated ventricular rhythm** and **slow ventricular tachycardia.**

Accelerated junctional rhythm. An arrhythmia originating in an ectopic pacemaker in the AV junction with a rate between 60 and 100 beats per minute.

Accelerated rhythm. Three or more consecutive beats originating in an ectopic pacemaker with a rate faster than the inherent rate of the ectopic pacemaker but less than 100 beats per minute. Examples are accelerated junctional rhythm and accelerated idioventricular rhythm (AIVR).

Accelerated ventricular rhythm. See *Accelerated idioventricular rhythm (AIVR).*

Acidosis. A disturbance in the acid-base balance of the body caused by excessive amounts of carbon dioxide (respiratory acidosis), lactic acid (metabolic acidosis), or both.

Actin. One of the contractile protein filaments in myofibrils which give the myocardial cells the property of contractility. The other is myosin.

Action potential. See *Cardiac action potential.*

Acute myocardial infarction (acute MI, AMI). A condition that is present when necrosis of the myocardium occurs because of prolonged and complete interruption of blood flow to the area. The area of the myocardium involved identifies the acute myocardial infarction:

Anterior MI
    Septal MI   Lateral MI
    Anterior (localized) MI   Anterolateral MI
    Anteroseptal MI   Extensive anterior MI
Inferior (diaphragmatic) MI
Inferolateral MI
Posterior MI

Adams-Stokes syndrome. Sudden attacks of unconsciousness, with or without convulsions, caused by a sudden slowing or stopping of the heart beat.

Adenosine. An antiarrhythmic used to convert paroxysmal atrial, junctional, and supraventricular tachycardias.

Adrenalin. Trade name for epinephrine. See *epinephrine.*

Adrenergic. Having the characteristics of the sympathetic nervous system; sympathomimetic.

Advanced life support. Emergency medical care beyond basic life support including one or more of the following: starting an IV, administering IV fluids, administering drugs, defibrillating, inserting an esophageal obturator airway or endotracheal tube, and monitoring and interpreting the ECG.

Afterdepolarization. An abnormal condition of latent pacemaker and myocardial cells (nonpacemaker cells) in which spontaneous depolarization occurs because of a spontaneous and rhythmic increase in the level of phase 4 membrane action potential following a normal depolarization. If afterdepolarization occurs early in phase 4, it is called early afterdepolarization; if late in phase 4, delayed afterdepolarization. This abnormal condition is also referred to as **triggered activity.**

Agonal. Occurring at the moment of or just before death.

Agonal rhythm. Cardiac arrhythmia present in a dying heart. Ventricular escape rhythm.

Amplitude (voltage). With respect to ECGs, the height or depth of a wave or complex measured in millimeters (mm).

Anion. An ion with a negative charge, e.g., Cl^-, PO_4^-, SO_4^-.

Anomalous AV conduction. See *Preexcitation syndrome.*

Anoxia. Absence or lack of oxygen.

Antegrade (or anterograde) conduction. Conduction of the electrical impulse in a forward direction, that is, from the SA node or atria to the ventricles or from the AV junction to the ventricles.

Anterior leads. Leads V_3 and V_4. The **midprecordial leads.**

Anterior (localized) MI. A myocardial infarction commonly caused by occlusion of the diagonal arteries of the left anterior descending (LAD) coronary artery and characterized by early changes in the ST segments and T waves (i.e., ST elevation and tall, peaked T waves) and the appearance later of abnormal Q waves in leads V_3-V_4.

Anterior MI. A myocardial infarction caused by the occlusion of the left anterior descending (LAD) coronary artery or the left circumflex coronary artery or any of their branches, singly or in combination. Anterior MI includes septal, anterior (localized), anteroseptal, lateral, anterolateral, and extensive anterior myocardial infarctions and is characterized by early changes in the ST segments and T waves (i.e., ST elevation and tall, peaked T waves) and the appearance early or later of abnormal Q waves in two or all of leads I, aVL, and V_1-V_4, depending on the site of the infarction.

Anterolateral MI. A myocardial infarction commonly caused by occlusion of the diagonal arteries of the left anterior descending (LAD) coronary artery alone or in conjunction with the anterolateral marginal artery of the left circumflex coronary artery and characterized by early changes in the ST segments and T waves (i.e., ST elevation and tall, peaked T waves) and the appearance later of abnormal Q waves in leads I, aVL, and V_3-V_6.

Anteroseptal MI. A myocardial infarction commonly caused by occlusion of the left anterior descending (LAD) coronary artery involving both the septal perforator and diagonal arteries and characterized by early changes in the ST segments and T waves (i.e., ST elevation and tall, peaked T waves) in leads V_1-V_4 and the appearance early of abnormal Q waves in leads V_1-V_2 and then later in leads V_3-V_4.

Aorta. The main trunk of the arterial system of the body consisting of the ascending aorta, the aortic arch, and the descending aorta. The descending aorta is further divided into the thoracic and abdominal aorta.

Aortic valve. The one-way valve located between the left ventricle and the ascending aorta.

Apex of the heart. The pointed lower end of the heart formed by the pointed lower ends of the right and left ventricles.

Arrhythmia. A rhythm other than a normal sinus rhythm when (1) the heart rate is less than 60 or greater than 100 beats per minute, (2) the rhythm is irregular, (3) premature contractions occur, or (4) the normal progression of the electrical impulse through the electrical conduction system is blocked. Also known as dysrhythmia, a more appropriate term but one not used as frequently.

Artifacts. Mechanically or electrically produced extraneous spikes and waves recorded on an ECG record. Common causes of artifacts are muscle tremor, alternating current (AC) interference, loose electrodes, interference related to biotelemetry, and external chest compression. Artifacts are also referred to as **electrical interference** or **noise.**

Artificial pacemaker. An electronic device used to stimulate the heart to beat when the electrical conduction system of the heart malfunctions, causing bradycardia or ventricular asystole. An artificial pacemaker consists of an electronic pulse generator, a battery, and a wire lead that senses the electrical activity of the heart and delivers electrical impulses to the atria or ventricles or both when the pacemaker senses an absence of electrical activity.

Asymptomatic bradycardia. A bradycardia with a systolic blood pressure greater than 90 to 100 mm Hg and stable and the absence of congestive heart failure, chest pain, dyspnea, signs and symptoms of decreased cardiac output, and premature ventricular contractions. Treatment may not be indicated even if the heart rate falls below 50 beats per minute.

Asystole. Absence of contractions of the ventricles or the entire heart.

Atrial and ventricular demand pacemaker. An artificial pacemaker that paces either the atria or ventricles when there is no appropriate spontaneous underlying atrial or ventricular rhythm.

Atrial arrhythmias. Arrhythmias originating in the atria, such as wandering atrial pacemaker (WAP), premature atrial contractions (PACs), atrial tachycardia (nonparoxysmal atrial tachycardia, paroxysmal atrial tachycardia [PAT]), atrial flutter, and atrial fibrillation.

Atrial demand pacemaker (AAI). An artificial pacemaker that senses spontaneously occurring P waves and paces the atria when they do not appear.

Atrial depolarization. The electrical process of discharging the resting (polarized) myocardial cells producing the P, P′, F, and f waves and causing the atria to contract.

Atrial dilatation. Distension of the atria because of increased pressure and/or volume within the atria; it may be acute or chronic.

Atrial enlargement. Includes atrial dilatation and hypertrophy. Common causes include heart failure, ventricular hypertrophy from whatever cause, pulmonary diseases, pulmonary or systemic hypertension, heart valve stenosis or insufficiency, and acute myocardial infarction. See *Left atrial enlargement (left atrial dilatation and hypertrophy), Right atrial enlargement (right atrial dilatation and hypertrophy).*

Atrial fibrillation. An arrhythmia arising in numerous ectopic pacemakers in the atria characterized by very rapid atrial fibrillation (f) waves and an irregular, often rapid ventricular response. Atrial fibrillation is "fast" if the ventricular rate is greater than 100 per minute, and, "slow" if it is less than 60. When fast, atrial fibrillation is considered uncontrolled (untreated atrial fibrillation); when slow, controlled (treated) atrial fibrillation.

Atrial fibrillation (f) waves. Irregularly shaped, rounded (or pointed), and dissimilar atrial waves originating in multiple ectopic pacemakers in the atria at a rate between 350 and 600 (average, 400) beats per minute. May be "fine" (less than 1 mm in height) or "coarse" (1 mm or greater in height).

Atrial flutter (AF). An arrhythmia arising in an ectopic pacemaker in the atria, characterized by abnormal atrial flutter waves with a sawtooth appearance and usually a regular ventricular response after every other or every fourth F wave. If the QRS complexes occur irregularly at varying F wave-to-QRS complex ratios, a variable AV block is present. Atrial flutter may be transient (paroxysmal) or chronic (persistent). When fast, atrial flutter is considered uncontrolled (untreated) atrial flutter; when slow, controlled (treated) atrial flutter.

Atrial flutter-fibrillation. An arrhythmia arising in the atria alternating between atrial flutter and atrial fibrillation.

Atrial flutter (F) waves. Regularly shaped, usually pointed atrial waves with a sawtooth appearance originating in an ectopic pacemaker in the atria at a rate between 240 and 360 (average, 300) beats per minute.

Atrial hypertrophy. Increase in the thickness of the atrial wall because of chronic increase in pressure and/or volume within the atria.

"Atrial kick." Refers to the complete filling of the ventricles brought on by the contraction of the atria during the last part of ventricular diastole just before the ventricles contract.

Atrial overload. Refers to increased pressure and/or volume within the atria.

Atrial repolarization. The electrical process by which the depolarized atria return to their polarized, resting state. Atrial repolarization produces the atrial T (Ta) wave.

Atrial standstill. Absence of electrical activity of the atria.

Atrial synchronous ventricular pacemaker (VDD). An artificial pacemaker that is synchronized with the patient's atrial rhythm and paces the ventricles when an AV block occurs.

Atrial tachycardia (AT). An arrhythmia originating in an ectopic pacemaker in the atria with a rate between 160 and 240 beats per minute. May or may not occur with AV block, which may be constant or variable. Includes nonparoxysmal atrial tachycardia, paroxysmal atrial tachycardia (PAT), and atrial tachycardia with AV block. When abnormal QRS complexes occur with the tachycardia because of aberrant ventricular conduction, the tachycardia is called atrial tachycardia with aberrant ventricular conduction (aberrancy).

Atrial T wave (Ta). Represents atrial repolarization; often buried in the following QRS complex.

Atrioventricular (AV) block. See *AV block and specific AV blocks.*

Atrioventricular (AV) dissociation. Occurs when the atria and ventricles beat independently.

Atrioventricular (AV) junction. The part of the electrical conduction system that normally conducts the electrical impulse from the atria to the ventricles. It consists of the AV node and the bundle of His.

Atrioventricular (AV) node. The part of the electrical conduction system, located in the posterior floor of the right atrium near the interatrial septum, through which the electrical impulses are normally conducted from the atria to the bundle of His.

Atrium. The thin-walled chamber into which venous blood flows before reaching the ventricle. The two atria form the upper part of the heart, or the base, and are separated from the ventricles by the mitral and tricuspid valves.

Atropine. A drug that counteracts parasympathetic activity in the heart thereby increasing the heart rate and enhancing the conduction of the electrical impulses through the AV node; used to treat bradycardias, second- and third- degree AV blocks, ventricular asystole, and pulseless electrical activity (PEA), such as electromechanical dissociation (EMD).

Augmented (unipolar) leads. Leads aVR, aVL, and aVF; each obtained using a positive electrode attached to one extremity and a negative electrode to a central terminal:

Lead aVR. The positive electrode attached to the right arm and the negative electrode to the central terminal.

Lead aVL. The positive electrode attached to the left arm and the negative electrode to the central terminal.

Lead aVF. The positive electrode attached to the left leg and the negative electrode to the central terminal.

Automaticity, property of. The property of a cell to reach a threshold potential and generate electrical impulses spontaneously. Also referred to as the **property of self-excitation.**

Autonomic nervous system. Part of the nervous system that is involved in the constant control of involuntary bodily functions, including the control of cardiac output (by regulating the heart rate and stroke volume) and blood pressure (by regulating blood vessel activity). It includes the sympathetic (adrenergic) and parasympathetic (cholinergic or vagal) nervous systems, each producing opposite effects when stimulated.

AV. Abbreviation for atrioventricular.

AV block. Delay or failure of conduction of electrical impulses through the AV junction.

AV block, first-degree. An arrhythmia in which there is a constant delay in the conduction of electrical impulses through the AV node. It is characterized by abnormally prolonged PR intervals (greater than 0.20 second).

AV block, second-degree, type I (Wenckebach). An arrhythmia in which progressive prolongation of the conduction of electrical impulses through the AV node occurs until conduction is completely blocked. It is characterized by progressive lengthening of the PR interval until a QRS complex fails to appear after a P wave. This phenomenon is cyclical.

AV block, second-degree, type II. An arrhythmia in which a complete block of conduction of the electrical impulses occurs in one bundle branch and an intermittent block in the other. It is characterized by regularly or irregularly absent QRS complexes (producing, commonly, an AV conduction ratio of 4:3 or 3:2) and a bundle branch block.

AV block, second-degree, 2:1 and high-degree (advanced). An arrhythmia caused by defective conduction of electrical impulses through the AV node or bundle branches or both. It is characterized by regularly or irregularly absent QRS complexes (producing, commonly, an AV conduction ratio of 2:1 or greater) with or without a bundle branch block.

AV blocks with wide QRS complexes. Second-degree AV block, type II and 2:1 and high-degree (advanced) AV block, and third-degree AV block with wide QRS complexes require a temporary transcutaneous pacemaker immediately, whether or not the bradycardia is symptomatic.

AV block, third-degree (complete AV block). An arrhythmia in which there is a complete block of the conduction of electrical impulses through the AV node, bundle of His, or bundle branches. It is characterized by independent beating of the atria and ventricles. Third-degree AV block may be transient and reversible or permanent (chronic).

AV conduction ratio. The ratio of P, P′, F, or f waves to QRS complexes. For example, an AV conduction ratio of 4:3 indicates that for every four P waves, three are followed by QRS complexes.

AV dissociation. Occurs when the atria and ventricles beat independently.

AV junction. See *Atrioventricular (AV) junction.*

AV node. See *Atrioventricular (AV) node.*

AV sequential pacemaker (DVI). An artificial pacemaker that paces either the atria or ventricles or both sequentially when spontaneous ventricular activity is absent.

Axis. Used alone, usually refers to the QRS axis—the single large vector representing the mean (or average) of all the ventricular vectors. Usually, graphically displayed as an arrow. **P axis, ST axis, and T axis.**

Axis of a lead (lead axis). A hypothetical line joining the poles of a lead. A lead axis has a direction and a polarity.

Bachmann's bundle. A branch of the internodal atrial conduction tracts that extends across the atria, conducting the electrical impulses from the SA node to the left atrium.

Baseline. The part of the ECG during which electrical activity of the heart is absent. Commonly the interval between the end of the T wave and the onset of the P wave (the TP segment) is considered the baseline and is used as the reference for the measurement of the amplitude of the ECG waves and complexes.

Base of the heart. The upper part of the heart formed by the right and left atria.

Beta blockers. A group of drugs that block sympathetic activity; used primarily to treat tachyarrhythmias, hypertension, and angina. **Propranolol.**

Bidirectional ventricular tachycardia. Ventricular tachycardia characterized by two distinctly different forms of QRS complexes alternating with each other, indicating the presence of two ventricular ectopic pacemakers.

Bigeminy. An arrhythmia in which every other beat is a premature contraction. The premature beat may be atrial, junctional, or ventricular in origin (i.e., atrial bigeminy, junctional bigeminy, ventricular bigeminy).

Biological death. Present when irreversible brain damage has occurred, usually within ten minutes after cardiac arrest, if untreated.

Biphasic deflection. A deflection having both a positive and a negative component (e.g., a biphasic P wave, a biphasic T wave).

Bipolar limb leads. Leads I, II, and III.

Block. Delay or failure of conduction of an electrical impulse through the electrical conduction system because of tissue damage or increased parasympathetic (vagal) tone.

Blocked PAC. A P′ wave not followed by a QRS complex.

Bolus. A single large dose of a drug that provides an initial high therapeutic blood level of the drug.

Bradycardia. An arrhythmia with a rate of less than 60 per minute.

Bradycardias. Arrhythmias with rates of less than 60 per minute, e.g., sinus bradycardia; sinus arrest and sinoatrial (SA) exit block; junctional escape rhythm; ventricular escape rhythm; second-degree, type I AV block (Wenckebach); second-degree, type II AV block; second-degree, 2:1 and high-degree (advanced) AV block; and third-degree AV block.

Bretylium tosylate. An antiarrhythmic used in the treatment of premature ventricular contractions (PVCs), ventricular fibrillation, and ventricular tachycardia.

Bundle branch block (BBB). Defective conduction of electrical impulses through the right or left bundle branch from the bundle of His to the Purkinje network causing a right or left bundle branch block. It may be complete or incomplete (partial) or permanent (chronic) or intermittent (transient). It may be present with or without an intact interventricular septum.

Bundle branches. The part of the electrical conduction system in the ventricles consisting of the right and left bundle branches that conducts the electrical impulses from the bundle of His to the Purkinje network of the myocardium.

Bundle of His. The part of the electrical conduction system located in the upper part of the interventricular septum that conducts the electrical impulses from the AV node to the right and left bundle branches. The bundle of His and the AV node form the AV junction.

Buried P wave. Refers to a P wave partially or completely hidden in a preceding T wave. This occurs when a sinus, atrial, or junctional P wave occurs during the repolarization of a previous beat as in a sinus, atrial, or junctional tachycardia or a premature atrial or junctional premature beat.

Bursts (or salvos). Refers to the occurrence of two or more consecutive premature atrial, junctional, or ventricular contractions.

Calcium channel blocker. A drug that blocks the entry of calcium ions (Ca^{++}) into cells, especially those of cardiac and vascular smooth muscle. Used as an antiarrhythmic, antihypertensive, and antianginal drug. **Diltiazem, verapamil.**

Calcium chloride. A calcium salt (electrolyte) used to replenish blood calcium levels following administration of excessive calcium channel blockers or to reverse the effects of hyperkalemia and hypermagnesemia on the heart.

Calibration (or standardization). Accomplished by inserting a standard 1-millivolt (mV) electrical signal to produce a 10-mm deflection (two large squares) on the ECG.

Capture. Refers to the ability of a pacemaker's electrical impulse to depolarize the atria or ventricles or both.

Capture beat. A normally conducted QRS complex of the underlying rhythm occurring within a ventricular tachycardia.

Cardiac action potential. Refers to the membrane potential of a myocardial cell and the changes it undergoes during depolarization and repolarization. The phases of the cardiac action potential are:

> Phase 0—**depolarization phase.**
> Phase 1—**early rapid repolarization phase.**
> Phase 2—**plateau phase of slow repolarization.**
> Phase 3—**terminal phase of rapid repolarization.**
> Phase 4—**period between action potentials.**

Cardiac arrest. The sudden and unexpected cessation of an adequate circulation to maintain life in a patient who was not expected to die.

Cardiac cells. Cells of the heart, consisting of the myocardial (or "working") cells and the specialized cells of the electrical conduction system of the heart.

Cardiac cycle. The interval from the beginning of one heart beat to the beginning of the next one. The cardiac cycle normally consists of a P wave, a QRS complex, and a T wave. It represents a sequence of atrial contraction and relaxation and ventricular contraction and relaxation, in that order.

Cardiac output. The amount of blood circulated by the heart in one minute, in liters per minute. Obtained by multiplying the amount of blood expelled by the left ventricle with each contraction (stroke volume) by the heart rate per minute.

Cardiac pacemaker. An artificial pacemaker. See *Artificial pacemaker.*

Cardiac standstill. Absence of atrial and ventricular contractions. This term is used interchangeably with ventricular asystole.

Cardiac tamponade. Acute compression of the heart because of effusion of fluid into the pericardial cavity (as occurs in pericarditis) or accumulation of blood in the pericardium from rupture of the heart or penetrating trauma.

Cardiac vector. A graphic presentation, using an arrow, representing the moment-to-moment electric current generated by depolarization or repolarization of a small segment of the atrial or ventricular wall.

Cardioaccelerator center. One of the nerve centers of the sympathetic nervous system, located in the medulla oblongata, a part of the brain stem. Impulses from the cardioaccelerator center reach the electrical conduction system of the heart and the atria and ventricles by way of the sympathetic nerves.

Cardiogenic. Originating in the heart.

Cardiogenic shock. A life-threatening complication of acute myocardial infarction caused by the inability of the damaged ventricles to maintain an adequate systemic circulation. One of the consequences of pump failure.

Cardioinhibitor center. One of the nerve centers of the parasympathetic nervous system, located in the medulla oblongata, a part of the brain stem. Impulses from the cardioinhibitor center by way of the right and left vagus nerves innervate the atria, SA node, and AV junction, and to a small extent the ventricles.

Cardiomyopathy. A primary disease of the myocardium affecting the bundle branches causing bundle branch and fascicular blocks, often of unknown etiology.

Cardioversion. Application of a synchronized countershock to convert certain arrhythmias—nonparoxysmal atrial tachycardia without block, paroxysmal atrial tachycardia (PAT), paroxysmal junctional tachycardia (PJT), paroxysmal supraventricular tachycardia (PSVT), atrial flutter, atrial fibrillation, and hemodynamically stable ventricular tachycardia (with pulse)—to an organized supraventricular rhythm.

Carotid artery disease. Primarily atherosclerotic in nature with progressive formation of lumen-narrowing (stenotic) atheromatous plaques. A carotid occlusive disease.

Carotid bruit. An abnormal sound or murmur heard by auscultation over a stenotic (narrowed) carotid artery, usually a sign of an atheromatous plaque.

Carotid sinus. A slightly dilated section of the common carotid artery at the point where it bifurcates, containing sensory nerve endings involved in the nervous reflexes regulating blood pressure and heart rate.

Carotid sinus massage. Application of pressure to one of the carotid sinuses with the fingertips to convert paroxysmal atrial tachycardia (PAT) and paroxysmal junctional tachycardia (PJT) to an organized supraventricular rhythm.

Catecholamines. Hormonelike substances such as epinephrine and norepinephrine that have a strong sympathetic action on the heart and peripheral blood vessels, increasing the cardiac output and blood pressure.

Cation. An ion with a positive charge, e.g., K^+, Na^+.

cc. Abbreviation for cubic centimeter. It is often substituted for ml.

Cell membrane potential. The difference in electrical potential across the cell membrane, that is, the difference between the electrical potential within the cell and a reference potential in the extracellular fluid surrounding the cell.

Central terminal. The central terminal, in the case of the augmented ECG leads, consists of connecting together two of the three electrodes used (the right and left arm electrodes and the left leg electrode) other than the positive electrode. In the case of the precordial leads, the central terminal consists of connecting all three extremity electrodes—the right and left arm electrodes and the left leg electrode. The central terminal is considered to be an **indifferent, zero reference point.**

Chronic obstructive pulmonary disease (COPD). A chronic disease of the lungs characterized by a chronic productive cough and dyspnea. Typical ECG pattern: Poor R-wave progression in the precordial leads V_1 through V_5 or V_6.

Circulatory system. The blood vessels in the body, including the systemic and pulmonary circulatory systems.

Clinical death. Present the moment the patient's cardiac output ceases, as evidenced by the absence of a pulse and blood pressure; occurs immediately after the onset of cardiac arrest. Common causes are ventricular fibrillation, pulseless ventricular tachycardia, ventricular asystole, and pulseless electrical activity.

Coarse atrial fibrillation. Atrial fibrillation with large fibrillatory waves—1 mm or greater in height.

Coarse ventricular fibrillation. Ventricular fibrillation with large fibrillatory waves—greater than 3 mm in height.

Compensatory pause. The R-R interval following a premature contraction. It may be full or incomplete depending on whether or not the SA node, for example, is depolarized by the premature contraction. If the SA node is not depolarized by the premature contraction, the compensatory pause is called "full" (or "fully"); the sum of a "full" compensatory pause and the preceding R-R interval is equal to the sum of two R-R intervals of the underlying rhythm. If the SA node is depolarized by the premature contraction, resetting the timing of the SA node, the compensatory pause is called "incomplete"; the sum of an "incomplete" compensatory pause and the preceding R-R interval is less than the sum of two R-R intervals of the underlying rhythm.

Complete atrioventricular (AV) block. See *AV block, third-degree.*

Complete bundle branch block (right, left). Complete disruption of the conduction of electrical impulses through the right or left bundle branch. The duration of the QRS complex is 0.12 second or greater.

Components of the electrocardiogram. Includes the P wave, PR interval, PR segment, QRS complex, ST segment, T wave, U wave, QT interval, TP segment, and R-R interval.

Conducted PAC. A positive P′ wave (in Lead II) followed by a QRS complex.

Conducted PJC. A negative P′ wave (in Lead II) followed by a QRS complex.

Conductivity, property of. The property of cardiac cells to conduct electrical impulses.

Congestive heart failure (CHF). Excessive blood or tissue fluid in the lungs or body or both caused by the inefficient pumping of the ventricles. One of the consequences of pump failure. May be of recent origin (acute) or of prolonged duration (chronic).

Contractile filament. See *Myofibril.*

Contractility, property of. The property of cardiac cells to contract when they are depolarized by an electrical impulse.

Controlled atrial flutter. A "treated" atrial flutter with a slow ventricular rate of about 60 to 75 beats per minute.

COPD. See *Chronic obstructive pulmonary disease (COPD).*

Coronary artery circulation. The coronary artery circulation consists of the left coronary artery (LCA) and the right coronary artery (RCA). The left coronary artery has a short main stem, the left main coronary artery, which branches into the left anterior descending (LAD) coronary artery and the left circumflex coronary artery. The arteries that commonly arise from the left anterior descending (LAD) coronary artery, the left circumflex coronary artery, and the right coronary artery are listed below.

Left anterior descending coronary artery	Left circumflex coronary artery	Right coronary artery
Diagonal arteries	Left atrial circumflex arteries	Conus artery
Septal perforator arteries	Anterolateral marginal artery	Sinoatrial node artery
Right ventricular arteries	Posterolateral marginal arteries	Anterior right ventricular artery
	Distal left circumflex artery	Right atrial artery
		Acute marginal artery
		Posterior descending coronary artery
		AV node artery
		Posterior left ventricular arteries

Coronary artery disease. Progressive narrowing and eventual obstruction of the coronary arteries by atherosclerosis.

Coronary circulation. Passage of blood through the coronary arteries and their branches and the capillaries in the heart and then back to the right atrium via the coronary venules and veins and the coronary sinus.

Coronary occlusion (or obstruction). Obstruction of a coronary artery, usually by a blood clot (coronary thrombus); the major cause of acute myocardial infarction.

Coronary sinus. The outlet in the right atrium draining the coronary venous system.

Coronary thrombosis. The formation of a blood clot (thrombus) within a coronary artery resulting in coronary artery obstruction; the major cause of acute myocardial infarction.

Coronary vasospasm. Coronary artery spasm. One of the causes of coronary artery obstruction.

Cor pulmonale. Right heart disease with right ventricular hypertrophy and right atrial dilatation due to pulmonary hypertension secondary to chronic lung disease.

Corrected QT interval (QTc). The average duration of the QT interval normally expected at a given heart rate.

Countershock. See *Synchronized countershock.*

Coupled beats. Atrial or ventricular ectopic beats occurring in groups of two. Also called **paired beats, couplet.**

Couplet. Two consecutive premature contractions. Also referred to as **coupled beats, paired beats.**

Coupling. Ventricular bigeminy with the premature ventricular contractions following the QRS complexes of the underlying rhythm at equal coupling intervals.

Coupling interval. The R-R interval between a premature contraction and the preceding QRS complex of the underlying rhythm.

Current of injury. The theoretical cause of ST segment elevation in acute myocardial infarction; an electrical manifestation of the inability of cardiac cells "injured" by severe ischemia to maintain a normal resting membrane potential during diastole.

Cyanosis. Slightly bluish, grayish, slatelike or purplish discoloration of the skin caused by the presence of unoxygenated blood.

Defibrillation shock. An unsynchronized direct-current (DC) shock used to terminate pulseless ventricular tachycardia and ventricular fibrillation.

Deflection. Refers to the waves in the ECG. A deflection may be positive (upright), negative (inverted), biphasic (both positive and negative), or equiphasic (equally positive and negative). When a series of waves, such as a QRS complex, is composed of positive and negative deflections, it may be (1) predominantly positive (the sum total of the positive and negative deflections is positive, no matter by how much); (2) predominantly negative (the sum total of the positive and negative deflections is negative, no matter by how much); or (3) equiphasic (the positive deflections are equal to the negative deflections).

Delayed afterdepolarization. See *Afterdepolarization.*

Delta wave. The initial slurring of the QRS complex found in anomalous AV conduction (preexcitation syndrome).

Demand pacemakers. Artificial pacemakers that have a sensing device that senses the heart's electrical activity and fires at a preset rate when the heart's electrical activity drops below a predetermined rate level.

Demand pacing. Refers to a mode of pacing by an artificial pacemaker in which the pacemaker is turned on when an appropriate underlying spontaneous atrial or ventricular rhythm fails to occur.

Depolarization. The electrical process by which the resting potential of a polarized, resting cell of the atria, ventricles, or electrical conduction system is reduced to a less negative value.

Depolarization waves. The parts of the ECG representing the depolarization of the atria and ventricles—the P wave (atrial depolarization) and the QRS complex (ventricular depolarization).

Depolarized state. The condition of the cell when it has been completely depolarized.

Diastole (electrical). Phase 4 of the action potential.

Diastole (mechanical). The period of atrial or ventricular relaxation.

Diazepam. An antianxiety agent used to produce amnesia in conscious patients before cardioversion of certain arrhythmias.

Digitalis. A drug used to decrease rapid ventricular rate in atrial fibrillation, atrial flutter, nonparoxysmal atrial tachycardia without block, paroxysmal atrial tachycardia (PAT), and paroxysmal junctional tachycardia (PJT) and to improve ventricular contraction in congestive heart failure.

Digitalis effect. The changes in the ECG caused by the administration of digitalis. They include prolongation of the PR interval over 0.2 second; depression of the ST segment by 1 mm or more in many of the leads, with a characteristic "scooped-out" appearance; alteration of the T waves so that they appear flattened, inverted, or biphasic; and shortening of the QT interval to less than normal for the heart rate.

Digitalis overdose. Excessive administration of digitalis, often accompanied by signs and symptoms of digitalis toxicity which includes the appearance of arrhythmias, such as accelerated idioventricular rhythm (AIVR), AV blocks, junctional tachycardia, nonparoxysmal atrial tachycardia with or without block, premature atrial contractions (PACs), premature junctional contractions (PJCs), ventricular fibrillation, and ventricular tachycardia. In fact, almost any arrhythmia may be caused by excess digitalis.

Digitalis toxicity. Digitalis overdose.

Digitalization. The process of administering an adequate amount of digitalis over a period of time in the treatment of certain arrhythmias. See *Digoxin.*

Digoxin. A drug used in the treatment of atrial fibrillation, atrial flutter, nonparoxysmal atrial tachycardia without block, paroxysmal atrial tachycardia (PAT), paroxysmal junctional tachycardia (PJT), and paroxysmal supraventricular tachycardia (PSVT).

Dilatation and hypertrophy. Refers to the two kinds of enlargement of the atria and ventricles.

Diltiazem hydrochloride. A calcium channel blocker drug used to treat atrial and junctional tachycardias in patients who are hemodynamically stable.

Direct-current (DC) shock. Used as defibrillation shock, synchronized countershock, and unsynchronized shock to terminate various arrhythmias. See *Defibrillation shock, Synchronized countershock,* and *Unsynchronized shock.*

Diuretic. A drug used in congestive heart failure to decrease excess body fluid by increasing the secretion of urine by the kidney.

Diving reflex. The technique of immersing the patient's face in ice water to elicit the parasympathetic reflex in an attempt to terminate a paroxysmal supraventricular tachycardia (PSVT), including paroxysmal atrial tachycardia (PAT) and paroxysmal junctional tachycardia (PJT), with narrow QRS complexes. It should only be tried if other vagal maneuvers are not effective and ischemic heart disease is not present or suspected.

Dominant coronary artery (right, left). Refers to the coronary artery, right or left, that gives rise to both the posterior left ventricular arteries and the posterior descending coronary artery.

Dominant (or primary) pacemaker of the heart. The SA node.

Dopamine hydrochloride. A sympathomimetic that increases blood pressure; used in the treatment of hypotension and shock.

Downsloping ST segment depression. A type of ST segment depression that is most specific for myocardial ischemia, including that present in subendocardial infarction.

Dropped beats. Nonconducted P waves in AV blocks.

Dropped P waves. Absent P waves in sinus arrest and sinoatrial (SA) exit block.

Dual-chamber pacemaker. An artificial pacemaker that paces the atria, ventricles, or both when appropriate.

Dying heart. A heart with feeble, ineffectual ventricular contractions and an ECG showing markedly abnormal QRS complexes, usually a ventricular escape rhythm.

Dysrhythmia. A rhythm other than a normal sinus rhythm. A term more correct than "arrhythmia" but less frequently used.

Early afterdepolarization. See *Afterdepolarization.*

ECG. Abbreviation for electrocardiogram.

ECG artifacts. See *Artifacts.*

ECG calipers. A device used in determining the heart rate and rhythm and measuring the various intervals and segments in an ECG tracing.

ECG grid. The grid on the ECG paper is formed by dark and light horizontal and vertical lines. It is used to measure the time in seconds (sec) and distance in millimeters (mm) along the horizontal lines, and voltage (amplitude) in millimeters (mm) along the vertical lines. The dark vertical lines are 0.20 second (5 mm) apart; the light vertical lines, 0.04 second (1 mm) apart. The dark horizontal lines are 5 mm apart; the light horizontal lines, 1 mm apart. A large square is 5 × 5 mm; a small square, 1 × 1 mm.

ECG lead. One of twelve ECG leads which measure the difference in electrical potential generated by the heart, obtained by using a positive and a negative electrode—the positive electrode attached to an extremity or the anterior chest wall and the negative electrode, to an extremity or a central terminal. Includes leads I, II, III, aVR, aVL, aVF, and V$_1$ through V$_6$.

ECG monitor. The screen of an oscilloscope used in viewing the ECG.

Ectopic beats. Premature beats originating in ectopic pacemakers in the atria, AV junction, and ventricles, e.g., premature atrial contractions (PACs), premature junctional contractions (PJCs), and premature ventricular contractions (PVCs).

Ectopic focus. A pacemaker other than the SA node.

Ectopic pacemakers. Abnormal pacemakers in the atria, AV junction, bundle branches, Purkinje network, and ventricular myocardium.

Ectopic P wave (P' wave). A P wave produced by the depolarization of the atria in an abnormal direction, initiated by an electrical impulse arising in an ectopic pacemaker in the atria, AV junction, or ventricles. The ectopic P wave may be either positive (upright) or negative (inverted) in lead II and may precede or follow the QRS complex.

Ectopic rhythms. Arrhythmias originating in ectopic pacemakers in the atria, AV junction, and ventricles.

Atrial. Wandering atrial pacemaker (WAP), premature atrial contractions (PACs), atrial tachycardia (nonparoxysmal atrial tachycardia, paroxysmal atrial tachycardia [PAT]), atrial flutter, atrial fibrillation.

Junctional. Premature junctional contractions (PJCs), nonparoxysmal junctional tachycardia (accelerated junctional rhythm, junctional tachycardia), paroxysmal junctional tachycardia (PJT).

Ventricular. Accelerated idioventricular rhythm (AIVR), premature ventricular contractions (PVCs), ventricular tachycardia (VT), ventricular fibrillation (VF).

Ectopic tachycardias. Abnormal rhythms originating in ectopic pacemakers having a rate of over 100 beats per minute, e.g., atrial tachycardia (nonparoxysmal atrial tachycardia, paroxysmal atrial tachycardia [PAT]), atrial flutter, atrial fibrillation, junctional tachycardia, paroxysmal junctional tachycardia (PJT), paroxysmal supraventricular tachycardia (PSVT), and ventricular tachycardia (VT).

Ectopic ventricular arrhythmias. Abnormal rhythms originating in ectopic pacemakers in the ventricles, e.g., accelerated idioventricular rhythm (AIVR), premature ventricular contractions (PVCs), ventricular tachycardia, and ventricular fibrillation.

Ectopy. A condition signifying the presence of ectopic beats and rhythms, e.g., ventricular ectopy.

Edema. A condition in which the body tissues have accumulated excessive tissue fluid or exudate (as in congestive heart failure).

Einthoven's equilateral triangle. An equilateral triangle depicted in the frontal plane using the lead axes of the three limb leads as the sides with the heart and its zero reference point in the center.

Einthoven's law. The sum of the electrical currents recorded in leads I and III equals the sum of the electrical currents recorded in lead **II**.

Electric current. The flow of electricity along a conductor in a closed circuit.

Electrical activity of the heart. The electric current generated by the depolarization and repolarization of the atria and ventricles, which can be graphically displayed on the ECG.

Electrical alternans. Periodic alternation in the size of the QRS complexes between normal and small, coincident with respiration; typically present in cardiac tamponade.

Electrical axis and vector. A graphic presentation, using an arrow, of the electric current generated by the depolarization and repolarization of the atria and ventricles.

Electrical conduction system of the heart. Includes the sinoatrial (SA) node, internodal atrial conduction tracts, interatrial conduction tract (Bachmann's bundle), atrioventricular (AV) node, bundle of His, right and left bundle branches, and Purkinje network.

Electrical conduction system of the ventricles. The His- Purkinje system which includes the bundle of His, the right and left bundle branches, and the Purkinje network.

Electrical impulse. The tiny electric current that normally originates in the SA node automatically and is conducted through the electrical conduction system to the atria and ventricles, causing them to depolarize and contract.

Electrical nonuniformity. A condition of the ventricles during the vulnerable period of ventricular repolarization, i.e., the relative refractory period of the ventricles coincident with the peak of the T wave, when the ventricular muscle fibers may be completely repolarized, partially repolarized, or completely refractory. Stimulation of the ventricles at this point by an intrinsic electrical impulse such as that generated by a PVC or by an extrinsic impulse from a cardiac pacemaker or an electrical countershock may result in nonuniform conduction of the electrical impulse through the muscle fibers, setting up a reentry mechanism that may precipitate repetitive ventricular contractions and result in ventricular tachycardia or fibrillation. Responsible for the "R-on-T phenomenon."

Electrical potential. Refers to the amount of electric current generated by the depolarization and repolarization of the heart and expressed as millivolts (mV). It ranges between 0 to ± 20 mV or more.

Electrocardiogram (ECG). The graphic display of the electrical activity of the heart generated by the depolarization and repolarization of the atria and ventricles. The ECG includes the QRS complex; the P, T, and U waves; the PR, ST, and TP segments; and the PR, QT, and R-R intervals.

Electrode. A sensing device that detects electrical activity such as that of the heart. May be positive or negative.

Electrolyte. A substance that when in solution dissociates into cations and anions, thus becoming capable of conducting electricity.

Electrolyte imbalance. Abnormal concentrations of serum electrolytes within the body caused by excessive intake or loss of such electrolytes as calcium, carbonate, chloride, potassium and sodium.

Electromechanical dissociation (EMD). A condition of the heart in which the electrical activity of the heart is present and can be recorded on the ECG, but effective ventricular contractions, blood pressure, and pulse are absent.

Embolism. Obstruction of a blood vessel by an embolus that reduces or stops blood flow, resulting in ischemia or necrosis of the tissue supplied by the blood vessel.

Embolus. A mass of solid, liquid, or gaseous material carried from one part of the circulatory system to another.

End-diastolic PVC. A PVC occurring at about the same time that a QRS complex of the underlying rhythm is expected to occur.

Endocardium. The thin membrane lining the inside of the heart.

Enhanced automaticity. An abnormal condition of latent pacemaker cells in which their firing rate is increased beyond their inherent rate because of a spontaneous increase in the slope of phase 4 depolarization. See *Slope of phase 4 depolarization.*

Epicardial surface. The outside surface of the heart.

Epicardium. The thin membrane lining the outside of the heart.

Epinephrine (Adrenalin). A hormone and drug produced by the adrenal gland and other tissues of the body. It is an alpha- and beta-stimulator causing an increase in blood pressure by means of peripheral artery vasoconstriction and an increase in cardiac output by increasing heart rate and force of ventricular contraction. Used in the treatment of bradycardia, hypotension and shock, ventricular fibrillation/pulseless ventricular tachycardia, ventricular asystole, and pulseless electrical activity (PEA).

Equiphasic deflection. A biphasic deflection in which the sum of the positive (upright) deflection or deflections in an ECG are equal to that of the negative (inverted) deflection or deflections.

Escape beat or complex. A QRS complex arising in an escape (or secondary pacemaker) in the AV junction or ventricles when the underlying rhythm slows to less than the escape or secondary pacemaker's inherent firing rate. Such rhythms are called junctional or ventricular escape beats or complexes.

Escape (or secondary) pacemaker. A latent pacemaker in the AV junction or ventricles that takes over pacing the heart when the pacemaker of the underlying rhythm slows to less than the latent pacemaker's inherent firing rate or stops functioning altogether.

Escape rhythm. Three or more consecutive QRS complexes that result when the underlying rhythm slows to less than the escape or secondary pacemaker's inherent firing rate or stops altogether and the escape pacemaker takes over. Examples of escape rhythms are junctional escape rhythm and ventricular escape rhythm.

Essentially regular rhythm. A rhythm in which the shortest and longest R-R interval varies by less than 0.16 seconds (four small squares) in an ECG tracing.

Excitability, property of. The ability of a cell to respond to stimulation.

Extensive anterior MI. A myocardial infarction commonly caused by occlusion of the left anterior descending (LAD) coronary artery alone or in conjunction with the anterolateral marginal artery of the left circumflex coronary artery and characterized by early changes in the ST segments and T waves (i.e., ST elevation and tall, peaked T waves) in leads I, aVL, and V_1-V_6 and the appearance early of abnormal Q waves in leads V_1-V_2 and then later in leads I, aVL, and V_3-V_6.

External cardiac pacing. A technique to treat bradycardias, ventricular asystole, and pulseless electrical activity (PEA), including electromechanical dissociation (EMD), using an external artificial pacemaker.

Extrasystole. A premature beat or contraction independent of the underlying rhythm caused by an electrical impulse originating in an ectopic focus in the atria, AV junction, or ventricles. Examples of extrasystoles are premature atrial contractions (PACs), premature junctional contractions (PJCs), and premature ventricular contractions (PVCs).

Facing ECG leads. Leads that view specific surfaces of the heart, e.g., leads V_1-V_4 are facing leads viewing the anterior of the heart.

Fascicular block. Absent conduction of electrical impulses through one of the fascicles of the left bundle branch, i.e., left anterior fascicular block, left posterior fascicular block.

Fascicular premature ventricular contraction (PVC). A PVC with an almost normal QRS complex originating in the ventricles near the bifurcation of the bundle of His.

Fast sodium channels. Structures in the cell membrane called "pores" which facilitate the rapid flow of sodium ions into the cell during depolarization, rapidly changing the electrical potential within the cell from negative to positive. Fast sodium channels are typically found in the myocardial cells and the cells of the electrical conduction system other than those of the SA and AV nodes.

Fibrillation. Chaotic, disorganized beating of the myocardium in which each myofibril contracts and relaxes independently, producing rapid, tremulous and ineffectual contractions. Fibrillation may occur in both the atria and ventricles.

Fibrillation (f) waves. On the ECG, these waves appear as numerous irregularly shaped, rounded (or pointed), and dissimilar waves originating in multiple ectopic foci in the atria or ventricles.

Fine atrial fibrillation. Atrial fibrillation with fine fibrillatory waves—less than 1 mm in height.

Fine ventricular fibrillation. Ventricular fibrillation with small fibrillatory waves—less than 3 mm in height.

Firing rate. The rate at which electrical impulses are generated in a pacemaker, whether it is the SA node or an ectopic or escape pacemaker.

First-degree AV block. An arrhythmia in which there is a constant delay in the conduction of electrical impulses through the AV node. It is characterized by abnormally prolonged PR intervals (greater than 0.20 second).

Fixed coupling. Equal intervals of time between each premature beat and the preceding QRS complex of the underlying rhythm, i.e., equal (constant) coupling intervals.

Fixed rate pacemakers. Artificial pacemakers designed to fire constantly at a preset rate without regard to the patient's own heart's electrical activity.

Fluid bolus. A rapidly administered predetermined volume of IV fluid, such as 0.9% saline or Ringer's lactate solution, to reverse hypotension and shock.

Flutter. Rapid, regular, repetitive beating of the atria or ventricles.

Flutter-fibrillation. Refers to the simultaneous occurrence of flutter and fibrillation as in atrial flutter-fibrillation.

Flutter (F) waves. On the ECG, these waves appear as numerous repetitive, similar, usually pointed waves originating in an ectopic pacemaker in the atria or ventricles.

Frequent PVCs. Five or more PVCs per minute.

Frontal plane. A flat surface passing through the body at right angles to a plane passing through the body from front to back in the midline (sagittal plane), as viewed from the front of the body.

Full (fully) compensatory pause. See *Compensatory pause.*

Furosemide. A rapid-acting diuretic used to treat congestive heart failure.

Fusion beat, ventricular. A ventricular complex unlike the QRS complexes of the underlying rhythm and those of the ventricular arrhythmia in a given ECG lead, having features of both. This results from the stimulation of the ventricles by two electrical impulses, one originating in the SA node or an ectopic focus in the atria or AV junction and the other in an ectopic focus in the ventricles. A fusion beat can occur in accelerated idioventricular rhythm (AIVR), pacemaker rhythm, premature ventricular contractions (PVCs), and ventricular tachycardia.

f waves. See *Atrial fibrillation (f) waves.*

F waves. See *Atrial flutter (F) waves.*

Gap junction. A structure within the intercalated disks located at the junctions of the branches of myocardial cells, permitting very rapid conduction of electrical impulses from one cell to another.

Gram (gm). Measurement of metric weight equal to about one cubic centimeter (cc) or one milliliter (ml) of water. 1,000 grams is equal to 1 kilogram.

Grid, ECG. See *ECG grid.*

Ground electrode. The ECG lead other than the positive and negative leads that grounds the input to prevent extraneous noise from entering the amplifier circuit.

Group beating. Repetitive sequence of two or more consecutive beats followed by a dropped beat as seen in second-degree AV block.

Group beats. Occurrence of two or more consecutive atrial, junctional, or ventricular premature contractions preceded and followed by the underlying rhythm.

Heart rate. The number of heart beats or QRS complexes per minute.

Heart rate calculator ruler. A rulerlike device used to calculate the heart rate.

Hemiblock. Blockage to the conduction of electrical impulses in one of the fascicles (anterior or posterior) of the left bundle branch. See *left anterior fascicular block (LAFB), left posterior fascicular block (LPFB).*

Hemodynamically stable (or unstable). Refers to a patient who is normotensive, without chest pain or congestive heart failure and not having an acute myocardial infarction or ischemic episode. A patient who is **hemodynamically unstable,** on the other hand, is hypotensive with evidence of poor peripheral perfusion, has chest pain or congestive heart failure, or is having an acute myocardial infarction or ischemic episode.

Hexaxial reference figure. A guide for determining the direction of the QRS axis in the frontal plane, formed by the lead axes of the three limb leads and three augmented leads, spaced 30° apart around a zero reference point.

His-Purkinje system (of the ventricles). The part of the electrical system consisting of the bundle of His, bundle branches, and Purkinje network.

"Hockey stick" pattern. The ventricular "strain" pattern in the QRS-ST-T complex produced by a downsloping ST segment depression and T wave inversion; characteristic of longstanding right or left ventricular hypertrophy. Synonymous with **left** or **right ventricular strain pattern.**

Horizontal plane. A flat surface passing through the body at right angles to the sagittal and frontal planes and, in the case of electrocardiography, dividing the chest into an upper and a lower half at the level of the heart.

Hypercalcemia. Elevated levels of calcium in the blood.

Hypercapnia. Excessive amount of carbon dioxide in the blood.

Hypercarbia. Hypercapnia.

Hyperkalemia. Excessive amount of potassium in the blood.

Hypertension. Blood pressure over 140/90 mm Hg.

Hypertrophy. See *Ventricular hypertrophy.*

Hyperventilation. Increased ventilation of the alveoli caused by abnormally rapid, deep, and prolonged respirations; the result is a loss of carbon dioxide from the body and eventually alkalosis.

Hypocalcemia. Low amount of calcium in the blood.

Hypocapnia. Low amount of carbon dioxide in the blood.

Hypocarbia. Hypocapnia.

Hypokalemia. Low amount of potassium in the blood.

Hypotension. Low blood pressure; generally considered to be a systolic blood pressure of 80 to 90 mm Hg or less.

Hypothermia. A state of low body temperature.

Hypoventilation. Decreased ventilation of the alveoli.

Hypovolemia. Decreased amount of blood in the body's cardiovascular system.

Hypoxemia. Reduced oxygenation of the blood.

Hypoxia. Reduced amount of oxygen. Hypoxia is used interchangeably with the term anoxia.

ICHD code. See *Intersociety Commission for Heart Disease Resources (ICHD) Code.*

Idioventricular. Pertaining to the ventricles.

Idioventricular rhythm. See *Ventricular escape rhythm.*

Idioventricular tachycardia. See *Accelerated idioventricular rhythm (AIVR).*

IM. Abbreviation for intramuscular.

Incomplete AV block (second-degree AV block). An arrhythmia in which one or more P waves are not conducted to the ventricles. See *Second-degree, type I AV block (Wenckebach); Second-degree, type II AV block; Second-degree, 2:1 and high-degree (advanced) AV block.*

Incomplete bundle branch block (right, left). Defective conduction of electrical impulses through the right or left bundle branch from the bundle of His to the Purkinje network in the myocardium, resulting in a slightly widened QRS complex, i.e., greater than 0.10 second but less than 0.12 second.

Incomplete compensatory pause. The R-R interval following a premature contraction that if added to the R-R interval preceding the premature complex would result in a sum less than the sum of two R-R intervals of the underlying rhythm. See *Compensatory pause.*

Indeterminate axis. A QRS axis between −90° and ±180°, i.e., **extreme right axis deviation.**

Indifferent, zero reference point. See *Central terminal.*

Infarction. Death (necrosis) of tissue caused by interruption of the blood supply to the affected tissue.

Inferior (diaphragmatic) MI. A myocardial infarction commonly caused by occlusion of the posterior left ventricular arteries of the right coronary artery or, less commonly, of the left circumflex coronary artery of the left coronary artery and characterized by early changes in the ST segments and T waves (i.e., ST elevation and tall, peaked T waves) and the appearance later of abnormal Q waves in leads II, III, and aVF.

Inferior vena cava. One of the two largest veins in the body that empty venous blood into the right atrium.

Inferolateral MI. A myocardial infarction that may be caused **(1)** by occlusion of **(a)** the laterally located diagonal arteries of the left anterior descending (LAD) coronary artery and/or the anterolateral marginal artery of the left circumflex coronary artery and **(b)** the posterior left ventricular arteries of the right coronary artery or, less commonly, of the left circumflex coronary artery of the left coronary artery or **(2)** by occlusion of the left circumflex artery of a dominant left coronary artery. The infarct is characterized by early changes in the ST segments and T waves (i.e., ST elevation and tall, peaked T waves) and the appearance later of abnormal Q waves in leads I, II, III, aVL, aVF, and V_5 or V_6.

Infranodal. Below the AV node.

Infrequent PVCs. Less than five PVCs per minute.

Infusion. Administration of a fluid other than blood into a vein.

Inherent firing rate. The rate at which a given pacemaker of the heart normally generates electrical impulses.

Instantaneous electrical axis or vector. A graphic presentation, using an arrow, of the electric current generated by the depolarization or repolarization of the atria and ventricles at any given moment.

Interatrial conduction tract. See *Bachmann's bundle.*

Interatrial septum. The membranous wall separating the right and left atria.

Intercalated disks. Specialized structures located at the junctions of the branches of myocardial cells that permit very rapid conduction of electrical impulses from one cell to another.

Internodal atrial conduction tracts. Part of the electrical conduction system of the heart consisting of three pathways of specialized conducting tissue located in the walls of the right atrium between the SA node and AV node.

Interpolated PVC. A PVC that occurs between two normally conducted QRS complexes without greatly disturbing the underlying rhythm. A full compensatory pause, commonly present with PVCs, is absent.

Intersociety Commission for Heart Disease Resources (ICHD) Code. A three letter code specifying the capabilities of an artificial pacemaker. The first letter of the code indicates which chamber is paced (A—atria, V—ventricles, D—both atria and ventricles); the second letter, which chamber is sensed (A—atria, V—ventricles, D—both atria and ventricles); the third letter, the response of the pacemaker to a P wave or QRS complex (I—pacemaker output inhibited by a P wave or QRS complex; D—pacemaker output inhibited by a QRS complex and triggered by a P wave).

Intervals. The sections of the ECG between waves and complexes of the ECG. Includes waves, complexes, and segments. See *P-P interval, PR interval, QT interval, and R-R interval.*

Interventricular septum. The membranous, muscular wall separating the right and left ventricles. The anterior portion of the interventricular septum is supplied by the left anterior descending (LAD) coronary artery, the posterior portion by the posterior descending coronary artery.

Intracardiac. Within the heart.

Intravenous (IV) drip. The very slow administration of fluid into a vein.

Intrinsicoid deflection. The downstroke of the R wave; the part of the QRS complex which begins at the peak of the last R wave and ends at the J point or tip of the following S wave. Follows the ventricular activation time (VAT) (or preintrinsicoid deflection).

Intrinsicoid deflection time (IDT). See *Ventricular activation time (VAT).*

Ion. An atom or group of atoms having a positive charge (cation) or a negative one (anion).

Ischemia. Reduced blood flow to tissue caused by narrowing or occlusion of the artery supplying blood to it. Ischemia results in tissue anoxia. Ischemia may be localized under the endocardium (subendocardial ischemia) or under the epicardium (subepicardial ischemia).

Ischemic heart disease. Heart disease caused by a deficiency of the blood supply to the heart (the myocardium, the electrical conduction system, and other structures), due to obstruction or constriction of the coronary arteries. Manifestations of ischemic heart disease include acute myocardial infarction, angina pectoris, bundle branch and fascicular blocks, and arrhythmias.

Ischemic T waves. Symmetrically positive and abnormally tall, peaked T waves or symmetrically and deeply inverted T waves that appear over an ischemic myocardium. Generally, the ischemic T waves are upright over subendocardial ischemia and inverted over subepicardial ischemia.

Isoelectric line. The flat (sometimes wavy) line in an ECG during which electrical activity is absent. Synonymous with **baseline.**

Isolated beat. A premature contraction occurring singly.

IV. Abbreviation for intravenous.

IV fluids. Sterile fluids such as 0.9% saline or Ringer's lactate solution administered intravenously.

IV line. A catheter or needle, a solution administration set, and an intravenous solution used to administer drugs and fluids intravenously.

Joules. Unit of electrical energy delivered for 1 second by an electrical source, such as a defibrillator. Used interchangeably with the term **Watt-seconds.**

J point. See *Junction (or "J") point.*

Junction (AV). See *Atrioventricular (AV) junction.*

Junctional arrhythmia. An arrhythmia arising in an ectopic or escape pacemaker in the AV junction, e.g., premature junctional contractions, junctional escape rhythm, nonparoxysmal junctional tachycardia (accelerated junctional rhythm, junctional tachycardia), and paroxysmal junctional tachycardia (PJT).

Junctional escape beats (complexes) and rhythms. Beats (or complexes) and rhythms originating in an escape pacemaker in the AV junction that occur when the rate of the underlying supraventricular rhythm drops to less than 40 to 60 beats per minute.

Junctional escape rhythm. An arrhythmia originating in an escape pacemaker in the AV junction with a rate of 40 to 60 beats per minute.

Junctional tachycardia. An arrhythmia originating in an ectopic pacemaker in the AV junction with a rate greater than 100 beats per minute. When abnormal QRS complexes occur with the tachycardia because of aberrant ventricular conduction, the tachycardia is called junctional tachycardia with aberrant ventricular conduction (aberrancy).

Junction (or "J") point. The point where the QRS complex becomes the ST segment or the ST-T wave.

K⁺. Symbol for potassium.

Kg. Abbreviation for kilogram.

Kilogram. A unit of metric weight measurement. One kilogram (kg) is equal to 1,000 grams, or 2.2 pounds.

KVO. Abbreviation for "keep the vein open."

L. Abbreviation for liter.

LAD. Left anterior descending coronary artery. See *Coronary circulation.*

Large squares. The areas on ECG paper enclosed by the dark horizontal and vertical lines of the grid.

Latent (or subsidiary) pacemaker cells. Cells in the electrical conduction system with the property of automaticity, located below the SA node. These cells hold the property of automaticity in reserve should the SA node fail to function properly or electrical impulses fail to reach them for any reason, such as a disruption in the electrical conduction system.

Lateral leads. Leads V₅ and V₆. The **left precordial leads.**

Lateral MI. A myocardial infarction commonly caused by occlusion of the laterally located diagonal arteries of the left anterior descending (LAD) coronary artery and/or the anterolateral marginal artery of the left circumflex coronary artery and characterized by early changes in the ST segments and T waves (i.e., ST elevation and tall, peaked T waves) and the appearance later of abnormal Q waves in leads I, aVL, and V₅ or V₆.

LBB. See *Left bundle branch (LBB).*

LBBB. See *Left bundle branch block (LBBB).*

Lead. A lead of the ECG. See *ECG lead.*

Lead axis. See *Axis of a lead (lead axis).*

Lead MCL₁, monitoring lead. See *Monitoring ECG lead MCL₁.*

Lead II, monitoring lead. See *Monitoring ECG lead II.*

Left anterior fascicular block (LAFB). Absent conduction of electrical impulses through the left anterior fascicle of the left bundle branch. Typical ECG pattern: q_1r_3 pattern. Also referred to as **left anterior hemiblock.**

Left atrial enlargement (left atrial dilatation and hypertrophy). This condition is usually caused by increased pressure and/or volume in the left atrium. It is found in mitral valve stenosis and insufficiency, acute myocardial infarction, left heart failure, and left ventricular hypertrophy from various causes, such as aortic stenosis or insufficiency, systemic hypertension, and hypertrophic cardiomyopathy.

Left axis deviation (LAD). A QRS axis greater than $-30°$ ($-30°$ to $-90°$).

Left bundle branch block (LBBB). Defective conduction of electrical impulses through the left bundle branch. Left bundle branch block may be complete or incomplete and be present with or without an intact interventricular septum.

Left bundle branch (LBB). Part of the electrical conduction system of the heart that conducts electrical impulses into the left ventricle. It consists of the left common bundle branch (or main stem), which divides into two bundles of fibers, the left anterior fascicle (LAF) and the left posterior fascicle (LPF).

Left posterior fascicular block (LPFB). Absent conduction of electrical impulses through the left posterior fascicle of the left bundle branch. Typical ECG pattern: q_3r_1 pattern. Also referred to as **left posterior hemiblock.**

Left precordial (or lateral) leads. Leads V_5 and V_6.

Left ventricular hypertrophy (LVH). Increase in the thickness of the left ventricular wall because of chronic increase in pressure and/or volume within the ventricle. Common causes include mitral insufficiency, aortic stenosis or insufficiency, and systemic hypertension.

Lenegre's disease/Lev's disease. Idiopathic degenerative disease of the electrical conduction system with fibrosis and/or sclerosis and disruption of the conduction fibers. A cause of bundle branch and fascicular blocks.

Lidocaine. An antiarrhythmic used to treat premature ventricular contractions (PVCs), ventricular fibrillation, and ventricular tachycardia.

Life-threatening arrhythmias. Include ventricular fibrillation, ventricular tachycardia, ventricular asystole, and pulseless electrical activity (PEA), such as electromechanical dissociation (EMD).

Limb or extremity leads. The three standard (bipolar) limb leads (leads I, II, and III) and the three augmented (unipolar) leads (leads aVR, aVL, and aVF).

Liter (L). A metric measurement of volume. One liter is equal to 1,000 milliliters (ml), or 1.1 quarts.

Loading dose. A single large dose of a drug that produces an initial high therapeutic blood level necessary to treat certain conditions.

Lower case letters. Lower case letters, such as q, r, s, are used to designate small deflections of the ECG.

LPF. See *Left posterior fascicle (LPF).*

LVH. See *Left ventricular hypertrophy (LVH).*

Magnesium sulfate. An electrolyte solution used to treat torsade de pointes.

Marked bradycardia. A bradycardia with a heart rate between 30 and 45 beats per minute or less accompanied by hypotension and signs and symptoms of decreased perfusion of the brain and other organs.

Marked sinus bradycardia. See *Marked bradycardia.*

MAT. See *Multifocal atrial tachycardia.*

MCL₁. See *Monitoring ECG lead MCL₁.*

Mean QRS axis. The average of all the ventricular vectors; the QRS axis, or simply, the axis.

Mean vector. An average of one or more vectors.

Medulla oblongata. Part of the brain stem connecting the cerebral hemispheres with the spinal cord; it contains specialized nerve centers for special senses, respiration, and circulation, including the sympathetic and parasympathetic nervous systems with their respective cardioaccelerator and cardioinhibitor centers.

Membrane potential. The electrical potential measuring the difference between the interior of a cell and the surrounding extracellular fluid.

mEq. Abbreviation for milliequivalents.

Meter. A metric unit of linear measurement. One meter is equal to 1,000 millimeters, or 39.37 inches.

mg. Abbreviation for milligrams.

μg. Abbreviation for microgram.

microgram (μg). A metric unit of measurement of weight. One thousand micrograms are equal to one milligram.

Midclavicular line. An imaginary line beginning in the middle of the left clavicle and running parallel to the sternum slightly inside the left nipple.

Midprecordial (or anterior) leads. Leads V_3 and V_4.

Mild bradycardia. A bradycardia with a heart rate between 50 and 59 beats per minute and absence of hypotension and signs and symptoms of decreased perfusion of the brain or other organs.

Mild sinus bradycardia. See *Mild bradycardia.*

Milliequivalents (mEq). The weight of a substance dissolved in one milliliter of solution.

Milligram (mg). A metric unit of weight. One thousand milligrams are equal to 1 kilogram, or 2.2 pounds.

Milliliter (ml). A metric unit of measurement of volume. One thousand milliliters are equal to 1 liter, or 1.1 quarts.

Millimeter (mm). A metric unit of linear measurement. One thousand millimeters are equal to 1 meter, or 39.37 inches.

Millimeter of mercury (mm Hg). A metric unit of weight used in the determination of blood pressure.

Millivolt (mV). A unit of electrical energy. One thousand millivolts are equal to 1 volt.

Mitral valve. The one-way valve located between the left atrium and the left ventricle.

ml. Abbreviation for milliliter.

mm. Abbreviation for millimeter.

mm Hg. Abbreviation for millimeters of mercury.

Monitored cardiac arrest. Cardiac arrest in a patient who is being monitored.

Monitoring ECG lead MCL₁. An ECG lead commonly used in the monitoring of arrhythmias in the hospital, particularly in differentiating supraventricular arrhythmias with aberrant ventricular conduction (aberrancy) from ventricular arrhythmias. Lead MCL₁ is obtained by attaching the positive electrode to the right side of the anterior chest in the fourth intercostal space just right of the sternum. The negative electrode is attached to left chest in the midclavicular line below the clavicle.

Monitoring ECG lead II. The single ECG lead commonly used for monitoring the heart solely for arrhythmias. Lead II is obtained by attaching the negative electrode to the right arm or the upper right anterior chest wall and the positive electrode to the left leg or the lower left anterior chest wall at the intersection of the fourth intercostal space and the midclavicular line.

Morphine sulfate. A narcotic analgesic used to produce amnesia in conscious patients before cardioversion of certain arrhythmias.

"M" (or rabbit ears) pattern. Refers to the rSR′ pattern of the QRS complex in V_1, representative of a right bundle branch block.

Multifocal. Indicates an arrhythmia originating in different pacemaker sites and having QRS complexes that differ in size, shape, and direction.

Multifocal atrial tachycardia (MAT). Atrial tachycardia originating in three or more different atrial ectopic pacemaker sites, characterized by P′ waves that differ in size, shape, and direction.

Multifocal premature ventricular contractions (PVCs). Different appearing premature ventricular contractions in the same tracing that originate from different ectopic pacemaker sites in the ventricles.

Multiform. Indicates an arrhythmia that originates in a single pacemaker site but has QRS complexes that differ in size, shape, and direction.

Multiform premature ventricular contractions (PVCs). Different appearing premature ventricular contractions in the same tracing that originate in the same ectopic pacemaker site in the ventricles.

Multiform ventricular tachycardia. Ventricular tachycardia with QRS complexes that differ markedly from beat to beat.

Muscle tremor. The cause of extraneous spikes and waves in the ECG brought on by voluntary or involuntary muscle movement or shivering; often seen in elderly persons or in a cold environment.

mV. Abbreviation for millivolt.

Myocardial. Pertaining to the muscular part of the heart.

Myocardial infarction (MI). See *Acute myocardial infarction (acute MI, AMI)*.

Myocardial injury. Reversible changes in the myocardial cells from prolonged lack of oxygen. ECG manifestations include ST segment elevation over injured myocardial cells.

Myocardial ischemia. Reversible changes in myocardial cells from a temporary lack of oxygen. ECG manifestations include symmetrical T wave elevation or inversion over ischemic myocardial cells.

Myocardial necrosis (infarction). Irreversible damage to myocardial cells causing their death, the result of prolonged lack of oxygen. ECG manifestations include abnormal Q waves over necrotic myocardial cells.

Myocardial (or "working") cells. Myocardial cells other than those in the electrical conduction system of the ventricles.

Myocardial rupture. Rupture of the myocardial wall, usually occurring in the left ventricle in the area of necrosis following an acute transmural myocardial infarction.

Myocardium. Cardiac muscle.

Myofibril. Tiny structure within a muscle cell that contracts when stimulated. Contains the contractile protein filaments actin and myosin.

Myosin. One of the contractile protein filaments in myofibrils which give the myocardial cells the property of contractility. The other is actin.

Na⁺. Symbol for sodium ion.

Necrosis. Death of tissue.

Nervous control of the heart. Emanates from the autonomic nervous system which includes the sympathetic (adrenergic) and parasympathetic (cholinergic or vagal) nervous systems, each producing opposite effects when stimulated.

Nitroglycerin. A vasodilator used to treat severe pulmonary edema.

Noise. Extraneous spikes, waves, and complexes in the ECG signal caused by muscle tremor, 60-cycle AC interference, improperly attached electrodes, and biomedical telemetry-related events, such as out-of-range ECG transmission and weak transmitter batteries.

Noncompensatory pause. The R-R interval following a premature contraction that, if added to the R-R interval preceding the premature complex, would result in a sum less than the sum of two R-R intervals of the underlying rhythm. Synonymous with **incomplete compensatory pause**. See *Compensatory pause*.

Nonconducted PAC. A positive P′ wave (in Lead II) not followed by a QRS complex. A blocked PAC.

Nonconducted PJC. A negative P′ wave (in Lead II) not followed by a QRS complex. A blocked PJC.

Nonconducted P wave. A P wave not followed by a QRS complex. A dropped beat.

Nonpacemaker cell. A cardiac cell without the property of automaticity.

Nonparoxysmal junctional tachycardia. See *Accelerated junctional rhythm* and *Junctional tachycardia*.

Nonparoxysmal atrial tachycardia. See *Atrial tachycardia*.

Non-Q wave MI. A myocardial infarction where abnormal Q waves are absent in the ECG; considered a nontransmural subendocardial myocardial infarction in this book.

Nonsustained ventricular tachycardia. Paroxysms of three or more PVCs separated by the underlying rhythm. Paroxysmal ventricular tachycardia.

Nontransmural. Not extending from the endocardium to the epicardium, i.e., partial involvement of the myocardial wall.

Nontransmural myocardial infarction. A myocardial infarction in which the ventricular wall is only partially involved by the infarction.

Norepinephrine base (Levophed, levarterenol). A sympathomimetic used in the treatment of hypotension and shock.

Normal QRS axis. A QRS axis between −30° and +90°.

Normal saline. Incorrect term for the intravenous saline solution containing 0.9 percent sodium chloride (0.9% saline).

Normal sinus rhythm (NSR). Normal rhythm of the heart, originating in the SA node with a rate of 60 to 100 beats per minute.

Notch. A sharply pointed upright or downward wave in the QRS complex or T wave that does not go below or above the baseline, respectively.

Opposite (or reciprocal) ECG leads. See *"Reciprocal" ECG changes*.

Optimal sequential pacemaker (DDD). An artificial pacemaker that paces the atria or ventricles or both when spontaneous atrial or ventricular activity is absent.

Overdrive suppression. The suppression of spontaneous depolarization of the SA node or an escape or ectopic pacemaker by a series of electrical impulses (from whatever source) that depolarize the pacemaker cells prematurely. Following termination of the electrical impulses, there may be a slight delay in the appearance of the next expected spontaneous depolarization of the affected pacemaker cells because of a depressing effect that premature depolarization has on their automaticity.

Overload. Refers to increased pressure, volume, or both within a chamber of the heart from various causes, resulting in chamber enlargement from dilatation, hypertrophy, or both. Examples are right atrial enlargement, left atrial enlargement, right ventricular hypertrophy, and left ventricular hypertrophy.

PAC. Abbreviation for premature atrial contraction.

Pacemaker, artificial. An electronic device used to stimulate the heart to beat when the electrical conduction system of the heart malfunctions causing bradycardia or ventricular asystole. An artificial pacemaker consists of an electronic pulse generator, a battery, and a wire lead that senses the electrical activity of the heart and delivers electrical impulses to the atria or ventricles or both when the pacemaker senses an absence of electrical activity.

Pacemaker cell. A cell with the property of automaticity.

Pacemaker of the heart. The SA node or an escape or ectopic pacemaker in the electrical system of the heart or in the myocardium. May be sinus nodal, atrial, AV junctional, or ventricular.

Pacemaker rhythm. An arrhythmia produced by an artificial pacemaker.

Pacemaker site. The site of the origin of an electrical impulse. It can be the SA node or an escape or ectopic pacemaker in any part of the electrical system of the heart or in the myocardium.

Pacemaker spike. The narrow sharp wave in the ECG caused by the electrical impulse generated by an artificial pacemaker.

Paired beats. Atrial or ventricular ectopic beats occurring in groups of two. Also called **coupled beats, couplet.**

Paired PVCs. Two consecutive PVCs.

Parasympathetic (cholinergic or vagal) activity. The inhibitory action on the heart, blood vessels, and other organs brought on by the stimulation of the parasympathetic nervous system. The effect on the heart and blood vessels results in an decrease in heart rate, cardiac output, and blood pressure and, sometimes, an AV block.

Parasympathetic (cholinergic or vagal) nervous system. Part of the autonomic nervous system involved in the control of involuntary bodily functions, including the control of cardiac and blood vessel activity. Activation of this system depresses cardiac activity and produces effects opposite to those of the sympathetic nervous system. Some effects of parasympathetic stimulation are slowing of the heart rate, decreased cardiac output, drop in blood pressure, nausea, vomiting, bronchial spasm, sweating, faintness and hypersalivation.

Parasympathetic (cholinergic or vagal) tone. Pertains to the degree of parasympathetic activity.

Paroxysm. Sudden occurrence; spasm or seizure.

Paroxysmal atrial tachycardia (PAT). An arrhythmia originating in an ectopic pacemaker in the atria with a rate between 160 and 240 beats per minute. It typically starts and ends abruptly, occurring in paroxysms which may last from a few seconds to many hours and recur for many years. May occur with narrow QRS complexes or abnormally wide QRS complexes because of preexisting bundle branch block, aberrant ventricular conduction, or anomalous AV conduction. When abnormal QRS complexes occur with the tachycardia because of aberrant ventricular conduction, the tachycardia is called paroxysmal atrial tachycardia (PAT) with aberrant ventricular conduction (aberrancy).

Paroxysmal junctional tachycardia (PJT). An arrhythmia originating in an ectopic pacemaker in the AV junction with a rate between 160 and 240 beats per minute. It typically starts and ends abruptly, occurring in paroxysms which may last from a few seconds to many hours and recur for many years. May occur with narrow QRS complexes or abnormally wide QRS complexes because of preexisting bundle branch block or aberrant ventricular conduction. When abnormal QRS complexes occur with the tachycardia because of aberrant ventricular conduction, the tachycardia is called paroxysmal junctional tachycardia (PJT) with aberrant ventricular conduction (aberrancy).

Paroxysmal supraventricular tachycardia (PSVT). A commonly used term to indicate a paroxysmal tachycardia with a rate between 160 and 240 beats per minute originating in the atria or AV junction when the origin of the tachycardia is not clearly evident. May occur with narrow QRS complexes or abnormally wide QRS complexes because of preexisting bundle branch block, aberrant ventricular conduction, or anomalous AV conduction. When abnormal QRS complexes occur with the tachycardia because of aberrant ventricular conduction, the tachycardia is called paroxysmal supraventricular tachycardia (PSVT) with aberrant ventricular conduction (aberrancy).

Paroxysmal ventricular tachycardia. A short burst of ventricular tachycardia consisting of three or more QRS complexes.

Paroxysms of beats. Bursts of three or more beats. Three or more beats are considered to be a tachycardia.

P axis. The mean of all the vectors generated during the depolarization of the atria.

PEA. See *Pulseless electrical activity (PEA).*

Peak of the T wave. Coincident with the vulnerable period of ventricular repolarization, during which a premature ventricular contraction (PVC) can initiate ventricular tachycardia or ventricular fibrillation.

Perfusion. Passage of a fluid such as blood through the vessels of a tissue or organ.

Pericardial effusion. Fluid within the pericardial cavity or sac.

Pericardial tamponade. Accumulation of fluid under pressure within the pericardial cavity.

Pericarditis. Inflammation of the pericardium accompanied by chest pain somewhat resembling that of acute myocardial infarction. The ECG in acute pericarditis mimics that of acute myocardial infarction because of marked ST segment elevation.

Pericardium. The tough fibrous sac containing the heart and origins of the superior vena cava, inferior vena cava, aorta, and pulmonary artery. The pericardium consists of an inner, two-layered, fluid-secreting membrane (serous pericardium) and an outer tough, fibrous sac (fibrous pericardium). The inner layer of the serous pericardium, the visceral pericardium or, as it is more commonly known, the epicardium, covers the heart itself and the outer layer, the parietal pericardium, lines the fibrous pericardium. Between the two layers of the serous pericardium is the pericardial space or cavity (or sac), containing the pericardial fluid.

Peripheral vascular resistance. The resistance to blood flow in the systemic circulation that depends on the degree of constriction or dilation of the small arteries, arterioles, venules, and small veins making up the peripheral vascular system.

Peripheral vasoconstriction. Constriction of blood vessels, especially the small arteries, arterioles, venules, and small veins, causing an increase in blood pressure and a decrease in the circulation of blood beyond the point of vasoconstriction.

Peripheral vasodilatation. Dilation of blood vessels, especially the small arteries, arterioles, venules, and small veins, causing a decrease in blood pressure.

Perpendicular of a lead axis (perpendicular axis). A line intersecting or connecting with the lead axis at ±90° (or a right angle), at its electrically "zero" point. Also referred to as simply as the **perpendicular.**

pH. Symbol for the concentration of hydrogen ions (H^+) in a solution.

Phases of acute MI.
Phase 1: 0 to 2 hours   **Phase 3:** 24 to 72 hours
Phase 2: 2 to 24 hours   **Phase 4:** 2 to 8 weeks

Phases of depolarization and repolarization. See *Cardiac action potential.*

Physiological AV block. An AV block that occurs only when an atrial arrhythmia, such as atrial fibrillation, atrial flutter, and atrial tachycardia, is present.

PJC. Abbreviation for premature junctional contraction.

Pleura. The serous membrane enveloping the lungs and lining the thoracic cavity, completely enclosing a space filled with fluid, the pleural cavity.

P mitrale. A wide notched P wave occurring in the presence of left atrial dilatation and hypertrophy. Typically associated with severe mitral stenosis.

Pneumothorax, tension. Accumulation of air under positive pressure within the pleural cavity.

Polarity. The condition of being positive or negative.

Polarized (or resting) state of the cell. The condition of the cell following repolarization when the interior of the cell is negative and the outside positive.

Poor R-wave progression. Refers to the presence of small R waves in the precordial leads V_1 through V_5 or V_6 characteristic of chronic obstructive pulmonary disease (COPD).

Post-defibrillation arrhythmia. An arrhythmia occurring following defibrillatory shocks, e.g., premature beats, bradycardias, and tachycardias.

Posterior MI. A myocardial infarction commonly caused by occlusion of the distal left circumflex artery and/or posterolateral marginal artery of the left circumflex artery and characterized by early changes in the ST segments and T waves (i.e., ST depression and inverted T waves) in leads V_1-V_4.

Potassium chloride. A potassium salt (electrolyte) used in the treatment of paroxysmal supraventricular tachycardia, including paroxysmal atrial and junctional tachycardia, if excessive administration of digitalis is suspected as the cause of the arrhythmia.

Potential (electrical). The difference in the concentration of ions across a cell membrane, for instance, measured in millivolts.

P-P interval. The section of the ECG between the onset of one P wave and the onset of the following P wave.

P prime (P′) wave. An abnormal P wave originating in an ectopic pacemaker in the atria or AV junction or, rarely, in the ventricles. Usually negative in lead II.

P pulmonale. A wide, tall P wave (greater than 2.5 mm in height) occurring in the presence of right atrial dilatation and hypertrophy. Typically associated with pulmonary disease such as COPD and increased pulmonary artery pressure.

Precordial. Pertaining to the precordium.

Precordial reference figure. An outline of the chest wall in the horizontal plane superimposed by the six precordial lead axes and their angles of reference in degrees, radiating out from the heart's zero reference point.

Precordial thump. A sharp brisk blow delivered to the midportion of the sternum with a clenched fist in an initial attempt to terminate ventricular fibrillation or pulseless ventricular tachycardia.

Precordial (unipolar) leads. Leads V_1, V_2, V_3, V_4, V_5, and V_6; each obtained using a positive electrode attached to a specific area of the anterior chest wall and a negative electrode to a central terminal. The positive electrode for each precordial lead is attached as follows:

V_1 Right side of the sternum in the fourth intercostal space.
V_2 Left side of the sternum in the fourth intercostal space.
V_3 Midway between V_2 and V_4.
V_4 Midclavicular line in the fifth intercostal space.
V_5 Anterior axillary line at the same level as V_4.
V_6 Midaxillary line at the same level as V_4.

V_1 and V_2 (the right precordial [or septal] leads) overlie the right ventricle.
V_3 and V_4 (the midprecordial [or anterior] leads) overlie the interventricular septum and part of the left ventricle.
V_5 and V_6 (the left precordial [or lateral] leads) overlie the left ventricle.

Precordium. The region of the thorax over the heart, the midportion of the sternum.

Preexcitation syndrome (anomalous AV conduction). An abnormal condition in which the electrical impulses enter the ventricles from the atria through an accessory pathway that bypasses the AV junction resulting in a short PR interval, a wide QRS complex with an initial slurring (delta wave) of the upward slope, and a tendency to atrial flutter and fibrillation with rapid ventricular rates and paroxysmal supraventricular tachycardia. A common type of preexcitation syndrome is the Wolff-Parkinson-White (WPW) syndrome.

Preintrinsicoid deflection. The part of the QRS complex measured from its onset to the peak of the R wave, or, if there is more than one R wave, to the peak of the last R wave. See *Ventricular activation time (VAT).*

Premature atrial contraction (PAC). An extra beat consisting of an abnormal P wave originating in an ectopic pacemaker in the atria followed by a normal or abnormal QRS complex. PACs with abnormal QRS complexes that occur only with the PACs are called PACs with aberrancy; such PACs resemble PVCs. Also called premature atrial beats (PABs) or complexes.

Premature ectopic beat (contraction). An extra beat or contraction originating in the atria, AV junction or ventricles, e.g., premature atrial contraction (PAC), premature junctional contraction (PJC), and premature ventricular contraction (PVC).

Premature junctional contraction (PJC). An extra beat that originates in an ectopic pacemaker in the AV junction, consisting of a normal or abnormal QRS complex with or without an abnormal P wave. If a P wave is present, the PR interval is shorter than normal. PJCs with abnormal QRS complexes that occur only with the PJCs are called PJCs with aberrancy. Such PJCs resemble PVCs.

Premature ventricular contraction (PVC). An extra beat consisting of an abnormally wide and bizarre QRS complex originating in an ectopic pacemaker in the ventricles.

Prinzmetal's angina. A severe form of angina pectoris occurring at rest, caused by coronary artery spasm.

Procainamide hydrochloride. An antiarrhythmic used to treat premature ventricular contractions and ventricular tachycardia.

Procainamide toxicity. Excessive administration of procainamide, manifested by wide QRS complexes, low and wide T waves, U waves, prolonged PR intervals, depressed ST segments, and prolonged QT intervals.

Prophylaxis. Preventive treatment.

Propranolol (Inderal). An antiarrhythmic used to treat atrial fibrillation, atrial flutter, nonparoxysmal atrial tachycardia without block, paroxysmal atrial tachycardia (PAT), and paroxysmal junctional tachycardia (PJT). Propranolol is one of several agents called beta blockers.

PR (P′R) interval. The section of the ECG between the onset of the P (or P′) wave and the onset of the QRS complex. Normal PR interval is 0.12 to 2.0 second.

PR segment. The section of the ECG between the end of the P wave and the onset of the QRS complex.

Pseudo-electromechanical dissociation. A life-threatening condition in which the ventricular contractions are too weak to produce a detectable pulse and blood pressure because of the failure of the myocardium or electrical conduction system or both from a variety of causes. A form of pulseless electrical activity (PEA).

Pulmonary circulation. Passage of blood from the right ventricle through the pulmonary artery, all of its branches, and capillaries in the lungs and then to the left atrium through the pulmonary venules and veins. The blood vessels within the lungs and those carrying blood to and from the lungs.

Pulmonary edema. Condition of the lungs where the pulmonary vessels are engorged and rigid with blood and the alveoli are filled with exudate and foam because of severe left heart failure. **Pulmonary congestion** is present when the pulmonary vessels are engorged and rigid with blood, but the alveoli are still clear.

Pulmonary embolism. Obstruction (occlusion) of pulmonary arteries by small amounts of solid, liquid, or gaseous material carried to the lungs through the veins. Typical ECG pattern: $S_1Q_3T_3$ pattern.

Pulmonary infarction. Localized necrosis of lung tissue caused by obstruction of the arterial blood supply, commonly caused by pulmonary embolism.

Pulmonic valve. The one-way valve located between the right ventricle and the pulmonary artery.

Pulseless electrical activity (PEA). The absence of a detectable pulse and blood pressure in the presence of electrical activity of the heart as evidenced by some type of an ECG rhythm other than ventricular fibrillation or ventricular tachycardia.

Pulseless ventricular tachycardia. A life-threatening arrhythmia equivalent to ventricular fibrillation and treated the same way, by immediate defibrillation.

Pump failure. Partial or total failure of the heart to pump blood forward effectively, causing congestive heart failure and cardiogenic shock. It is a complication of acute myocardial infarction, occurring more frequently in the presence of a bundle branch block.

Purkinje fibers. Tiny, immature muscle fibers forming an intricate web, the Purkinje network, spread widely throughout the subendocardial tissue of the ventricles, whose ends finally terminate at the myocardial cells.

Purkinje network of the ventricles. The part of the electrical conduction system between the bundle branches and the ventricular myocardium consisting of the Purkinje fibers and their terminal branches.

PVC. Abbreviation for premature ventricular contraction.

P wave. Normally, the first wave of the P-QRS-T complex representing the depolarization of the atria. The P wave may be positive (upright), symmetrically tall and peaked, or wide and notched; negative (inverted); biphasic (partially upright, partially inverted); or flat.

q_1r_3 pattern. Typical ECG pattern of an initial small q wave in lead I and an initial small r wave in lead III indicative of a left anterior fascicular block.

q_3r_1 pattern. Typical ECG pattern of an initial small q wave in lead III and an initial small r wave in lead I indicative of a left posterior fascicular block.

QRS axis. The single large vector representing the mean (or average) of all the ventricular vectors.

QRS complex. Normally, the wave following the P wave, consisting of the Q, R and S waves, and representing ventricular depolarization. May be normal (narrow), 0.10 second or less, or abnormal (wide), greater than 0.10 second.

qRS pattern. The QRS pattern present in leads V_5-V_6 typical of right bundle branch block with an intact interventricular septum. An example of a QRS complex with a "terminal S" wave.

QRS-ST-T pattern. Refers to the abnormally wide, "sine-wave" appearing QRS-ST-T complex that occurs in hyperkalemia.

QSR pattern. The QRS pattern present in leads V_1-V_2 typical of right bundle branch block with a damaged interventricular septum.

QS wave. A QRS complex that consists entirely of a single, large negative deflection.

QTc. See *Corrected QT interval (QTc).*

QT interval. The section of the ECG between the onset of the QRS complex and the end of the T wave, representing ventricular depolarization and repolarization.

Quadrants. Refers to the four quadrants of the hexaxial reference figure—quadrants I, II, III, and IV.

Quadrigeminy. A series of groups of four beats, usually consisting of three normally conducted QRS complexes followed by a premature contraction which may be atrial, junctional, or ventricular in origin (i.e., atrial quadrigeminy, junctional quadrigeminy, ventricular quadrigeminy).

Quinidine sulfate. An antiarrhythmic used to treat premature atrial and junctional contractions.

Quinidine toxicity. Excessive administration of quinidine, manifested electrocardiographically by wide, often notched P waves, wide QRS complexes, low, wide T waves, U waves, prolonged PR intervals, depressed ST segments, and prolonged QT intervals.

Q wave. The first negative deflection of the QRS complex not preceded by an R wave.

Q wave MI (infarction). A myocardial infarction where abnormal Q waves are present in the ECG. Considered a **transmural myocardial infarction.**

Rabbit ears pattern. See *rSR' pattern.*

Rate conversion table. A table converting the number of small squares between two adjacent R waves into the heart rate per minute.

Rate of impulse formation (the firing rate). See *Slope of phase 4 depolarization.*

R double prime (R''). The third R wave in a QRS complex.

"Reciprocal" ECG changes. ECG changes of evolving acute myocardial infarction present in opposite ECG leads, being, for the most part, opposite in direction to those in the facing ECG leads, i.e., a mirror image. For example, an elevated ST segment and a symmetrically tall, peaked T wave in a facing ECG lead is mirrored as a depressed ST segment and a deeply inverted T wave in an opposite ECG lead.

Reentry mechanism. A mechanism by which an electrical impulse repeatedly exits and reenters an area of the heart causing one or more ectopic beats.

Refractory. Inability to respond to a stimulus.

Refractory period. The time during which a cell or fiber may or may not be depolarized by an electrical stimulus depending on the strength of the electrical impulse. It extends from phase 0 to the end of phase 3 and is divided into the **absolute refractory period (ARP)** and **relative refractory period (RRP).** The absolute refractory period extends from phase 0 to about midway through phase 3. The relative refractory period extends from about midway through phase 3 to the end of phase 3.

Relative refractory period (RRP) of the ventricles. The period of ventricular repolarization during which the ventricles can be stimulated to depolarize by an electrical impulse stronger than usual. It begins at about the peak of the T wave and ends with the end of the T wave.

Repolarization. The electrical process by which a depolarized cell returns to its polarized, resting state.

Repolarization wave. The progression of the repolarization process through the atria and ventricles that appears on the ECG as the atrial and ventricular T waves.

Repolarized state. The condition of the cell when it has been completely repolarized.

Resting membrane potential. Electrical measurement of the difference between the electrical potential of the interior of a fully repolarized, resting cell and that of the extracellular fluid surrounding it.

Resting state of a cell. The condition of a cell when a layer of positive ions surrounds the cell membrane and an equal number of negative ions lines the inside of the cell membrane directly opposite each positive ion. A cell in such a condition is called a **polarized cell.**

Resuscitation. The restoration of life by artificial respiration and external chest compression.

Retrograde atrial depolarization. Abnormal depolarization of the atria that begins near the AV junction, producing a negative P' wave in Lead II. Typically associated with junctional arrhythmias.

Retrograde AV block. Delay or failure of backward conduction through the AV junction into the atria of electrical impulses originating in the bundle of His or ventricles.

Retrograde conduction. Conduction of an electrical impulse in a direction opposite to normal, that is, from the AV junction or ventricles (through the AV junction) to the atria or SA node. Same as **retrograde AV conduction.**

Right atrial enlargement (right atrial dilatation and hypertrophy). This condition is usually caused by increased pressure and/or volume in the right atrium. It is found in pulmonary valve stenosis, tricuspid valve stenosis and insufficiency (relatively rare), and pulmonary hypertension and right ventricular hypertrophy from various causes. These include chronic obstructive pulmonary disease (COPD), status asthmaticus, pulmonary embolism, pulmonary edema, mitral valve stenosis or insufficiency, and congenital heart disease.

Right axis deviation (RAD). A QRS axis greater than $+90°$. Extreme right axis deviation:—a QRS axis between $-90°$ and $\pm 180°$.

Right bundle branch block (RBBB). Defective conduction of electrical impulses through the right bundle branch. It may be complete or incomplete and be present with or without an intact interventricular septum. Typical ECG patterns:

- **rSR' pattern** in lead V_1, the so-called **"M" (or rabbit ears) pattern.**
- **Tall "terminal" R waves** in leads aVR and V_1-V_2.
- **Deep and slurred "terminal" S waves** in leads I, aVL, and V_5-V_6.
- **qRS pattern** in leads V_5-V_6—typical of right bundle branch block with an intact interventricular septum.
- **QSR pattern** in leads V_1-V_2—typical of right bundle branch block without an intact interventricular septum.

Right bundle branch (RBB). Part of the electrical conduction system of the heart that conducts electrical impulses into the right ventricle.

Right precordial (or septal) leads. Leads V_1-V_2.

Right ventricular hypertrophy (RVH). Increase in the thickness of the right ventricular wall because of chronic increase in pressure and/or volume within the ventricle. It is found in pulmonary valve stenosis and other congenital heart defects (e.g., atrial and ventricular septal defects), tricuspid valve insufficiency (relatively rare), and pulmonary hypertension from various causes. These include chronic obstructive pulmonary disease (COPD), status asthmaticus, pulmonary embolism, pulmonary edema, and mitral valve stenosis or insufficiency.

Ringer's lactate solution. Frequently used sterile IV solution containing sodium, potassium, calcium and chloride ions in about the same concentrations as present in blood, in addition to lactate ions.

R-on-T phenomenon. An ominous type of premature ventricular contraction that falls on the T wave of the preceding QRS-T complex. This can cause ventricular tachycardia or ventricular fibrillation.

RP' interval. The section of the ECG between the onset of the QRS complex and the onset of the P' wave following it. This is present in junctional arrhythmias and occasionally in ventricular arrhythmias.

R prime (R'). The second R wave in a QRS complex.

R-R interval. The section of the ECG between the onset of one QRS complex and the onset of an adjacent QRS complex or between two adjacent R waves.

RS pattern. Refers to the appearance of a QRS complex in which there is an initial tall R wave followed by a deep S wave.

rSR' pattern. A typical QRS complex pattern in V₁ present in right bundle branch block. Also referred to as the **"M" or rabbit ears pattern.**

R wave. The positive wave or deflection in the QRS complex. An upper case "R" indicates a large R wave; a lower case "r," a small R wave. May be tall or small; narrow or wide, slurred, or notched; biphasic, equiphasic, or triphasic.

Salvos. Refers to two or more consecutive premature contractions. Bursts.

SA node. The dominant pacemaker of the heart located in the wall of the right atrium near the inlet of the superior vena cava.

Saw tooth appearance. Description given atrial flutter waves.

Scooped-out appearance. Description given to the depression of the ST segment caused by digitalis. Also referred to as the **"digitalis effect."**

S double prime (S"). The third S wave in the QRS complex.

Secondary pacemaker of the heart. A pacemaker in the electrical system of the heart other than the SA node; an escape or ectopic pacemaker.

Second-degree AV block. An arrhythmia in which one or more P waves are not conducted to the ventricles. **Incomplete AV block.** See *AV block, second-degree, type I (Wenckebach); AV block, second-degree, type II;* and *AV block, second-degree, 2:1 and high-degree (advanced).*

Second-degree, type I AV block (Wenckebach). An arrhythmia in which progressive prolongation of the conduction of electrical impulses through the AV node occurs until conduction is completely blocked. It is characterized by progressive lengthening of the PR interval until a QRS complex fails to appear after a P wave. This phenomenon is cyclical.

Second-degree, type II AV block. An arrhythmia in which a complete block of conduction of the electrical impulses occurs in one bundle branch and an intermittent block in the other. It is characterized by regularly or irregularly absent QRS complexes (producing, commonly, an AV conduction ratio of 4:3 or 3:2). The QRS complexes, typically, are abnormally wide (greater than 0.12 second in duration).

Second-degree, 2:1 and high-degree (advanced) AV block. An arrhythmia caused by defective conduction of the electrical impulses through the AV node or the bundle branches or both. It is characterized by regularly or irregularly absent QRS complexes (producing, commonly, an AV conduction ratio of 2:1 or greater). The QRS complexes may be narrow (0.10 second or less) or abnormally wide (greater than 0.12 second in duration).

Segment. A section of the ECG between two waves, e.g., PR segment, ST segment, and TP segment. A segment does not include waves or intervals.

Self-excitation, property of. The property of a cell to reach a threshold potential and generate electrical impulses spontaneously without being externally stimulated. Also referred to as the **property of automaticity.**

Septal depolarization. Refers to the depolarization of the interventricular septum early in ventricular depolarization, producing the septal q and r waves.

Septal leads. Leads V₁-V₂. The **right precordial leads.**

Septal MI. A myocardial infarction commonly caused by occlusion of the left anterior descending (LAD) coronary artery beyond the first diagonal branch, involving the septal perforator arteries, and characterized by early changes in the ST segments and T waves (i.e., ST elevation and tall, peaked T waves) and the early appearance of abnormal Q waves in leads V₁-V₂.

Septal q waves. The small q waves produced by the normal left to right depolarization of the interventricular septum early in ventricular depolarization. Present in leads I, II, aVF, and the left precordial leads V₄, V₅, and V₆.

Septal r waves. The small r waves produced by the normal left to right depolarization of the interventricular septum early in ventricular depolarization. Present in the right precordial leads V₁ and V₂.

Septum. A wall separating two cavities.

Shock. A state of cardiovascular collapse caused by numerous factors such as severe AMI, hemorrhage, anaphylactic reaction, severe trauma, pain, strong emotions, drug toxicity, or other causes. A patient in decompensated shock typically has dulled senses and staring eyes, a pale and cyanotic color, cold and clammy skin, systolic blood pressure of 80 to 90 mm Hg or less, a feeble rapid pulse (over 110 beats per minute), and a urinary output of less than 20 milliliters per hour.

Short vertical lines. The vertical lines inscribed at every three-second interval along the top of the ECG paper.

Sick sinus syndrome. A clinical entity manifested by syncope or near-syncope, dizziness, increased congestive heart failure, angina, and/or palpitations as a result of a dysfunctioning sinus node, especially in the elderly. The ECG may show marked sinus bradycardia, sinus arrest, sinoatrial (SA) block, chronic atrial fibrillation or flutter, AV junctional escape rhythm, or tachyarrhythmias interspersing with the bradycardias (sinus-tachyarrhythmia syndrome).

Single-chamber pacemaker. Artificial pacemaker that paces either the atria or the ventricles when appropriate.

Sinoatrial (SA) exit block. An arrhythmia caused by a block in the conduction of the electrical impulse from the SA node to the atria, resulting in bradycardia, episodes of asystole, or both.

Sinoatrial (SA) node. See *SA node.*

Sinus arrest. An arrhythmia caused by a decrease in the automaticity of the SA node resulting in bradycardia, episodes of asystole, or both.

Sinus arrhythmia. Irregularity of the heart rate caused by fluctuations of parasympathetic activity on the SA node during breathing.

Sinus bradycardia. An arrhythmia originating in the SA node with a rate of less than 60 beats per minute.

Sinus node arrhythmias. Arrhythmias arising in the sinus (SA) node include: sinus arrhythmia, sinus bradycardia, sinus arrest and sinoatrial (SA) exit block, and sinus tachycardia.

Sinus P wave. A P wave produced by the depolarization of the atria initiated by an electrical impulse arising in the SA node.

Sinus tachycardia. An arrhythmia originating in the SA node with a rate of over 100 beats per minute.

Site of origin. Pacemaker site.

Six-second count method. A method of determining the heart rate by counting the number of QRS complexes within a six-second interval and multiplying this number by 10 to get the heart rate per minute.

Six-second intervals. The period of time between every third three-second interval mark.

Slope of phase 4 depolarization. Refers to the rate at which a cell membrane depolarizes spontaneously, becoming progressively less negative, during Phase 4—the period between action potentials. As soon as the threshold potential is reached, rapid depolarization of the cell (Phase 0) occurs. The rate of spontaneous depolarization is dependent on the degree of sloping of phase 4 depolarization. The steeper the slope of phase 4 depolarization, the faster is the rate of spontaneous depolarization and the rate of impulse formation (the firing rate). The flatter the slope, the slower is the firing rate.

Slow calcium-sodium channels. A mechanism in the membrane of certain cardiac cells, predominantly those of the SA and AV nodes, by which positively charged calcium and sodium ions enter the cells slowly during depolarization, changing the potential within these cells from negative to positive. The result is a slower rate of depolarization as compared to the depolarization of cardiac cells with fast sodium channels.

Slow ventricular tachycardia. See *Accelerated idioventricular rhythm (AIVR).*

Slurring of the QRS complex. The delta wave.

Small squares. The areas on ECG paper enclosed by the light horizontal and vertical lines of the grid.

Sodium bicarbonate. Chemical substance with alkaline properties used to increase the pH or alkalinity of the body when acidosis is present; considered in the treatment of electromechanical dissociation (EMD), ventricular asystole, ventricular fibrillation, and ventricular tachycardia.

Sodium-potassium pump. A mechanism in the cell membrane, activated during Phase 4—the period between action potentials, that transports excess sodium out of the cell and potassium back in to help maintain a stable membrane potential between action potentials.

Specialized cells of the electrical conduction system of the heart. One of two kinds of cardiac cells in the heart, the other being the myocardial (or "working") cells. The specialized cells conduct electrical impulses extremely rapidly (six times faster than do the myocardial cells), but do not contract. Some of these cells, the pacemaker cells, are also capable of generating electrical impulses spontaneously, having the property of automaticity.

Spikes. Artifacts in the ECG. If numerous and occurring randomly, they are most likely caused by muscle tremor, AC interference, loose electrodes, or biotelemetry-related interference. If they are regular, occurring at a rate of about 60 to 80/minute, they are most likely caused by an artificial pacemaker.

Spontaneous depolarization. Property possessed by pacemaker cells allowing them to achieve threshold potential and depolarize without external stimulation.

S prime (S′). The second S wave in the QRS complex.

$S_1Q_3T_3$ pattern. Typical ECG changes in lead I and lead III that occur in acute pulmonary embolism, i.e., large S wave in lead I and a Q wave and inverted T wave in lead III.

Standard (bipolar) limb leads. Standard limb leads I, II, and III; each obtained using a positive electrode attached to one extremity and a negative electrode to another extremity as follows:

Lead I. The positive electrode attached to the left arm and the negative electrode to the right arm.

Lead II. The positive electrode attached to the left leg and the negative electrode to the right arm. Commonly used as a monitoring lead in prehospital emergency cardiac care.

Lead III. The positive electrode attached to the left leg and the negative electrode to the left arm.

Standardization of the ECG tracing. A means of standardizing the amplitude of the waves and complexes of the ECG using a one millivolt/10 mm standardization impulse.

Standard Leads. Usually refers to the twelve ECG leads—**leads I, II, III, aVR, aVL, aVF, and V_1 through V_6.**

Standard paper speed. A rate of 25 mm per second.

ST axis. The mean of all the vectors generated during the ST segment.

Strain pattern. Refers to the combination of a downsloping ST segment depression and a T wave inversion, characteristic of longstanding right or left ventricular hypertrophy. Along with the R wave, gives the so-called "hockey stick" appearance to the QRS-ST-T complex.

ST segment. The section of the ECG between the end of the QRS complex and onset of the T wave. May be flat (horizontal), downsloping, or upsloping.

ST segment depression. An ECG sign of severe myocardial ischemia. An ST segment is considered to be depressed when it is ≥1 mm (≥0.1 mV) below the baseline, measured 0.08 second (2 small boxes) after the J point of the QRS complex. It may be downsloping, horizontal, and upsloping.

ST segment elevation. An ECG sign of severe widespread myocardial injury in the evolution of an acute myocardial infarction, usually indicating a transmural involvement. An ST segment is considered to be elevated when it is ≥1 mm (≥0.1 mV) above the baseline, measured 0.08 second (2 small boxes) after the J point of the QRS complex. ST segments may be elevated in leads opposite the leads with ST segment depression, that is, the leads facing ischemic tissue.

ST-T wave. The section of the ECG between the end of the QRS complex and the end of the T wave that includes the ST segment and T wave.

Subendocardial. Located under the endocardium.

Subendocardial, non-Q wave MI (infarction). A myocardial infarction localized in the subendocardial area of the myocardium with absent Q waves in the ECG. See *Non-Q wave myocardial infarction.*

Subepicardial. Located under the epicardium.

Sublingual. Under the tongue.

Substernal. Under the sternum (retrosternal).

Sudden death. Sudden and unexpected death usually from coronary artery disease in patients with relatively minor or vague premonitory symptoms, who appear well and are not expected to die.

Superior vena cava. One of the two largest veins in the body that empty venous blood into the right atrium.

Supernormal period of ventricular repolarization. The last phase of repolarization during which the cell can be stimulated to depolarize by an electrical stimulus smaller than usual, i.e., a subthreshold stimulus.

Supraventricular. Refers to the part of the heart above the bundle branches; includes the SA node, atria and AV junction.

Supraventricular arrhythmia. An arrhythmia originating above the bifurcation of the bundle of His.

Supraventricular tachycardia. An arrhythmia originating above the bifurcation of the bundle of His with a rate of over 100 beats per minute.

Sustained ventricular tachycardia. Prolonged ventricular tachycardia.

S wave. The first negative or downward wave of deflection of the QRS complex that is preceded by an R wave. An upper case "S" indicates a large S wave; a lower case "s," a small S wave. May be deep and narrow or wide and slurred.

Sympathetic (adrenergic) activity. The excitatory action on the heart, blood vessels, and other organs brought on by the stimulation of the sympathetic nervous system. The effect on the heart and blood vessels results in an increase in heart rate, cardiac output, and blood pressure.

Sympathetic (adrenergic) nervous system. Part of the autonomic nervous system involved in the control of involuntary bodily functions, including the control of cardiac and blood vessel activity. This system stimulates cardiac activity and produces effects opposite to those of the parasympathetic nervous system, which depresses cardiac activity. Some effects of sympathetic stimulation are an increase in heart rate, cardiac output, and blood pressure.

Sympathetic tone. Pertains to the degree of sympathetic activity.

Sympathomimetic drugs. Drugs that mimic the effects of stimulation of the sympathetic nervous system, e.g., epinephrine and norepinephrine.

Symptomatic bradycardia. A bradycardia with one or more of the following signs or symptoms: (1) hypotension (systolic blood pressure less than 80 to 90 mm Hg), (2) congestive heart failure, (3) chest pain, (4) dyspnea, (5) signs and symptoms of decreased cardiac output, or (6) premature ventricular contractions. Requires treatment immediately.

Symptomatic "relative" bradycardia. Normal sinus rhythm or an arrhythmia with a heart rate somewhat above 60 beats per minute with signs or symptoms associated with a symptomatic bradycardia because of the heart rate being too slow relative to the existing metabolic needs. Requires treatment immediately.

Synchronized countershock. A direct-current (DC) shock synchronized with the QRS complex used to terminate:
- **Atrial flutter** (hemodynamically stable or unstable)
- **Atrial fibrillation** (hemodynamically unstable)
- **Nonparoxysmal atrial tachycardia without block** (hemodynamically stable or unstable)
- **Paroxysmal atrial tachycardia (PAT), paroxysmal junctional tachycardia (PJT), paroxysmal supraventricular tachycardia (PSVT) with narrow QRS complexes** (hemodynamically stable or unstable), and
- **Ventricular tachycardia (with pulse)** (hemodynamically stable).

Syncytium. A branching and anastomosing network of cells, such as that formed by the interconnection of the cardiac cells to form the myocardium.

Systemic circulation. Passage of blood from the left ventricle through the aorta, all its branches, and capillaries in the tissue of the body and then to the right atrium through the venules, veins, and vena cavae. The blood vessels in the body (except those in the lungs) and those carrying blood to and from the body.

Systole (electrical). The period of time from phase 0 to the end of phase 3 of the cardiac action potential.

Systole (mechanical). The period of atrial or ventricular contraction.

Tachycardia. Considered to be three or more beats occurring at a rate exceeding 100 beats per minute.

Ta wave. Atrial T wave; usually buried in the following QRS complex.

T axis. The mean of all the vectors generated during the repolarization of the ventricles (i.e., during the T wave).

Temporary transvenous pacemaker. Delivery of electrical impulses generated by an external artificial pacemaker through a catheter threaded through a vein and positioned in the right ventricle.

Terminal. The final wave of the QRS complex.

Terminal R and S waves. Typical ECG findings in right bundle branch block—tall "terminal" R waves in leads aVR and V_1-V_2; deep and slurred "terminal" S waves in leads I, aVL, and V_5-V_6.

Third-degree AV block (complete AV block). Complete absence of conduction of electrical impulses from the atria to the ventricles through the AV junction. May be transient and reversible or permanent (chronic). Usually associated with abnormally wide QRS complexes, but the QRS complexes may be narrow. See *AV block, third-degree.*

Three-second interval. The time period between two adjacent three-second interval lines.

Threshold potential. The value of intracellular negativity at which point a cardiac cell can be depolarized after being electrically stimulated.

Thrombolysis. Disintegration of a blood clot.

Torsade de pointes. A form of ventricular tachycardia characterized by QRS complexes that gradually change back and forth from one shape and direction to another over a series of beats. A French expression meaning "twisting around a point."

TP segment. The section of the ECG between the end of the T wave and the onset of the P wave. Used as the baseline reference for the measurement of the amplitude of the ECG waves and complexes.

Transcutaneous overdrive pacing. The use of a transcutaneous pacemaker to terminate certain arrhythmias, such as, premature ventricular contractions; paroxysmal supraventricular tachycardia, including paroxysmal atrial and junctional tachycardia; wide-QRS-complex tachycardia of unknown origin; ventricular tachycardia (with pulse); and torsade de pointes. This is done by adjusting the pacemaker's rate to one that is greater than that of the arrhythmia.

Transcutaneous pacing. The delivery of electrical impulses through the skin.

Transmural. Extending from the endocardium to the epicardium.

Transmural, Q wave MI (infarction). An infarction where the zone of infarction involves the entire full thickness of the ventricular wall, from the endocardium to the epicardial surface.

Trendelenburg position. One in which the patient is supine on the backboard, the head of which is tilted downward 30 to 40 degrees, and the patient's knees bent.

Triaxial reference figure. A guide for determining the direction of the QRS axis in the frontal plane, formed by the lead axes of the three limb leads or the three augmented leads, spaced 60° apart around a zero reference point. The two triaxial reference figures, one formed by the standard limb leads and the other by the augmented leads, superimposed, form the hexaxial reference figure.

Tricuspid valve. The one-way valve located between the right atrium and the right ventricle.

Trigeminy. A series of groups of three beats, usually consisting of two normally conducted QRS complexes followed by a premature contraction. The premature contraction may be atrial, junctional, or ventricular in origin (i.e., atrial trigeminy, junctional trigeminy, ventricular trigeminy).

Triggered activity. See *Afterdepolarization.*

Triphasic rSR' pattern of RBBB. See *"M" (or rabbit ears) pattern.*

Triplicate method. A method used to determine the heart rate.

T wave. The part of the ECG representing repolarization of the ventricles that follows the QRS complex from which it is separated by the ST segment if it is present. It may be positive (symmetrically tall and peaked) or negative (deeply inverted).

T wave elevation/inversion. See *Ischemic T waves.*

12-lead electrocardiogram (ECG). The routine (or conventional) ECG consisting of three standard (bipolar) limb leads (leads I, II, and III), three augmented (unipolar) leads (leads aVR, aVL, and aVF), and six precordial (unipolar) leads (leads V_1, V_2, V_3, V_4, V_5, and V_6).

Uncontrolled. Refers to arrhythmias such as atrial flutter and atrial fibrillation that are untreated and, consequently, have rapid ventricular rates.

Underlying rhythm. The basic rhythm upon which certain arrhythmias are superimposed, e.g., sinus arrest and sinoatrial (SA) exit block, AV blocks, pacemaker rhythm, and premature atrial, junctional, and ventricular contractions.

Unifocal. Pertains to a single ectopic pacemaker.

Unifocal PVCs. PVCs originating in the same ventricular ectopic pacemaker site.

Uniform PVCs. PVCs having the same appearance and configuration, presumably arising from the same ventricular ectopic pacemaker site.

Unipolar chest ("V") leads. Leads V_1 to V_6.

Unipolar limb leads. Leads aVR, aVL and aVF.

Unmonitored cardiac arrest. Cardiac arrest that is witnessed by the resuscitation team or that has occurred before the arrival of the team and the patient is not being monitored.

Unsynchronized shock. A direct-current (DC) shock not synchronized with the QRS complex, used to treat (1) ventricular tachycardia with a pulse in a hemodynamically unstable patient and (2) torsade de pointes with or without a pulse.

Upper case letters. Upper case letters, such as Q, R, S, are used to designate large deflections of the ECG.

U wave. The positive wave superimposed on or following the T wave. Possibly represents the final phase of repolarization of the ventricles.

Vagal maneuvers. Methods to increase the vagal (parasympathetic) tone to convert paroxysmal atrial and junctional tachycardias. See *Valsalva maneuver.*

Vagal (parasympathetic) tone. See *Parasympathetic (vagal) tone.*

Vagus nerve. The parasympathetic nerve. Consists of the right and left vagus nerves.

Valsalva maneuver. Forceful act of expiration with the mouth and nose closed producing a bearing down on the abdomen. Used to increase the parasympathetic tone to convert paroxysmal atrial and junctional tachycardias.

Variable AV block. Refers to an AV block with varying AV conduction ratios, i.e., the ratio of P, P', F, or f waves to QRS complexes varies.

Vasoconstriction. Narrowing the diameter of blood vessels.

Vasoconstrictor. A drug, hormone, or substance that constricts the diameter of blood vessels.

Vasodilatation. Widening the diameter of blood vessels.

Vasodilator. A drug, hormone, or substance that dilates or widens the diameter of blood vessels.

Vasopressor. A drug that causes vasoconstriction.

Vasovagal. Pertaining to a vascular and neurogenic cause.

VAT. See *Ventricular activation time (VAT).*

Vector. A graphic presentation, using an arrow, of the electric current generated by the depolarization or repolarization of the atria and ventricles at any one moment of time.

Ventricle. The thick-walled muscular chamber which receives blood from the atrium and pumps it into the pulmonary or systemic circulation. The two ventricles form the larger lower part of the heart and the apex. They are separated from the atria by the mitral and tricuspid valves.

Ventricular activation time (VAT). The time it takes for depolarization of the interventricular septum, the right ventricle, and most of the left ventricle, up to and including the endocardial to epicardial depolarization of the left ventricular wall under the facing lead. Also called the **preintrinsicoid deflection** or **intrinsicoid deflection time (IDT).**

Ventricular arrhythmia. An arrhythmia originating in an ectopic pacemaker in the ventricles. Also referred to as **ventricular ectopy.**

Ventricular asystole (cardiac standstill). Cessation of ventricular contractions.

Ventricular demand pacemaker (VVI). An external pacemaker that senses spontaneously occurring QRS complexes and paces the ventricles when they do not appear.

Ventricular diastole. The interval or period during which the ventricles are relaxed and filling with blood. The period between ventricular contractions.

Ventricular dilatation. Distension of the ventricle because of increased pressure and/or volume within the ventricle; it may be acute or chronic.

Ventricular enlargement. Ventricular enlargement includes ventricular dilatation and hypertrophy. Common causes include heart failure, pulmonary diseases, pulmonary or systemic hypertension, heart valve stenosis or insufficiency, congenital heart defects, and acute myocardial infarction. See *Left ventricular hypertrophy (LVH)*, *Right ventricular hypertrophy (RVH)*.

Ventricular escape rhythm. An arrhythmia arising in an escape or ectopic pacemaker in the ventricles with a rate of less than 40 beats per minute.

Ventricular fibrillation/pulseless ventricular tachycardia. Two ventricular life-threatening arrhythmias that are treated alike by immediate defibrillation.

Ventricular fibrillation (VF, V-FIB). An arrhythmia originating in multiple ectopic pacemakers in the ventricles characterized by numerous ventricular fibrillatory waves and no QRS complexes.

Ventricular fibrillation (VF) waves. Bizarre, irregularly shaped, rounded or pointed, and markedly dissimilar waves originating in multiple ectopic pacemakers in the ventricles.

Ventricular fusion beat. See *Fusion beat, ventricular.*

Ventricular hypertrophy. Enlargement of the ventricular myocardium, the result of an increase in the size of the muscle fibers because of chronic increase in pressure and/or volume within the ventricle. Common causes include heart failure, pulmonary diseases, pulmonary or systemic hypertension, heart valve stenosis or insufficiency, and congenital heart defects. See *Left ventricular hypertrophy (LVH), Right ventricular hypertrophy (RVH).*

Ventricular overload. Refers to increased pressure and/or volume within the ventricles.

Ventricular repolarization. The electrical process by which the depolarized ventricles return to their polarized, resting state. Ventricular depolarization is represented by the T wave on the ECG.

Ventricular "strain" pattern. The changes in the QRS-ST-T complex produced by a downsloping ST segment depression and T wave inversion, characteristic of longstanding right or left ventricular hypertrophy. Also known as the **"hockey stick" pattern.**

Ventricular systole. The interval or period during which the ventricles are contracting and emptying of blood.

Ventricular tachycardia (VT, V-TACH). An arrhythmia originating in an ectopic pacemaker in the ventricles with a rate between 110 and 250 beats per minute.

Ventricular T wave (T wave). Represents ventricular repolarization.

Verapamil. An antiarrhythmic used to treat paroxysmal atrial and junctional tachycardias.

V leads. Leads V_1, V_2, V_3, V_4, V_5, and V_6. See *Precordial (unipolar) leads.*

Voltage (amplitude). See *Amplitude (voltage).*

Vulnerable period of ventricular repolarization. The part of the last phase of repolarization during which the ventricles can be stimulated to depolarize prematurely by a greater than normal electrical stimulus. This corresponds to the downslope of the T wave.

Wandering atrial pacemaker (WAP). An arrhythmia originating in pacemakers that shift back and forth between the SA node and an ectopic pacemaker in the atria or AV junction. It is characterized by P waves varying in size, shape, and direction in any given lead.

Warning arrhythmias. PVCs that are more prone than others to initiate life-threatening arrhythmias, particularly following an acute myocardial infarction or ischemic episode:
- **PVCs falling on the T wave** (the **R-on-T phenomenon**)
- **Multiform** and **multifocal PVCs**
- **Frequent PVCs** of more than five or six per minute
- **Ventricular group beats** with bursts or salvos of two, three, or more

Watt/seconds. Units of electrical energy delivered by a source of energy, such as a defibrillator. One watt/second equals **1 joule.**

Waves. Refers to various components of the ECG—the P, Q, R, S, T, and U waves. Waves may be large or small.

Wenckebach block. See *Second-degree, type I AV block (Wenckebach).*

Wenckebach phenomenon. A progressive prolongation of the conduction of electrical impulses through the AV junction until conduction is completely blocked, occurring in cycles.

Wide-QRS-complex tachycardia. A tachycardia with abnormally wide QRS complexes (0.12 second or greater) which may be ventricular tachycardia or a supraventricular tachycardia with wide QRS complexes resulting from a preexisting bundle branch block, aberrant ventricular conduction, or anomalous AV conduction.

"Window" theory. Refers to the popular theory of why Q waves occur over infarcted myocardium. According to the theory, the facing leads over electrically inert infarcted myocardium (or "window") view the endocardium of the opposite noninfarcted ventricular wall, and detect the R waves generated by the opposite wall as large Q waves.

Wolff-Parkinson-White (WPW) syndrome. See *Preexcitation syndrome.*

"Zero" center of the heart. Refers to the hypothetical reference point with an electrical potential of zero, located in the electrical center of the heart—left of the interventricular septum and below the AV junction. Formed by connecting the extremity electrodes together, the "indifferent," zero reference point is used as the central terminal for the unipolar leads. It also represents the central point for the hexaxial reference figure.

Zones of infarction (necrosis), injury, and ischemia. A myocardial infarction at its height typically consists of a central area of dead, necrotic tissue—the **zone of infarction** (or **necrosis**), surrounded immediately by a layer of injured myocardial tissue—the **zone of injury,** and, lastly, by an outer layer of ischemic tissue—the **zone of ischemia.**

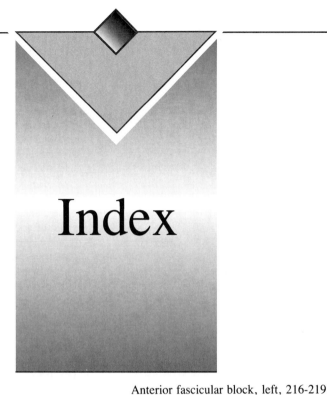

Index

A

439

Jabuuuuu punch
back fist uuuu punch
front snap kick stepping
forward

(Kick back leg - put down in front)

Round house kick

Round house kick step forward

Back leg kick - put down

Back hammer fist

step out → elbow

Back Kick - hands up → kick

Step up kick - reverse punch